Handbook of Probiotics

Handbook of Probiotics

Edited by **Ricky Parks**

hayle
medical

New York

Published by Hayle Medical,
30 West, 37th Street, Suite 612,
New York, NY 10018, USA
www.haylemedical.com

Handbook of Probiotics
Edited by Ricky Parks

International Standard Book Number: 978-1-63241-242-3 (Hardback)

Printed in the United States of America.

Contents

Preface

Over the last few decades, the prevalence of research regarding probiotics strains has significantly grown in most regions of the world. Probiotics are particular strains of microorganisms, which when served to animals or humans in suitable amount, have an advantageous impact, enhancing health or decreasing the risk of getting sick and the probiotics are employed in production of functional foods and pharmaceutical products. The book contains complete information regarding issues relating to probiotics in food which will serve extremely helpful for the people engaged in this field across the world.

The information shared in this book is based on empirical researches made by veterans in this field of study. The elaborative information provided in this book will help the readers further their scope of knowledge leading to advancements in this field.

Finally, I would like to thank my fellow researchers who gave constructive feedback and my family members who supported me at every step of my research.

Editor

Use of Probiotic in Food

Recent Application of Probiotics in Food and Agricultural Science

Danfeng Song, Salam Ibrahim and Saeed Hayek

Additional information is available at the end of the chapter

1. Introduction

Probiotic foods are a group of functional foods with growing market shares and large commercial interest [1]. Probiotics are live microorganisms which when administered in adequate amounts confer a beneficial health benefit on the host [2]. Probiotics have been used for centuries in fermented dairy products. However, the potential applications of probiotics in nondairy food products and agriculture have not received formal recognition. In recent times, there has been an increased interest to food and agricultural applications of probiotics, the selection of new probiotic strains and the development of new application has gained much importance. The uses of probiotics have been shown to turn many health benefits to the human and to play a key role in normal digestive processes and in maintaining the animal's health. The agricultural applications of probiotics with regard to animal, fish, and plants production have increased gradually. However, a number of uncertainties concerning technological, microbiological, and regulatory aspects exist [3].

1.1. Definition of probiotics

Probiotics are live microbes that can be formulated into many different types of products, including foods, drugs, and dietary supplements. Probiotic is a relatively new word that is used to name the bacteria associated with the beneficial effects for the humans and animals. The term probiotic means "for life" and it was defined by an Expert Committee as "live microorganisms which upon ingestion in certain numbers exert health benefits beyond inherent general nutrition" [4]. FAO/WHO Expert Consultation believes that general guidelines need to provide to how these microorganisms can be tested and proven for safety and potential health benefits when administered to humans.

Lactobacillus and *Bifidobacterium* are most commonly used probiotics in food and feed (Table 1). Other microorganisms such as yeast *Saccharomyces cerevisiae* and some *Escherichia coli* and *Bacillus* species are also used as probiotics. Lactic acid bacteria (LAB) which have been used for food fermentation since the ancient time, can serve a dual function by acting as food fermenting agent and potentially health benefits provider. LAB are GRAS (general recognized as safe) with no pathogenic, or virulence properties have been reported. For the use of LAB as probiotics, some desirable characteristics such as low cost, maintaining its viability during the processing and storage, facility of the application in the products, resistance to the physicochemical processing must be considered.

Lactobacillus species	Bifidobacterium species	Others
L. acidophilus	*B. adolescentis*	*Bacillus cereus*
L. amylovorus	*B. animalis*	*Clostridium botyricum*
L. brevis	*B. breve*	*Enterococcus faecalis*[a]
L. casei	*B. bifidum*	*Enterococcus faecium*[a]
L. rhamnosus	*B. infantis*	*Escherichia coli*
L. crispatus	*B. lactis*	*Lactococcus lactis* subsp. *cremoriss*
L. delbrueckii subsp. *bulgaricus*	*B. longum*	*Lactococcus lactis* subsp. *lactis*
L. fermentum		*Leuconostoc mesenteroides* subsp. *dextranicum*
L. gasseri		*Pediococcus acidilactici*
L. helveticus		*Propionibacterium freudenreichii*[a]
L. johnsonii		*Saccharomyces boulardii*
L. lactis		*Streptococcus salivarius* subsp. *thermophilus*
L. paracasei		*Sporolactobacillus inulinus*[a]
L. plantarum		
L. reuteri		
L. salivarius		
L. gallinarum[a]		

[a] mainly applied in animals

Table 1. Probiotic microorganisms. Adapted from [5, 6]

1.2. Characteristics of probiotics

Characteristics of probiotics will determine their ability to survive the upper digestive tract and to colonize in the intestinal lumen and colon for an undefined time period. Probiotics are safe for human consumption and no reports have found on any harmfulness or production of any specific toxins by these strains [7, 8]. In addition, some probiotics could produce antimicrobial substances like bacteriocins. Therefore, the potential health benefit will depend on the characteristic profile of the probiotics. Some probiotic strains can reduce intestinal transit time, improve the quality of migrating motor complexes [9], and temporarily increase the rate of mitosis in enterocytes [10, 11].

The most common probiotics are *Lactobacillus* and *Bifidobacterium*. In general most probiotics are gram-positive, usually catalase-negative, rods with rounded ends, and occur in pairs, short, or long chains [7]. They are non-flagellated, non-motile and non-spore-forming, and are intolerant to salt. Optimum growth temperature for most probiotics is 37°C but some strains such as *L. casei* prefer 30 °C and the optimum pH for initial growth is 6.5-7.0 [7]. *L. acidophilus* is microaerophilic with anaerobic referencing and capability of aerobic growth. *Bifidobacterium* are anaerobic but some species are aero-tolerant. Most probiotics bacteria are fastidious in their nutritional requirements [12, 13]. With regard to fermentation probiotics are either obligate homofermentative (ex. *L. acidophilus*, *L. helvelicas*), obligate heterofermentative (ex. *L. brevis*, *L. reuteri*), or facultative heterofermentative (ex. *L. casei*, *L. plantarum*) [14]. Additionally, probiotics produce a variety of beneficial compounds such as antimicrobials, lactic acid, hydrogen peroxide, and a variety of bacteriocins [15, 16] . Probiotics should have the ability to interact with the host microflora and competitive with microbial pathogens, bacterial, viral, and fungal [16].

2. Probiotics health benefits

Probiotic research suggests a range of potential health benefits to the host organism. The potential effects can only be attributed to tested strains but not to the whole group of probiotics. Probiotics have shown to provide a diverse variety of health benefits to human, animal, and plans. However, viability of the microorganisms throughout the processing and storage play an important role in transferring the claimed health effects. Therefore, the health benefits must be documented with the specific strain and specific dosage [17].

2.1. Human health

Probiotics display numerous health benefits beyond providing basic nutritional value [4]. These evidences have been established by the scientific testing in the humans or animals, performed by the legitimate research groups and published in peer-reviewed journals [16, 18]. Some of these benefits have been well documented and established while the others have shown a promising potential in animal models, with human studies required to substantiate these claims [18]. Health benefits of probiotic bacteria are very strain specific; therefore, there is no universal strain that would provide all proposed benefits and not all strains of the same species are effective against defined health conditions [18].

Probiotics have been used in fermented food products for centuries. However, nowadays it has been claimed that probiotics can serve a dual function by their potentially importing health benefits. The health benefit of fermented foods may be further enhanced by supplementation of   *Lactobacillus* and *Bifidobacterium* species [19]. *L. acidophilus*, *Bifidobacterium* spp. and *L. casei* species are the most used probiotic cultures with established human health in dairy products, whereas the yeast *Saccharomyces cerevisiae* and some *E. coli* and *Bacillus* species are also used as probiotics [20].

Several studies have documented probiotic effects on a variety of gastrointestinal and extraintestinal disorders, including prevention and alleviation symptoms of traveler's diarrhea and antibiotic associated diarrhea [21], inflammatory bowel disease [21], lactose intolerance [22], protection against intestinal infections [23], and irritable bowel syndrome. Some probiotics have also been investigated in relation to reducing prevalence of atopic eczema later in life [24], vaginal infections, and immune enhancement [25], contributing to the inactivation of pathogens in the gut, rheumatoid arthritis, improving the immune response of in healthy elderly people [26], and liver cirrhosis.

In addition, probiotics are intended to assist the body's naturally occurring gut microbiota. Some probiotic preparations have been used to prevent diarrhea caused by antibiotics, or as part of the treatment for antibiotic-related dysbiosis. Although there is some clinical evidence for the role of probiotics in lowering cholesterol but the results are conflicting. Probiotics have a promising inhibitory effect on oral pathogens especially in childhood but this may not necessarily lead to improved oral health [27]. Antigenotoxicity, antimutagenicity and anticarcinogenicity are important potential functional properties of probiotics, which have been reported recently. Observational data suggest that consumption of fermented dairy products is associated with a lower prevalence of colon cancer, which is suggested that probiotics are capable of decreasing the risk of cancer by inhibition of carcinogens and pro-carcinogens, inhibition of bacteria capable of converting pro-carcinogens to carcinogens [18].

2.2. Animal health

Probiotics which are traditional idea in the human food have been extended to animals by developing fortified feed with intestinal microbiota to benefit the animals. The microflora in the gastrointestinal tracts of animals plays a key role in normal digestive processes and in maintaining the animal's health. Probiotics can beneficially improve the intestinal microbial balance in host animal. Commercial probiotics for animal use are claimed to improve animal performance by increasing daily gain and feed efficiency in feedlot cattle, enhance milk production in dairy cows, and improve health and performance of young calves [28] and in improving growth performance of chickens [29]. Probiotics can attach the mucosal wall, adjust to immune responses [30], and compete the pathogenic bacteria for attachment to mucus [31, 32]. Probiotics provide the animal with additional source of nutrients and digestive enzymes [33, 34]. They can stimulate synthesis vitamins of the B-group and enhancement of growth of nonpathogenic facultative anaerobic and gram positive bacteria by producing inhibitory compounds like volatile fatty acids and hydrogen peroxide that inhibit the growth of harmful bacteria enhancing the host's resistance to enteric pathogens [32, 35]. Probiotics stimulate the direct uptake of dissolved organic material mediated by the bacteria, and enhance the immune response against pathogenic microorganisms [36, 37]. Finally, probiotics can inhibit pathogens by competition for a colonization sites or nutritional sources and production of toxic compounds, or stimulation of the immune system.

2.3. Plant health

The more beneficial the bacteria and fungi are, the more "fertile" the soil is. These microorganisms break down organic matter in the soil into small, usable parts that plants can uptake through their roots. The healthier the soil, the lower the need for synthetic herb/pesticides and fertilizers.The concept that certain microorganisms 'probiotics' may confer direct benefits to the plant acting as biocontrol agents for plants. The plant probiotic bacteria have been isolated and commercially developed for use in the biological control of plant diseases or biofertilization [38]. These microorganisms have fulfilled important functions for plant as they antagonize various plant pathogens, induce immunity, or promote growth [38-40]. The interaction between bacteria and fungi with their host plants has shown their ability to promote plant growth and to suppress plant pathogens in several studies [41-44].

3. Food applications of probiotics

Today an increase in knowledge of functional foods has led to develop foods with health benefits beyond adequate nutrition. The last 20 years have shown an increased interest among consumers in functional food including those containing probiotics. The presence of probiotics in commercial food products has been claimed for certain health benefits. This has led to industries focusing on different applications of probiotics in food products and creating a new generation of 'probiotic health' foods. This section will summarize the common applications of probiotics in food products.

3.1. Dairy-based probiotic foods

Milk and its products is good vehicle of probiotic strains due to its inherent properties and due to the fact that most milk and milk products are stored at refrigerated temperatures. Probiotics can be found in a wide variety of commercial dairy products including sour and fresh milk, yogurt, cheese, etc. Dairy products play important role in delivering probiotic bacteria to human, as these products provide a suitable environment for probiotic bacteria that support their growth and viability [45-48]. Several factors need to be addressed for applying probiotics in dairy products such as viability of probiotics in dairy [19, 48], the physical, chemical and organoleptic properties of final products [49-51], the probiotic health effect [52, 53], and the regulations and labeling issues [4, 54].

3.1.1. Drinkable fresh milk and fermented milks

Among probiotics carrier food products, dairy drinks were the first commercialized products that are still consumed in larger quantities than other probiotic beverages. Functional dairy beverages can be grouped into two categories: fortified dairy beverages (including probiotics, prebiotics, fibers, polyphenols, peptides, sterol, stanols, minerals, vitamins and fish oil), and whey-based beverages [55]. Among the probiotic bacteria used in the manufacture of dairy beverages, *L. rhamnosus* GG is the most widely used. Owing to *L. rhamnosus* GG acid and bile resistance [56], this probiotic is very suitable for industrial applications. Özer and Avnikirmaci have reported several examples of commercial probiotic dairy beverages showing that *L. acidophilus, L. casei, L. rhamnosus*, and *L. plantarum* as most applied probiotics [55].

Several factors have been reported to affect the viability of probiotic cultures in fermented milks. Acidity, pH, dissolved oxygen content, redox potential, hydrogen peroxide, starter microbes, potential presence of flavoring compounds and various additives (including preservatives) affect the viability of probiotic bacteria and have been identified as having an effect during the manufacture and storage of fermented milks [19, 48, 57]. Today, a wide range of dairy beverages that contain probiotic bacteria is available for consumers in the market including: Acidophilus milk, Sweet acidophilus milk, Nu-Trish A/B, Bifidus milk, Acidophilus buttermilk, Yakult, Procult drink, Actimel, Gaio, ProViva, and others [55].

Probioticts such as *Lactobacillus* and *Bifidobacterium* strains grow weakly in milk due to their low proteolytic activity and inability to utilize lactose [47, 57]. These bacteria also need certain compounds for their growth which is missing in milk [19, 58, 59]. To improve growth and viability of probiotics in dairy beverages various substances have been tested in milk. Citrus fiber presence in fermented milks was found to enhance bacterial growth and survival of probiotic bacteria in fermented milks [60]. Addition of soygerm powder has shown certain positive effects on producing fermented milk with *L. reuteri*. Soygerm powder may release important bioactive isoflavones during fermentation that could protect *L. reuteri* from bile salt toxicity in the small intestine [61]. Other substances include fructooligosaccahrides (FOS), aseinomacropeptides (CMP), whey protein concentrate (WPC), tryptone, yeast extracts, certain amino acids, nucleotide precursors and an iron source were also documented [59, 63, 64]. Additionally, the selection of probiotic strains and optimization of the manufacturing conditions (both formulation properties and storage conditions) are of utmost importance in the viability of probiotic bacteria in fermented milk [47, 65].

3.1.2. Yogurt

Yogurt is one of the original sources of probiotics and continues to remain a popular probiotic product today. Yogurt is known for its nutritional value and health benefits. Yogurt is produced using a culture of *L. delbrueckii* subsp. *bulgaricus* and

Streptococcus salivarius subsp. *thermophilus* bacteria. In addition, other lactobacilli and bifidobacteria are also sometimes added during or after culturing yogurt. The probiotic characteristics of these bacterial strains that form the yogurt culture are still debatable. The viability of probiotics and their proteolytic activities in yoghurt must be considered. Numerous factors may affect the survival of *Lactobacillus* and *Bifidobacterium* spp. in yogurt. These include strains of probiotic bacteria, pH, presence of hydrogen peroxide and dissolved oxygen, concentration of metabolites such as lactic acid and acetic acids, buffering capacity of the media as well as the storage temperature [19, 66, 67].

Although yogurt has been widely used as probiotics vehicle, most commercial yogurt products have low viable cells at the consumption time [19, 68]. Viability of probiotics in yogurt depends on the availability of nutrients, growth promoters and inhibitors, concentration of solutes, inoculation level, incubation temperature, fermentation time and storage temperature. Survival and viability of probiotic in yogurt was found to be strain dependant. The main factors for loss of viability of probiotic organisms have been attributed to the decrease in the pH of the medium and accumulation of organic acids as a result of growth and fermentation. Among the factors, ultimate pH reached at the end of yogurt fermentation appears to be the most important factor affecting the growth and viability of probiotics. Metabolic products of organic acids during storage may further affect cell viability of probiotics [66]. The addition of fruit in yogurt may have negative effect on the viability of probiotics, since fruit and berries might have antimicrobial activities. Inoculation with very high level of probiotics with attempts to compensate the potential viability loss, might result in an inferior quality of the product. The present of probiotic was found to affect some characteristics of yogurt including: acidity, texture, flavor, and appearance [69]. However, encapsulation in plain alginate beads, in chitosancoated alginate, alginate-starch, alginate-prebiotic, alginate-pectin, in whey protein-based matrix, or by adding prebiotics or cysteine into yogurt, could improve the viability and stability of probiotics in yogurt [70-79].

3.1.3. Cheese

Yogurt and milk are the most common vehicles of probiotics among dairy products. However, alternative carriers such as cheese seem to be well suited. Cheeses have a number of advantages over yogurt and fermented milks because they have higher pH and buffering capacity, highly nutritious, high energy, more solid consistency, relatively higher fat content, and longer shelf life [80, 81]. Several studies have demonstrated a high survival rate of probiotics in cheese at the end of shelf life and high viable cells [45, 48, 82, 83]. Probiotics in cheese were found to survive the passage through the simulated human gastrointestinal tract and significantly increase the numbers of probiotic cells in the gut [82]. However, comparing the serving size of yogurt to that of cheese, cheese needs to have higher density of probiotic cells and higher viability to provide the same health benefits. Cheese was introduced to probiotic industry in 2006 when Danisco decided to test the growth and survival of probiotic strains in cheese [84]. At that time, only few probiotic cheese products were found on the market. The test showed that less than 10% of the bacteria were lost in the cheese whey. Based on the process, a commercial probiotic cheese was first developed by the Mills DA, Oslo, Norway. Nowadays, there are over 200 commercial probiotic cheeses in various forms, such as fresh, semi-hard, hard cheese in the marketplaces. Semi-hard and hard cheese, compared to yogurt as a carrier for probiotics, has relatively low recommended daily intake and need relatively high inoculation level of probiotics (about 4 to 5 times). Fresh cheese like cottage cheese has high recommended daily intake, limited shelf life with refrigerated storage temperature. It may, thus, serve as a food with a high potential to be applied as a carrier for probiotics.

3.1.4. Other dairy based products

Other dairy products including quark, chocolate mousse, frozen fermented dairy desserts, sour cream, and ice cream can be good vehicles of probiotics. Quark was tested with two probiotic cultures to improve its nutrition characteristics and the results showed that probiotics can ensure the highest level of utilization of fat, protein, lactose, and phosphorus partially in skimmed milk [85]. Chocolate mousse with probiotic and prebiotic ingredients were developed [86]. Probiotic chocolate mousse was supplemented with *L. paracasei* subsp. *paracasei* LBC 82, solely or together with inulin and the results showed that chocolate mousse is good vehicle for *L. paracasei* [86]. Sour cream was investigated as probiotic vehicle and the results showed that using sour cream as a probiotic carrier is proved feasible [87]. Ice creams are among the food products with high potential for use as probiotic vehicles. Cruz and others have reviewed the technological parameters involved in the production of probiotic ice creams [88]. They have pointed several factors that need to be controlled, including the appropriate selection of cultures, inoculums concentration, the appropriate processing stage for the cultures to be added, and the processing procedures and transport and storage temperatures. They concluded that probiotic cultures do not modify the sensory characteristics of the ice-creams and frozen desserts also these products hold good viability for probiotics during the product storage period.

3.2. Non dairy based probiotic products

Dairy products are the main carriers of probiotic bacteria to human, as these products provide a suitable environment for probiotic bacteria that support their growth and viability. However, with an increase in the consumer vegetarianism throughout the developed countries, there is also a demand for the vegetarian probiotic products. Nondairy probiotic products have shown a big interest among vegetarians and lactose intolerance customers. According to the National Institute of Diabetes and Digestive and Kidney Diseases (NIDDK) of the U.S. National Institutes of Health, about 75% of the world population is lactose intolerant. The development of new nondairy probiotic food products is very much challenging, as it has to meet the consumer's expectancy for healthy benefits [89, 90]. Granato and others have overview of functional food development, emphasizing nondairy foods that contain probiotic bacteria strains [91]. From their review, some nondairy probiotic products recently developed are shown in Table 2.

3.2.1. Vegetable-based probiotic products

Fermentation of vegetables has been known since ancient time. Fermented vegetables can offer a suitable media to deliver probiotics. However, it shows that the low incubation temperature of vegetable fermentation is a problem for the introduction of the traditional *L. acidophilus* and *Bifidobacterium* probiotic bacteria. Probiotic of *L. rhamnosus*, *L. casei* and *L. plantarum* are better adapted to the vegetable during fermentation [94]. Nevertheless, when the temperature is adjusted at 37°C, probiotic bacteria grow quite rapidly in plant-based substrates [95].

Category	Product
Fruit and vegetable based	Vegetable-based drinks
	Fermented banana pulp
	Fermented banana
	Beets-based drink
	Tomato-based drink
	Many dried fruits
	Green coconut water
	Peanut milk
	Cranberry, pineapple, and orange juices
	Ginger juice
	Grape and passion fruit juices
	Cabbage juice
	Carrot juice
	Noni juice
	Onion
	Probiotic banana puree
	Nonfermented fruit juice beverages
	Blackcurrant juice
Soy based	Nonfermented soy-based frozen desserts
	Fermented soymilk drink
	Soy-based stirred yogurt-like drinks
Cereal based	Cereal-based puddings
	Rice-based yogurt
	Oat-based drink
	Oat-based products
	Yosa (oat-bran pudding)
	Mahewu (fermented maize beverage)
	Maize-based beverage
	Wheat, rye, millet, maize, and other cereals fermented probiotic beverages
	Malt-based drink
	Boza (fermented cereals)
	Millet or sorghum flour fermented probiotic beverage
Other nondairy foods	Starch-saccharified probiotic drink
	Probiotic cassava-flour product
	Meat products
	Dosa (rice and Bengal gram)

Table 2. Some nondairy probiotic products recently developed. Adapted from [91]

To develop new probiotic vegetable products, many studies have been carried out. The suitability of carrot juice as a raw material for the production of probiotic food with Bifidobacterium strains was investigated [96]. Kun and others have found that Bifidobacteria were capable of having biochemical activities in carrot juice without any nutrient supplementation [96]. Yoon and others studied the suitability of tomato juice for the production of a probiotic product by L. acidophilus, L. plantarum, L. casei and L. delbrueckii. They reported that the four LAB were capable of rapidly utilizing tomato juice for cell synthesis and lactic acid production without nutrient supplementation and pH adjustment [109]. Yoon and others also tested the suitability of cabbage to produce probiotic cabbage juice and suggested that fermented cabbage juice support the viability of probiotics and serve as a healthy beverage [97]. The viability of various bifidobacteria in kimchi was investigated under various conditions and the results show the acceptable levels of probiotics in kimchi [98]. In addition, sauerkraut-type products such as fermented cabbage, carrots, onions, and cucumbers based on a lactic fermentation by L. plantarum could be good probiotic carrier. Yoon and others have evaluated the potential of red beets as substrate for the production of probiotic beet juice by four strains of lactic acid bacteria and all strains were capable of rapidly utilizing the beet juice for the cell synthesis and lactic acid production [99]. However, traditional methods of production might result in inactivation of the probiotic cultures and the use of probiotics in fermented vegetables would require low temperature storage of the products [94].

Moreover, soybean has received attention from the researchers due to its high protein and quality. Soymilk is suitable for the growth of LAB and bifidobacteria [100, 101]. Several studies have focused on developing fermented soymilk with different strains of LAB and Bifidobacteria to produce a soymilk product with improved health benefits [62, 101-103]. Soymilk is now known for their health benefits such as prevention of chronic diseases such as menopausal disorder, cancer, atherosclerosis, and osteoporosis, therefore, soymilk fermented with bifidobacteria may be a unique functional food [62, 104]. In probiotic soy products, fermentation by probiotics has the potential to (1) reduce the levels of some carbohydrates possibly responsible for gas production in the intestinal system, (2) increase the levels of free isoflavones, which has many beneficial effects on human health, and (3) favor desirable changes in bacterial populations in the gastrointestinal tract. Supplementing soymilk with prebiotics such as, fructooligosaccharides (FOS), mannitol, maltodextrin and pectin, was found to be a suitable medium for the viability of probiotic bacteria [105].

3.2.2. Fruit-based probiotic products

Nowadays, there is increasing interest in the development of fruit-juice based probiotic products. The fruit juices contain beneficial nutrients that can be an ideal medium for probiotics [106, 107]. Fruit juices have pleasing taste profiles to all age groups and they are perceived as being healthy and refreshing. The fruits are rich in several nutrients such as minerals, vitamins, dietary fibers, antioxidants, and do not contain any dairy allergens that might prevent usage by certain segments of the population [107, 108]. Those characteristics allow the selection of appropriate strains of probiotics to manufacture enjoyable healthy fruit juice. However, the sensory impact of probiotic cultures would have different taste profiles compared to the conventional, nonfunctional products. The different aroma and flavors have been reported when *L. plantarum* was added to orange juices which consumers do not prefer. But if their health benefits information is provided the preference increases over the conventional orange juices. Different attempts have been made to reduce the sensations of unpleasant aromas and flavors in probiotic fruit juice. Luckow and others reported that the perceptible off-flavors caused by probiotics that often contribute to consumer dissatisfaction may be masked by adding 10% (v/v) of tropical fruit juices, mainly pineapple, but also mango or passion fruit [108].

To develop probiotic fruits, many studies have been carried out. The suitability of noni juice as a raw material for the production of probiotics was studied by Wang and others and found that *B. longum* and *L. plantarum* can be optimal probiotics for fermented noni juice [109]. Suitability of fermented pomegranate juice was tested using *L. plantarum, L. delbruekii, L. paracasei, L. acidophilus.* Pomegranate juice was proved to be a suitable probiotic drink as results have shown desirable microbial growth and viability for *L. plantarum* and *L. delbruekii* [110]. Optimized growth conditions of *L. casei* in cashew apple juice were studied. *L. casei* has shown suitable survival ability in cashew apple juice during 42 days of refrigerated storage. It was observed that *L. casei* grew during the refrigerated storage and cashew apple juice showed to be suitable probiotic product [111]. Tsen and others reported that *L. acidophilus* immobilized in Ca-alginate can carry out a fermentation of banana puree, resulting in a novel probiotic banana product with higher number of viable cells [112]. Kourkoutas and others reported that *L. casei* immobilized on apple and quince pieces survived for extended storage time periods and adapted to the acidic environment, which usually has an inhibitory effect on survival during lactic acid production [113].

3.2.3. Cereal-based probiotic products

Cereal-based probiotic products have health-benefiting microbes and potentially prebiotic fibers. The development of new functional foods which combine the beneficial effects of cereals and health promoting bacteria is a challenging issue. Nevertheless, cereal-based products offer many possibilities. Indeed, numerous cereal-based products in the world require a lactic fermentation, often in association with yeast or molds. Cereals are good substrates for the growth of probiotic strains and due to the presence of non-digestible components of the cereal matrix may also serve as prebiotics [114, 115]. Due to the complexity of cereals, a systematic approach is required to identify the factors that enhance the growth of probiotic in cereals [116]. Champagne has listed number of cereal-based products that require a lactic fermentation, often in association with yeast or molds. We have found it useful to include part of these products in Table 3.

Food	Country	Ingredients	Microorganisms
Adai	India	Cereal, legume	*Pediococcus* spp., *Streptococcus* spp., *Leuconostoc* spp.
Anarshe	India	Rice	Lactic acid bacteria
Aya-bisbaya	Mexico	Rice	Lactic acid bacteria
Bhatura	India	Wheat	Lactic acid bacteria, yeasts
Burukutu	Nigeria	Sorghum, cassava	Lactic acid bacteria, *Candida* spp., *S. cerevisiae*
Fermented oatmeal (ProViva)	Sweden	Oatmeal	*L. plantarum*
Llambazi, lakubilisa	Zimbabwe	Maize	Lactic acid bacteria, yeasts, molds
Injera	Ethiopia	Sorghum, tef, corn, millet, barley, wheat	*L. plantarum, Aspergillus* spp., *Penicillium* spp., *Rhodotorula* spp., *Candida* spp.
Kishk, kushuk, trahanas	Egypt, Syria, Lebanon	Milk (yoghurt), wheat	*L. casei, L. plantarum, L. brevis, B. subtilis, B. licheniformis, B. megaterium,* yeasts
Kisra	Sudan, Irak, Arabian Gulf	Sorghum, millet	*Lactobacillu.* spp., *L. brevis, L. fermentum, E. faecium, Acetobacter* spp., *S. cerevisiae*
Togwa	Tanzania	Maize, sorghum	*L. plantarum, L. brevis, L. fermentum, L. cellobiosus P. pentosaceus, W. confusa, S. cerevisiae, C. tropicalis*

Table 3. Fermented cereal products that carry a lactic fermentation [94]

A multitude of fermented cereal products have been created, but only recently probiotic microorganisms involved in traditional fermented cereal foods have been reported. Strains of *L. plantarum,Candida rugosa* and *Candida lambica* isolated from a traditional Bulgarian cereal-based fermented beverage exhibited probiotic properties, being resistant up to 2% bile concentration, which enables them to survive bile toxicity during their passage through the gastrointestinal system [117]. More studies are being done to demonstrate that cereals are suitable substrates for the growth of some probiotic bacteria. Rozada-Sa'nchez and others have studied the growth and metabolic activity of four different *Bifidobacterium* spp. in a malt hydrolisate using four *Bifidobacterium* strains with the aim of producing a potentially probiotic beverage [92]. The study has reported potential use for malt hydrolysate as probiotic beverage with the addition of a growth and yeast extract. Angelov and others have used a whole-grain oat substrate to obtain a drink with probiotics and oat prebiotic beta-glucan. They have found that viable cell counts reached at the end of the process were about 7.5×10^{10} cfu/ ml. Also the addition of sweeteners aspartame, sodium cyclamate, saccharine and Huxol (12% cyclamate and 1.2% saccharine) had no effect on the dynamics of the fermentation process and on the viability of the starter culture during product storage [93]. Charalapompoulos and others have done experiments with different cereals to determine the main parameters that need to be considered in the growth of probiotic microorganisms, defining them as follows: the composition and processing of cereal grains, the substrate formulation, the growth capability and productivity of the starter culture, the stability of the probiotic strain during storage, the organoleptic properties and the nutritional value of the final product [114]. They reported that many cereals supported the growth of probiotics with some differences. Malt medium supported the growth of all examined strains (*L. plantarum, L. fermentum, L. acidophilus* and *L. reuteri*) better than barley and wheat media due to its chemical composition. Also, wheat and barley extracts were found to exhibit a significant protective effect on the viability of *L. plantarum, L. acidophilis* and *L. reuteri* under acidic conditions (pH 2.5).

Oat is often used in studies of cereal fermented by probiotic bacteria. Several studies have evaluated the potential of oat as substrates for the development of a probiotic product. Kedia and others have explored the potential of using mixed culture fermentation to produce cereal-based foods with high numbers of probiotic bacteria. In this study, LAB growth was enhanced by the introduction of yeast and the production of lactic acid and ethanol were increased in comparison against pure LAB culture. They have fermented whole oat flour with *L. plantarum* along with white flour and bran in order to compare the suitability of these substrates for the production of a probiotic beverage. Those substrates were found to enhance probiotic viability at the end of fermentation above the minimum required in a probiotic product [118]. Martensson and others have studied the development of nondairy fermented product based on oat [119]. Yosa is a snack food made from oat bran pudding cooked in water and fermented with LAB and Bifidobacteria. It is mainly consumed in Finland and other Scandinavian countries. It has a texture and a flavor similar to yogurt but it is totally free from milk or other animal products. It is lactose-free, low in fat, contains beta-glucan and it is suitable for vegetarians [120]. Yosa is therefore considered a healthy food due to its content of oat fiber and probiotic LAB, which combine the effect of beta-glucan for cholesterol reduction and the effect of LAB benefits to maintain and improve the intestinal microbiota balance of the consumer.

Other cereals and cereal components that can be used as fermentation substrates for probiotics have been studied. Survival of probiotics in a corn-based fermented substrate was reported [121]. Autoclaved maize porridge was fermented with probiotic strains (grown separately): *L. reuteri, L. acidophilus* and *L. rhamnosus* for 24h at 37 °C. All strains examined showed good growth in maize porridge with added barley malt. Probiotic fermented maize products could have a good world-wide acceptance, since maize fermentation induces fruity flavors in traditional Mexican foods. Prado and others have summarized some of the international cereal based probiotic beverages including: *Boza* made from wheat, rye, millet and other cereals in Bulgaria, Albania, Turkey and Romania, *Bushera* made from sorghum, or millet flour in Western highlands of Uganda, *Mahewu* (amahewu) made from corn meal in Africa and some Arabian Gulf countries, *Pozol* made from maize in the Southeastern Mexico, and *Togwa* made from maize flour and millet malt in Africa [5].

Normally sourdoughs are the cereal products fermented by LAB cultures. However, baking will kills most probiotic bacteria and only probiotics which synthesize a thermostable bioactive compound during leavening can be of use in bread making. Different studies have shown the ability of human derived strains of L. reuteri to resist simulated gastric acidity and bile acid, and also to grow well in a number of cereal substrates [89, 116]. In this perspective, L. reuteri has potential use in bread making due to reuterin synthesis [122]. The L. reureri cells might be inactivated by heating, but the bioactive compound might remain active. Probiotic Bacillus strains could better adapt to bread making due to their spore-forming characteristics.

3.2.4. Meat-based probiotic foods

Probiotic applications are restricted to fermented meats, such as dry sausages. The idea of using probiotic bacteria in fermenting meat products has introduced the idea of using antimicrobial peptides, i.e. bacteriocins, or other antimicrobial compounds as an extra hurdle for meat products. Meat starter culture was defined as preparations which contain living or resting microorganisms that develop the desired metabolic activity in the meat [123]. LAB are the most common used starter culture in meat which produce lactic acid from glucose or lactose. As meat content of these sugars are low, sugar is added at 0.4–0.7% (w/w) for glucose and 0.5–1.0% (w/w) for lactose to the sausage matrix [124]. Some LAB strains such as L. rhamnosus GG are not able to utilize lactose, therefore, the starter culture properties have to be taken into account for successful applications. From pentoses, such as arabinose and xylose, meat starter LAB produce both lactic acid and acetic acid [125]. As indicated in commercial catalogues LAB strains currently most employed in meat starter cultures are L. casei, L. curvatus, L. pentosus, L. plantarum, L. sakei, Pediococcus acidilactici and Pediococcus pentosaceus [124].

LAB have been used for dry sausage manufacturing process since 1950s in order to ensure the safety and quality of the end product. Dry sausages are non heated meat products, which may be suitable carriers for probiotics into the human gastrointestinal tract [124]. Dry sausage is made from a mixture of frozen pork, beef and pork fat with the addition of sugars, salt, nitrite, and nitrate, ascorbates and spices. The raw sausage material is stuffed into casing material of variable diameters and hung vertically in fermentation and ripening chambers for several weeks. Salt, nitrite, and added spices are the main contributors in the inhibition of different bacteria on the surface of the sausages. Lactic acid bacteria and staphylococci used as starter cultures to ferment the sausage. Salt decreases the initial water activity inhibiting or at least delaying the growth of many bacteria while favoring the growth of starter LAB and starter staphylococci. During the first day of fermentation the growth of microbes in sausage material uses up all the oxygen mixed in the sausage matrix during the chopping. After few days of fermentation, LAB decrease the pH to about 5.0 which acts as a hurdle for several Gram-negative bacterial species [126, 127]. The presence LAB in the food suggests that bacteriocins may be active in the human small intestine against food pathogens as long as they are able to survive the environment of gastrointestinal tract [27]. Likewise, probiotic strains with antimicrobial effects on food act similarly and therefore might be more successful than commonly used food fermenting bacteria. It could be concluded that dry sausage is suitable carrier for probiotics. However, human clinical studies are needed before the final answer concerning the health promoting effects of probiotic dry sausage.

Some traditional Indian fermented fish products such as Ngari, Hentak and Tungtap have been analyzed for microbial load [128]. LAB were identified as *Lactococcus lactis* subsp. *cremoris*, *Lactococcus plantarum*, *Enterococcus faecium*, *L. fructosus*, *L. amylophilus*, *L. coryniformis* subsp. *torquens*, and *L. plantarum*. Most strains of LAB had a high degree of hydrophobicity, indicating that these microorganisms have a probiotic potential.

4. Agricultural applications of probiotics

Probiotics applications have been extended from human applications to diversity of agricultural application. Agricultural applications include animal and plants.

4.1. Animal

Probiotics, with regard to animal applications, were defined as live microbial feed supplements beneficially improve the intestinal microbial balance in host animal [26]. They have been approved to provide many benefits to the host animal and animal products production. They are used as animal feed to improve the animal health and to improve food safety with examples of the application in poultry, ruminant, pig and aquaculture.

The microflora in the gastrointestinal tracts of poultry plays a key role in normal digestive processes and in maintaining the animal's health. Some feed additives can substantially affect this microbial population and their health promoting effects. Recently, concerns about some unwanted harmful side effects caused by antibiotics [129] has grown in many countries, so that there is an increasing interest in finding alternatives to antibiotics in poultry production. Probiotic has provided a possible natural alternative to antibiotics in poultry production to produce foods of reliable quality and safety [130]. In addition, the application of probiotic to chicken feed was shown to increase the internal and external quality of eggs. Addition of probiotic to chicken feed increased egg weight shell thickness, shell weight, albumen weight, and specific gravity and decreased shape index [131]. Farm animals are often subjected to environmental stresses which can cause imbalance in the intestinal ecosystem and could be a risk factor for pathogen infections. Applications of probiotics in feed have decreased the pathogen load in the farm animals. Feeding probiotic LAB and yeast to calve was found to promote the growth and suppress diarrhea in Holstein calve [132]. Gaggia and others have reviewed the applications of probiotics and prebiotics in animal feeding that can introduce to safe food production [133]. Probiotics has been used to intervene in decreasing pathogen load and in ameliorating gastrointestinal disease symptoms in pigs. Beside the in vitro test to identify the best potential probiotics, several studies are conducted in vivo utilizing different probiotic microorganisms. Most of the studies showed a beneficial role of improving the number of beneficial bacteria, decreasing the load of pathogens, stimulating the immune cell response towards pathogens in comparison to control, and increasing defensive tools against pathogenic invasion. In contrast, some authors reported an enhancement of the course of infection or a partial alleviation of diarrhea.

Applications of probiotics in aquaculture generally depend on producing antimicrobial metabolites and their ability to attach to intestinal mucus. *Aeromonas hydrophila* and *Vibrio alginolyticus* are common pathogens in fish, however, addition of probiotics strains (isolated from the clownfish, *Amphiprion percula*) were found capable to prevent the adhesion of these microbes to fish intestinal mucus and to compete with the pathogens [31]. Feeding probiotics to shrimp was found to reduce disease caused by *Vibrio parahaemolyticus* in shrimp [36]. Balcazar and others have reviewed the use of probiotics for prevention of bacterial diseases in aquaculture [134].

4.2. Plant

A strong growing market for plant probiotics for the use in agricultural biotechnology has been shown worldwide with an annual growth rate of approximately 10%. Based on the mode of action and effects, the plant probiotics products can be used as biofertilizers, plant strengtheners, phytostimulators, and biopesticides [38]. Berg has reported several advantages of using plant probiotics over chemical pesticides and fertilizers including: more safe, reduced environmental damage, less risk to human health, much more targeted activity, effective in small quantities, multiply themselves but are controlled by the plant as well as by the indigenous microbial populations, decompose more quickly than conventional chemical pesticides, reduced resistance development due to several mechanisms, and can be also used in conventional or integrated pest management systems [38]. Plant growth promotion can be achieved by the direct interaction between beneficial microbes and their host plant and also indirectly due to their antagonistic activity against plant pathogens. Several model organisms for plant growth promotion and plant disease inhibition are well-studied including: the bacterial genera *Azospirillum* [44, 135], *Rhizobium* [136], *Serratia* [137], *Bacillus* [138, 139], *Pseudomonas* [140, 141], *Stenotrophomonas* [142], and *Streptomyces* [143] and the fungal genera *Ampelomyces*, *Coniothyrium*, and *Trichoderma* [144]. Some examples of commercial products that have plant probiotics are listed in Table 4.

Several mechanisms are involved in the probiotics-plant interaction. It is important to specify the mechanism and to colonize plant habitats for successful application. Steps of colonization include recognition, adherence, invasion, colonization and growth, and several strategies to establish interactions. Plant roots initiate crosstalk with soil microbes by producing signals that are recognized by the microbes, which in turn produce signals that initiate colonization [43, 51]. Colonizing bacteria can penetrate the plant roots or move to aerial plant parts causing a decreasing in bacterial density in comparison to rhizosphere or root colonizing populations [43]. Furthermore, in the processes of plant growth, probiotic bacteria can influence the hormonal balance of the plant whereas phytohormones can be synthesized by the plant themselves and also by their associated microorganisms [38].

Microorganism	Name of the product	Plant pathogens, or pathosystem	Company
Ampelomyces quisqualis M-10	AQ10 Biofungicide	Powdery mildew on apples, cucurbits, grapes, ornamentals, strawberries, and tomatoes.	Ecogen
Azospirillum spp.	Biopromoter	Paddy, millets, oilseeds, fruits, vegetables, sugarcane, banana	Manidharma Biotech
Bacillus subtilis GB03	Kodiak	Growth promotion; *Rhizoctonia* and *Fusarium* spp.	(Gustafson); Bayer CropScience
Bradyrhizobium japonicum	Soil implant	Soy bean	Nitragin
Bacillus pumilus GB34	YiedShield	Soil-born fungal pathogens	(Gustafson); Bayer CropScience
Coniothyrium minitans	Contans WG, Intercept WG	*Sclerotinia sclerotiorum, S. minor*	Prophyta Biologischer Pflanzenschutz
Delftia acidovorans	BioBoost	Canola	Brett-Young Seeds Limited
Phlebiopsis gigantea	Rotex	*Heterobasidium annosum*	E~nema Biologischer Pflanzenschutz
Pseudomonas chlororaphis	Cedomon	Leaf stripe, net blotch, *Fusarium* sp., sot blotch, leaf spot, etc. on barley and oats	BioAgri AB
Streptomyces griseoviridis K61	Mycostop	*Phomopsis* spp., *Botrytis* spp., *Pythium* spp.,*Phythophora* spp.	Kemira Agro Oy
Trichoderma harzianum T22	RootShield, PlantShield T22, Planter box	*Pythium spp., Rhizoctonia solani, Fusarium* spp	Bioworks
Pseudomonas spp.	Proradix	*Rhizoctonia solani*	Sourcon Padena

Table 4. Examples of commercial products that have plant probiotics. Adapted from [38]

Besides these mechanisms, probiotic bacteria can supply macronutrients and micronutrients. They metabolize root exudates and release various carbohydrates, amino acids, organic acids, and other compounds in the rhizosphere [43]. Bacteria may contribute to plant nutrition by liberating phosphorous from organic compounds such as phytates and thus indirectly promote plant growth [145]. Furthermore, probiotic can reduce the activity of pathogenic microorganisms through microbial antagonisms and by activating the plant to better defend itself, a phenomenon termed "induced systemic resistance" [146, 147]. Microbial antagonism includes the inhibition of microbial growth, competition for colonization sites and nutrients, competition for minerals, and degradation of pathogenicity factors [38, 43]. In Japanese composting, at least three groups of compositing bacteria were used individually, or in combination. The following species were used: *Bacillus* bacteria groups, Lactic acid bacteria groups and *Actinomycetous* groups. These bacteria species can protect plant products from cropping hazards. They do this by expelling against various bad worms and insects, such as nematodes with potatoes and some types of insects with soybeans and maize. They are also effective in controlling fungi such as powdery mildew, downy mildew, *phythium* (damping off with many plants), *plasmodipophora brosscae* (club-root with the cabbage Jamily); *Crucijertle* (plants. and fusarium of wilt with tomato and banana) [148].

5. Probiotics application challenges

From a technological standpoint, Champagne has listed many challenges in the development of a probiotic food product including: strain selection, inoculation, growth and survival during processing, viability and functionality during storage, assessment the viable counts of the probiotic strains particularly when multiple probiotic strains are added and when there are also starter cultures added, and the effects on sensory properties [94]. Champagne has focused in his chapter on three of these challenges: inoculation, processing and storage issues. Other challenges such as: maintaining of probiotics, diversity and origin of probiotics, probiotic survival and being active, dealing with endogenous microbiota, and proving health benefits have also been discussed [149]. This section will focus on the viability and sensory acceptance as we have found these are the most important challenges to ensure transferring the health benefits and the commercial success.

5.1. Viability and survival

Probiotics have been proved to provide many health benefits. However, the claimed health benefits can't be achieved without high number of viable cells. Many probiotic bacteria have shown to die in the food products after exposure to low pH after fermentation, oxygen during refrigeration distribution and storage of products, and/or acid in the human stomach [150, 151]. Probiotic products need to be supplemented with additional ingredients to support the viability throughout processing, storage, distribution, and gastrointestinal tract to reach the colon. Several reports have shown that survival and viability of probiotic bacteria is often low in yogurt. The efficiency of added probiotic bacteria depends on dose level and their viability must be maintained throughout storage, products shelf-life and they must survive the gut environment [151]. Several studies have focused on the effect of adding certain compounds to enhance the probiotic viability. Many evidences have shown that inulin, oligosaccharides, and fructooligosaccharides (FOS) have good impacts on the probiotics viability. However, the effect of these compounds are strain specific. Martinez-Villaluenga and others have examined the influence of raffinose on the survival of *Bifidobacteria* and *L. acidophilus* in fermented milk. The results showed that retention of viability of *Bifidobacteria* and *L. acidophilus* greater in fermented milk with raffinose [65]. Supplementing probiotic products with FOS, mannitol, maltodextrin and pectin were found to provide a suitable viability for probiotic bacteria [105]. Inulin and FOS were found to support the growth and viability of *L. acidophilus* but did not significantly affect growth and viability of *Bifidobacterium* and *L. casei* [152]. During food formulation step several things need to be considered such as the composition (nutrients, antimicrobials), structure (oxygen permeability, water activity) and pH of the food matrix, and possible interactions with starter microbes in fermented food matrices. Growth of probiotics in non-fermented foods is not desirable (due to possible off flavor formation), but their growth during the production of fermented foods can lower process costs and increase the adaptation of probiotics leading to enhanced viability. The starter microbes in fermented foods can sometimes inhibit probiotics but they can also enhance their survival by producing beneficial substances or by lowering the oxygen pressure. In beverages the most important factor affecting probiotic viability is probably the pH. Shelf-stable beverages typically have pH values below 4.4 to ensure their microbial stability and this low pH value combined with long storage periods is very demanding for most probiotic strains, especially those representing bifidobacteria. The packaging material should be a good oxygen barrier to promote the survival of especially anaerobic probiotic bacteria (bifidobacteria) [153]. Transportation and storage temperature is an important determinant of the shelf-life; with increasing temperatures viability losses can occur rapidly [154].

The viability and survival of probiotics are strain specific. To maintain the viability of very sensitive strains, encapsulation is often the only option, especially microcapsulation that do not affect the sensory properties of the food produced. Microencapsulation technologies have been developed and successfully applied using various matrices to protect the bacterial cells from the damage caused by the external environment [155]. Overall microencapsulation improved the survival of probiotic bacteria when exposed to acidic conditions, bile salts, and mild heat treatment [156]. The immobilization of probiotics using microencapsulation may improve the survival of these microorganisms in products, both during processing and storage, and during digestion [157, 158].

Some probiotic bacteria, such as the spore-forming bacteria, GanedenBC[30] provides better viability and stability, making it an ideal choice for product development, compared to other probiotic bacteria strains, such as *L. acidophilus* and bifidobacteria. This spore safeguards the cell's genetic material from the heat and pressure of manufacturing processes, challenges of shelf life and the acid and bile it is exposed to during transit to the digestive system. GanedenBC^{30} can withstand manufacturing processes. and survive through high temperature processes such as baking and boiling, low temperature processes such as freezing and refrigeration and high pressure applications like extrusion and roll forming. GanedenBC^{30} requires no refrigeration and can be formulated into products to have up to a two-year. Once it is safely inside the small intestine, the viable spore is then able to germinate and produce new vegetative cells or good bacteria [159].

5.2. Sensory acceptance

Probiotic foods must show, at least, the same performance in any sensory test as conventional foods. In most probiotic foods sensory tests are aiming to determine acceptance of the products, without, obtaining details concerning the addition of the probiotics to the food and their interaction with the consumer. Therefore, it is important to development sensory tests for probiotic foods that can be accompanied by specific sensory analyses. Sensory testing must cover all characteristics with regard to change over time during storage. Some studies have reported the possibility of obtaining similar, or even better, performance with probiotic products as compared to conventional products such as: functional yogurt supplemented with *L. reuteri* RC-14 and *L. rhamnosus* GR-1 [160], chocolate mousse with added inulin and *L. paracasei* [86] , curdled milk with inulin, and *L. acidophilus* [152], and milk fermented with *B. animalis* and *L. acidophilus* La-5, and supplemented with inulin [161].

Sensory methodology will allow obtaining important data for developing the probiotic foods. In most cases the developed products need to match similar commercial products in parallel. In general, metabolism of the probiotic culture can result in the production of components that may contribute negatively to the aroma and taste of the food product, probiotic off-flavor. For example, acetic acid produced by *Bifidobacterium* spp. can result in a vinegary flavor in the product, prejudicing the performance in sensory assessments.

Masking is one technique that has been used to reduce the off flavors in foods and it has been performed successfully through the addition of new substances or flavors to reduce the negative sensory attributes contributed by probiotic cultures. The addition of tropical fruit juices, mainly pineapple, but also mango or passion fruit, might positively contribute to the aroma and flavor of the final product and might avoid the identification of probiotic off-flavors by consumers [162]. The influence of exposure has been identified in many consumer studies [91, 163] that the frequency of exposure to a food stimulus is increased, food stimuli have been shown to be better liked. Therefore, repeated exposure and increased familiarity to sensory off-flavors, may influence consumer attitudes in a positive way, therefore increasing willingness to consume probiotic juices. Nonsensory techniques have proven useful in enhancing the sensory quality of products, such as providing consumers with health benefit information associated with probiotic cultures. Health information has been shown to be a vital tool in the consumer acceptance of a variety of probiotic food products [164-166]. Finally, microcapsules of probiotics may help prevent the off flavor of cultures [167].

6. The future of probiotics

Dairy based products containing live bacteria are the main vehicles of probiotics to human. Non-dairy beverages would be the next food category where the healthy bacteria will make their mark. Microencapsulation technologies have provided the necessary protection for probiotics and moved them outside the pharmaceutical and supplemental use to become food ingredients.

6.1. Nanotechnology, encapsulation, and probiotics

The word "nano" comes from the Greek for "dwarf ". A nanometer is a thousandth of a thousandth of a thousandth of a meter (10^{-9} m). Nanoparticles are usually sized below 100 nanometers which will enable novel applications and benefits. Nanotechnology of probiotics is an area of emerging interest and opens up whole new possibilities for the probiotics applications. Their applications to the agriculture and food sector are relatively recent compared with their use in drug delivery and pharmaceuticals. The basic of probiotic nanotechnology applications is currently in the development of nano-encapsulated probiotics. The nanostructured food ingredients are being developed with the claims that they offer improved taste, texture and consistency. Applications of nanotechnology in organic food production require precaution, as little is known about their impact on environment and human health. Some recent food applications of nanotechnology, safety and risk problems of nanomaterials, routes for nanoparticles entering the body, existing regulations of nanotechnology in several countries, and a certification system of nanoproducts were reported [168, 169]. Currently, no regulations exist that specifically control or limit the production of nanosized particles and this is mainly owing to a lack of knowledge about the risks [169]. Nanoencapsulation is defined as a technology to pack substances in miniature using techniques such as nanocomposite, nanoemulsification, and nanoestructuration and provides final product functionality and control the release of the core [170]. Encapsulation of food ingredients may extend the shelf life of the product. Nanoencapsulation of probiotic is desirable technique that could deliver the probiotic bacteria to certain parts of the gastrointestinal tract where they interact with specific receptors [170]. These nanoencapsulated probiotic bacterial may also act as *de novo* vaccines, with the capability of modulating immune responses [171].

Microencapsulation with alginate can be applied to many different probiotic strains and results show better survival than free cells at low pH of 2.0, high bile salt concentrations, and moderate heat treatment of up to 65 °C [156]. Microencapsulation may prove to be an important method of improving the viability of probiotic bacteria in acidic food products and help deliver viable bacteria to the host's gastrointestinal tract. Furthermore, microencapsulation appeared to be effective in protecting cells from mild heat treatment and thus could stimulate research in functional food products that receive a mild heat treatment [156]. The microencapsulation allows the probiotic bacteria to be separated from its environment by a protective coating. Several studies have reported the technique of the microencapsulation by using gelatin, or vegetable gum to provide protection to acid-sensitive *Bifidobacterium* and *Lactobacillus* [172-176].

6.2. Biotechnology and probiotics

With the revolution in sequencing and bioinformatic technologies well under way it is timely and realistic to launch genome sequencing projects for representative probiotic microorganisms. The rapidly increasing number of published lactic acid bacterial genome sequences will enable utilizing this sequence information in the studies related to probiotic technology. If genome sequence information is available for the probiotic species of interest, this can be utilized, e.g. to study the gene expression (transcription) profile of the strain during fermenter growth. This will enable better control and optimization of the growth than is currently possible. Transcription profiling during various production steps will allow following important genes for probiotic survival during processing (e.g., stress and acid tolerance genes) and identifying novel genes important for the technological functionality of probiotics [177].

Increasing knowledge of genes important for the technological functionality and rapid development of the toolboxes for the genetic manipulation of *Lactobacillus* and *Bifidobacterium* species will in the future enable tailoring the technological properties of probiotic strains. However, before wide application of tailored strains in probiotic food products, safety issues are of utmost importance and have to be seriously considered for each modified strain [178].

7. Regulations and guidelines for probiotics

Depending on intended use of a probiotic (drug *vs.* dietary supplement), regulatory requirements differ greatly. If a probiotic is intended for use as a drug, then it must undergo the regulatory process as a drug, which is similar to that of any new therapeutic agent. An Investigational New Drug application must be submitted and authorized by the Food and Drug Administration before an investigational or biological product can be administered to humans. The probiotic drug must be proven safe and effective for its intended use before marketing [14]. In the United States, probiotic products are marketed to a generally healthy population as foods or dietary supplements. For dietary supplements, premarketing demonstration of safety and efficacy and approval by the Food and Drug Administration are not required; only premarket notification is required. The law allows that in addition to nutrient content claims, manufacturers of dietary supplements may make structure/function or health claims for their products. The "health claims" must be defensible when placed under the scrutiny by the controlling authorities. Efforts are being made to establish meaningful standards or guideline for probiotic products worldwide (Table 5). The Joint Food and Agriculture Organization of the United Nations/World Health Organization Expert Consultation on Evaluation of Health and Nutritional Properties of Probiotics developed guidelines could be used as the global standards for evaluating probiotics in food that could lead to the substantiation of health claims.

Organization	Region of impact	Action
Food Agriculture Organization (FAO)/ World Health Organization (WHO)	Worldwide	Developed guidelines for the evaluation of probiotics in foods.
International Dairy Federation	Worldwide	Has begun working on methods to determine certain functional and safety properties outlined in the FAO guidelines for the evaluation of probiotics in food.
European Food and Feed Culture Association	Europe	Developed guidelines for use of probiotics in foods.
Codex Standard for Fermented Milks (Codex Stan 243-2003)	Worldwide	Among other composition stipulations, this standard specifies minimum numbers of characterizing and additional labeled microbes in yoghurt, acidophilus milk, kefir, kumys and other fermented milks.
National Yogurt Association	USA	Petition under consideration by the FDA which would change the standard of identity of yoghurt, including the requirement of minimum levels of live cultures in yoghurt, but not specifically levels for any additional probiotic cultures.
International Scientific Association for Probiotics and Prebiotics	Worldwide	Industry Advisory Committee and Board of Directors to consider method validation and establishment of laboratory sites to assess microbiological content of probiotic products.

Table 5. Organizations involved in attempting to establish standards for probiotics in commercial products. Adapted from [179]

8. Conclusion

The uses of probiotics and their applications have shown tremendous increase in the last two decades. Probiotics can turn many health benefits to the human, animals, and plants. Applications of probiotics hold many challenges. In addition to the viability and sensory acceptance, it must be kept in mind that strain selection, processing, and inoculation of starter cultures must be considered. Probiotics industry also faces challenges when claiming the health benefits. It cannot be assumed that simply adding a given number of probiotic bacteria to a food product will transfer health to the subject. Indeed, it has been shown that viability of probiotics throughout the storage period in addition to the recovery levels in the gastrointestinal tract are important factors [3, 48, 83]. For this purpose, new studies must be carried out to: test ingredients, explore more options of media that have not yet been industrially utilized, reengineer products and processes, and show that lactose-intolerant and vegetarian consumers demand new nourishing and palatable probiotic products.

Author details

Danfeng Song*, Salam Ibrahim and Saeed Hayek
Department of Family and Consumer Science,
North Carolina Agricultural and Technical State University, Greensboro, NC, USA

9. References

[1] Arvanitoyannis IS, Van Houwelingen-Koukaliaroglou M (2005) Functional Foods: a Survey of Health Claims, Pros and Cons, and Current Legislation. Crit. rev. food sci. nutr. 45:385-404.

[2] Joint Food and Agriculture Organization of the United Nations/ World Health Organization Working Group report on drafting guidelines for the evaluation of probiotics in food, London, Ontario, Canada, April 30 and May, 2002 [cited 2010 Aug 25]. ftp://ftp.fao.org/es/esn/food/wgreport2.pdf

[3] Kröckel L (2006) Use of Probiotic Bacteria in Meat Products. Fleischwirtschaft. 86:109-113.

[4] FAO/WHO. (2001) Health and Nutritional Properties of Probiotics in Food including Powder Milk with Live Lactic Acid Bacteria. Cordoba, Argentina: Food and Agriculture Organization of the United Nations and World Health Organization Expert Consultation Report.

[5] Prado FC, Parada JL, Pandey A, Soccol CR (2008) Trends in Non-dairy Probiotic Beverages. Food res. int. 41:111-123.

[6] Leroy F, Falony G, Vuyst L (2008) Latest Developments in Probiotics. In: Toldra F, editor. Meat Biotechnology. Brussels, Belgium: Springer. pp. 217-229.

[7] Von Wright A, Axelsson L (2000) Lactic Acid Bacteria: An Introduction. In: Lahtinne S, Salminen, S, Von Wright A, Ouwehand A, editor. Lactic Acid Bacteria: Microbiological and Functional Aspects. London: CRC Press. pp. 1-16.

[8] Salminen S, von Wright A, Morelli L, Marteau P, Brassart D, de Vos WM, et al (1998) Demonstration of Safety of Probiotics—a Review. Int. j. food microbiol. 44:93-106.

[9] Husebye E, Hellström PM, Sundler F, Chen J, Midtvedt T (2001) Influence of Microbial Species on Small Intestinal Myoelectric Activity and Transit in Germ-free Rats. Am. j. physiol-gast. l. 280:G368-G380.

[10] Banasaz M, Norin E, Holma R, Midtvedt T (2002) Increased Enterocyte Production in Gnotobiotic Rats Mono-associated with *Lactobacillus rhamnosus* GG. Appl. environ. microb. 68:3031-3034.

[11] Halvorsen R, Berstad A, Lassen J, Midtvedt T, Narvhus J (2000) The Use of Probiotics for Patients in Hospitals: A Benefit and Risk Assessment. Norwegian Scientific Committee for Food Safety. 07/112-FINAL: 1-29. ISBN: 978-82-8082-291-8.

* Corresponding Author

[12] Desmazeaud M (1983) Nutrition of Lactic Acid Bacteria: State of the Art. Le lait. 63:267-316.

[13] Marshall V, Law B (1984) The Physiology and Growth of Dairy Lactic-Acid Bacteria. In: Davies FL, Law BA, editors. Advances in the Microbiology and Biochemistry of Cheese and Fermented Milk. London: Elsevier Applied Science Publishers Ltd. pp. 67-98.

[14] Barrangou R, Lahtinen SJ, Ibrahim F, Ouwehand AC (2011) Genus *Lactobacillus*. In: Lactic Acid Bacteria: Microbiological and Functional Aspects. London: CRC Press. pp. 77-91.

[15] Holzapfel WH, Haberer P, Geisen R, Björkroth J, Schillinger U (2001) Taxonomy and Important Features of Probiotic Microorganisms in Food and Nutrition. Am. j. clin. nutr. 73:365S-373S.

[16] Gorbach S (2002) Probiotics in the Third Millennium. Digest liver dis. 34:S2-S7.

[17] Guarner F, Khan AG, Garisch J, Eliakim R, Gangl A, Thomson A, et al (2009) World Gastroenterology Organisation Practice Guideline: Probiotics and prebiotics. Arab j. gastroenterol. 10:33-42.

[18] Vasiljevic T, Shah N (2008) Probiotics—from Metchnikoff to Bioactives. Int. dairy j. 18:714-728.

[19] Shah N (2000) Probiotic Bacteria: Selective Enumeration and Survival in Dairy Foods. J. dairy sci. 83:894-907.

[20] de Vrese M, Schrezenmeir J (2008) Probiotics, Prebiotics, and Synbiotics. Adv. biochem. engin/biotechnol. 111:1-66.

[21] Marteau P, Seksik P, Jian R (2002) Probiotics and Intestinal Health Effects: a Clinical Perspective. Brit. j. nutr. 88:51-58.

[22] de Vrese M, Stegelmann A, Richter B, Fenselau S, Laue C, Schrezenmeir J (2001) Probiotics—Compensation for Lactase Insufficiency. Am. j. clin. nutr. 73:421S-429S.

[23] Reid G, Howard J, Gan B (2001) Can Bacterial Interference Prevent Infection? Trends microbiol. 9:424-428.

[24] Gueimonde M, Kalliomäki M, Isolauri E, Salminen S (2006) Probiotic Intervention in Neonates--Will Permanent Colonization Ensue? J. pediatr. gastroenterol. nutr. 42(5):604-606.

[25] Isolauri E, Sütas Y, Kankaanpää P, Arvilommi H, Salminen S (2001) Probiotics: Effects on Immunity. Am. j. clin. nutr. 73:444S-450S.

[26] Ibrahim F, Ruvio S, Granlund L, Salminen S, Viitanen M, Ouwehand AC (2010) Probiotics and Immunosenescence: Cheese as a Carrier. FEMS immunol. med. microbiol. 59(1):53-59.

[27] Twetman S, Stecksen-Blicks C (2008) Probiotics and Oral Health Effects in Children. Int. j. paediatr. dent. 18:3-10.

[28] Krehbiel CR, Rust SR, Zhang G, & Gilliland SE (2003) Bacterial Direct-fed Microbials in Ruminant Diets: Performance Response and Mode of Action. J. anim. sci. 81(14). Electronic Supplement (2), E120.

[29] Kalavathy R, Abdullah N, Jalaludin S, & Ho YW (2003) Effects of *Lactobacillus* Cultures on Growth Performance, Abdominal Fat Deposition, Serum Lipids and Weight of Organs of Broiler Chickens. Br. poult. sci. 44(1), 139-144.

[30] Patterson J, Burkholder K (2003) Application of Prebiotics and Probiotics in Poultry Production. Poult. sci. 82:627-631.

[31] Vine N, Leukes W, Kaiser H, Daya S, Baxter J, Hecht T (2004) Competition for Attachment of Aquaculture Candidate Probiotic and Pathogenic Bacteria on Fish Intestinal Mucus. J. fish dis. 27:319-326.

[32] Jin L, Marquardt R, Zhao X (2000) A strain of Enterococcus faecium (18C23) Inhibits Adhesion of Enterotoxigenic Escherichia coli K88 to Porcine Small Intestine Mucus. Appl. environ. microb. 66:4200-4204.

[33] Wang YB (2007) Effect of Probiotics on Growth Performance and Digestive Enzyme Activity of the Shrimp Penaeus vannamei. Aquacult. 269:259-264.

[34] Hooper LV, Midtvedt T, Gordon J (2002) How Host-microbial Interactions Shape the Nutrient Environment of the Mammalian Intestine. Annu. rev. nutr. 22:283-307.

[35] Musa H, Wu S, Zhu C, Seri H, Zhu G (2009) The Potential Benefits of Probiotics in Animal Production and Health. J. anim. vet. adv. 8:313-321.

[36] Balcázar JL, Rojas-Luna T, Cunningham DP (2007) Effect of the Addition of Four Potential Probiotic Strains on the Survival of Pacific White Shrimp (Litopenaeus vannamei) Following Immersion Challenge with Vibrio parahaemolyticus. J. invertebr. pathol. 96:147-150.

[37] Balcázar JL, De Blas I, Ruiz-Zarzuela I, Vendrell D, Gironés O, Muzquiz JL (2007) Enhancement of the Immune Response and Protection Induced by Probiotic Lactic Acid Bacteria against Furunculosis in Rainbow Trout (Oncorhynchus mykiss). FEMS immunol. med. microbiol. 51:185-193.

[38] Berg G (2009) Plant–microbe Interactions Promoting Plant Growth and Health: Perspectives for Controlled Use of Microorganisms in Agriculture. Appl. microbiol. biot. 84:11-18.

[39] Bloemberg GV, Lugtenberg BJJ (2001) Molecular Basis of Plant Growth Promotion and Biocontrol by rhizobacteria. Curr. opin. plant biol. 4:343-350.

[40] Nelson LM (2004) Plant Growth Promoting Rhizobacteria (PGPR): Prospects for New Inoculants. Crop manage. doi.:10.1094/CM-2004-0301-05-RV.

[41] Saleem M, Arshad M, Hussain S, Bhatti AS (2007) Perspective of Plant Growth Promoting Rhizobacteria (PGPR) Containing ACC Deaminase in Stress Agriculture. J. ind. microbial. biot. 34:635-648.

[42] Sheng XF, Xia JJ, Jiang CY, He LY, Qian M (2008) Characterization of Heavy Metal-resistant Endophytic Bacteria from Rape (Brassica napus) Roots and Their Potential in Promoting the Growth and Lead Accumulation of Rape. Environ pollut. 156(3):1164-1170.

[43] Compant S, Clément C, Sessitsch A (2010) Plant Growth-promoting Bacteria in the Rhizo-and Endosphere of Plants: Their Role, Colonization, Mechanisms Involved and Prospects for Utilization. Soil biol. biochem. 42:669-678.

[44] Perrig D, Boiero M, Masciarelli O, Penna C, Ruiz O, Cassán F, et al (2007) Plant-growth-promoting Compounds Produced by Two Agronomically Important Strains of Azospirillum brasilense, and Implications for Inoculant Formulation. Appl. microbiol. biot. 75:1143-1150.

[45] Gardiner G, Stanton C, Lynch P, Collins J, Fitzgerald G, Ross R (1999) Evaluation of Cheddar Cheese as a Food Carrier for Delivery of a Probiotic Strain to the Gastrointestinal Tract. J. dairy sci. 82:1379-1387.

[46] Ross R, Fitzgerald G, Collins K, Stanton C (2002) Cheese Delivering Biocultures: Probiotic Cheese. Aust. j. dairy technol. 57:71-78.

[47] Saarela M, Virkajärvi I, Alakomi HL, Sigvart-Mattila P, Mättö J (2006) Stability and Functionality of freeze-dried Probiotic Bifidobacterium Cells during Storage in Juice and Milk. Int. dairy i. 16:1477-1482.

[48] Phillips M, Kailasapathy K, Tran L (2006) Viability of Commercial Probiotic Cultures (*L. acidophilus, Bifidobacterium* sp., *L. casei, L. paracasei,* and *L. rhamnosus*) in Cheddar Cheese. Int i. food microbiol. 108:276-280.

[49] Akın M, Akın M, Kırmacı Z (2007) Effects of Inulin and Sugar Levels on the Viability of Yogurt and Probiotic Bacteria and the Physical and Sensory Characteristics in Probiotic Ice-cream. Food chem. 104:93-99.

[50] Akin MS (2005) Effects of Inulin and Different Sugar Levels on Viability of Probiotic Bacteria and the Physical and Sensory Characteristics of Probiotic Fermented Ice-cream. Milchwissenschaft. 60:297-301.

[51] Bais HP, Weir TL, Perry LG, Gilroy S, Vivanco JM (2006) The role of Root Exudates in Rhizosphere Interactions with Plants and Other Organisms. Annu. rev. plant biol. 57:233-266.

[52] Parvez S, Malik K, Ah Kang S, Kim HY (2006) Probiotics and Their Fermented Food Products are Beneficial for Health. J. appl. microbiol. 100:1171-1185.

[53] Sanders ME, Klaenhammer T (2001) Invited Review: The Scientific Basis of *Lactobacillus acidophilus* NCFM Functionality as a Probiotic. J. dairy sci. 84:319-331.

[54] Sanders ME, Huis in't Veld J (1999) Bringing a Probiotic-containing Functional Food to the Market: Microbiological, Product, Regulatory and Labeling Issues. Anton leeuw. 76:293-315.

[55] Özer BH, Kirmaci HA (2010) Functional Milks and Dairy Beverages. Int. j. dairy technol. 63:1-15.

[56] Succi M, Tremonte P, Reale A, Sorrentino E, Grazia L, Pacifico S, et al (2005) Bile Salt and Acid Tolerance of *Lactobacillus rhamnosus* Strains Isolated from Parmigiano Reggiano Cheese. Fems. microbiol. lett. 244:129-137.

[57] Saarela M, Paquin P (2009) Probiotics as Ingredients in Functional Beverages. In: Paquin P, editer. Functional and Speciality Beverage Technology. New York: CRC Press. pp. 55-70.

[58] Roy D (2005) Technological Aspects Related To the Use of Bifidobacteria in Dairy Products. Le lait. 85:39-56.

[59] Østlie HM, Helland MH, Narvhus JA (2003) Growth and Metabolism of Selected Strains of Probiotic Bacteria in Milk. Int. i. food microbiol. 87:17-27.

[60] Sendra E, Fayos P, Lario Y, Fernández-López J, Sayas-Barberá E, Pérez-Alvarez JA (2008) Incorporation of Citrus Fibers in Fermented Milk Containing Probiotic Bacteria. Food microbiol. 25:13-21.

[61] De Boever P, Wouters R, Verstraete W (2001) Combined Use of *Lactobacillus reuteri* and Soygerm Powder as Food Supplement. Lett. appl. microbiol. 33:420-424.

[62] Shimakawa Y, Matsubara S, Yuki N, Ikeda M, Ishikawa F (2003) Evaluation of *Bifidobacterium breve* Strain Yakult-Fermented Soymilk as a Probiotic Food. Int. i. food microbial. 81:131-136.

[63] Stephenie W, Kabeir B, Shuhaimi M, Rosfarizan M, Yazid A (2007) Growth Optimization of a Probiotic Candidate, *Bifidobacterium pseudocatenulatum* G4, in Milk Medium Using Response Surface Methodology. Biotechnol. bioproc. eng. 12:106-113.

[64] Janer C, Pelaez C, Requena T (2004) Caseinomacropeptide and Whey Protein Concentrate Enhance *Bifidobacterium lactis* Growth in Milk. Food chem. 86:263-267.

[65] Martinez-Villaluenga C, Frías J, Gómez R, Vidal-Valverde C (2006) Influence of Addition of Raffinose Family Oligosaccharides on Probiotic Survival in Fermented Milk during Refrigerated Storage. Int. dairy i. 16:768-774.

[66] Donkor O, Henriksson A, Vasiljevic T, Shah N (2006) Effect of Acidification on the Activity of Probiotics in Yoghurt during Cold Storage. Int. dairy j. 16:1181-1189.

[67] Talwalkar A, Kailasapathy K (2004) A Review of Oxygen Toxicity in Probiotic Yogurts: Influence on the Survival of Probiotic Bacteria and Protective Techniques. Compr. rev. food sci. f. 3:117-124.

[68] Donkor O, Nilmini S, Stolic P, Vasiljevic T, Shah N (2007) Survival and Activity of Selected Probiotic Organisms in Set-type Yoghurt during Cold Storage. Int. dairy j. 17:657-665.

[69] Aryana KJ, McGrew P (2007) Quality Attributes of Yogurt with *Lactobacillus casei* and Various Prebiotics. LWT-Food sci technol. 40:1808-1814.

[70] Dave RI, and Shah NP (1997) Effect of Cysteine on the Viability of Yoghurt and Probiotic Bacteria in Yoghurts Made with Commercial Starter Cultures. Int. dairy j. 7(8-9): 537-545.

[71] Sultana K, Godward G, Reynolds N, Animugaswainy R, Peiris P, and Kailasapathy K (2000) Encapsulation of Probiotic Bacteria with Alginate-starch and Evaluation of Survival in Simulated Gastrointestinal Conditions and In Yoghurt. Int. j. food microbiol. 62(1-2): 47-55.

[72] [72]Kailasapathy K, and Sureeta BS (2004) Effect of Storage on Shelf Life and Viability of Freeze-dried and Microencapsulated *Lactobacillus acidophilus* and *Bifidobacterium infantis* cultures. Aust. j. dairy technol. 59(3): 204-208.

[73] Picot A, and Lacroix C (2004) Encapsulation of Bifidobacteria in Whey Proteinbased Microcapsules and Survival in Simulated Gastrointestinal Conditions and in Yoghurt. Int. dairy j. 14 (6):505-515.

[74] Iyer C, and Kailasapathy K (2005) Effect of Co-encapsulation of Probiotics with Prebiotics on Increasing the Viability of Encapsulated Bacteria under in vitro Acidic and Bile Salt Conditions and in Yogurt. J. food sci. 70 (1): 18-23.

[75] Capela P, Hay TKC, and Shah NP (2006) Effect of Cryoprotectants, Prebiotics and Microencapsulation on Survival of Probiotic Organisms in Yogurt and Freeze-dried Yogurt. Food res. int. 39 (2): 203-211.

[76] Kailasapathy K (2006) Survival of Free and Encapsulated Probiotic Bacteria and Their Effect on the Sensory Properties of Yogurt. LWT- Food sci technol. 39(10):1221-1227.

[77] Oliveira RPS, Florence ACR, Silva RC, Perego P, Converti A, Gioeilli LA, Oliveria MN (2009) Effect of Different Prebiotics on the Fermentation Kinetics, Probiotic Survival and Fatty Acids Profiles in Nonfat Symbiotic Fermented Milk. Int. i. food microbio.128 (3): 467-472.

[78] Paseephol T, and Sherkat F (2009) Probiotic Stability of Yoghurts Containing *Jerusalem artichoke* Insulin during Refrigerated Storage. J. funct. foods. 1(3): 311-318.

[79] Sandoval-Castilla O, Lobato-Calleros C, Garcia-Galllido HS, Alvarez-Rainirez J, and Venion-Carter EJ (2010) Textural Properties of Alginate-pectin Beads and Survivability of Entrapped *Lb. casei* in Simulated Gastrointestinal Conditions and in Yogurt. Food res. int. 43(1): 111-117.

[80] Ong L, Henriksson A, Shah NP (2007) Chemical Analysis and Sensory Evaluation of Cheddar Cheese Produced with *Lactobacillus acidophilus, Lb. casei, Lb. paracasei* or Bifidobacterium sp. Int dairy j. 17:937-945.

[81] Heller KJ, Bockelmann W, Schrezenmeir J, DeVRESE M (2003) Cheese and Its Potential as a Probiotic Food. In: Farnworth E, editore. Handbook of Fermented Functional Foods. Boca Raton, CRC Press. pp. 203-225.

[82] Mäkeläinen H, Forssten S, Olli K, Granlund L, Rautonen N, Ouwehand A (2009) Probiotic Lactobacilli in a Semi-soft Cheese Survive in the Simulated Human Gastrointestinal Tract. Int. dairy j. 19:675-683.

[83] Vinderola C, Prosello W, Ghiberto D, Reinheimer J (2000) Viability of Probiotic (*Bifidobacterium, Lactobacillus acidophilus* and *Lactobacillus casei*) and Nonprobiotic Microflora in Argentinian Fresco Cheese. J. dairy sci. 83:1905-1911.

[84] Mäkeläinen H, Ibrahim F, Forssten S, Jorgensen P, Ouwehand AC (2010) Probiotic Cheese Devlopment and Functionality. Nutra. foods. 9(3):15-19.

[85] Đurić MS, Iličić MD, Milanović SD, Carić MĐ, Tekić MN (2007) Nutritive Characteristics of Probiotic Quark as Influenced by Type of Starter. Acta periodica technologica. 38:11-19.

[86] Aragon-Alegro LC, Alarcon Alegro JH, Roberta Cardarelli H, Chih Chiu M, Isay Saad SM (2007) Potentially Probiotic and Synbiotic Chocolate Mousse. LWT-Food Sci. technol. 40:669-675.

[87] Wilson E, Seo C, Shahbazi A, Ibrahim S (2004) Survival and Growth of Probiotic Cultures in Sour Cream Products. IFT Annual Meeting. 17A.

[88] Cruz AG, Antunes AEC, Sousa ALOP, Faria JAF, Saad SMI (2009) Ice-cream As a Probiotic Food Carrier. Food res. int. 42:1233-1239.

[89] Charalampopoulos D, Wang R, Pandiella S, Webb C (2002) Application of Cereals and Cereal Components in Functional Foods: a Review. Int. j. food microbiol. 79:131-141.

[90] Stanton C, Desmond C, Coakley M, Collins JK, Fitzgerald G, Ross RP (2003) Challenges Facing Development of Probiotic-Containing Functional Foods. In: Farnworth E, editor. Handbook of Fermented Functional Foods. Boca Raton: CRC Press. 27-58.

[91] Granato D, Branco GF, Nazzaro F, Cruz AG, Faria JAF (2010) Functional Foods and Nondairy Probiotic Food Development: Trends, Concepts, and Products. Compr. rev. food sci. f. 9:292-302.

[92] [92] Rozada-Sánchez R, Sattur AP, Thomas K, Pandiella SS (2008) Evaluation of *Bifidobacterium* spp. for the Production of a Potentially Probiotic Malt-based Beverage. Process biochem. 43:848-854.

[93] Angelov A, Gotcheva V, Kuncheva R, Hristozova T (2006) Development of a New Oat-based Probiotic Drink. Int. j. food microbiol. 112:75-80.

[94] Champagne CP (2009) 19 Some Technological Challenges in the Addition of Probiotic Bacteria to Foods. In: Charalampopoulos D, Rastall RA, editors. Prepiotics and Probiotics Science and Technology. New York: Springer. pp. 761-804.

[95] Savard T, Gardner N, Champagne C (2003) Growth of Lactobacillus and Bifidobacterium Cultures in a Vegetable Juice Medium, and Their Stability during Storage in a Fermented Vegetable Juice. Sci. aliment. 23(2): 273-283.

[96] Kun S, Rezessy-Szabó JM, Nguyen QD, Hoschke Á (2008) Changes of Microbial Population and Some Components in Carrot Juice during Fermentation with Selected Bifidobacterium Strains. Process biochem. 43: 816-821.

[97] Yoon KY, Woodams EE, Hang YD (2006) Production of Probiotic Cabbage Juice by Lactic Acid Bacteria. Bioresource technol. 97:1427-1430.

[98] Lee S, Ji G, Park Y (1999) The Viability of Bifidobacteria Introduced into Kimchi. Lett. appl. microbiol. 28: 153-156.

[99] Yoon KY, Woodams EE, Hang YD (2005) Fermentation of Beet Juice by Beneficial Lactic Acid Bacteria. LWT-Food sci. technol. 38: 73-75.

[100] Chou CC, Hou JW (2000) Growth of Bifidobacteria in Soymilk and Their Survival in the Fermented Soymilk Drink during Storage. Int. j. food microbiol. 56:113-121.

[101] Wang YC, Yu RC, Chou CC (2002) Growth and Survival of Bifidobacteria and Lactic Acid Bacteria during the Fermentation and Storage of Cultured Soymilk Drinks. Food microbiol. 19: 501-508.

[102] Lin FM, Chiu CH, Pan TM (2004) Fermentation of a Milk–soymilk and *Lycium chinense* Miller Mixture using a New Isolate of *Lactobacillus paracasei* subsp. *paracasei* NTU101 and *Bifidobacterium longum*. J. ind. microbiol biot. 31:559-564.

[103] Tsai J, Lin Y, Pan B, Chen T (2006) Antihypertensive Peptides and γ-aminobutyric Acid from Prozyme 6 Facilitated Lactic Acid Bacteria Fermentation of Soymilk. Process biochem. 41:1282-1288.

[104] Fotiou F, Goulas A, Fountoulakis K, Koutlas E, Hamlatzis P, Papakostopoulos D, et al (1998) Characterization of Bifidobacterium Strains for Use in Soymilk Fermentation. Int. j. food microbiol. 39:213-219.

[105] Yeo SK, Liong MT (2010) Effect of Prebiotics on Viability and Growth Characteristics of Probiotics in Soymilk. J. sci. food agr. 90:267-275.

[106] Verbeke W (2006) Functional Foods: Consumer Willingness to Compromise on Taste for Health? Food qual. prefer. 17:126-131.

[107] Tuorila H, Cardello AV (2002) Consumer Responses to an Off-flavor in Juice in the Presence of Specific Health Claims. Food qual. prefer. 13:561-569.

[108] Luckow T, Delahunty C (2004) Consumer Acceptance of Orange Juice Containing Functional Ingredients. Food res. int. 37:805-814.

[109] Wang CY, Ng CC, Su H, Tzeng WS, Shyu YT (2009) Probiotic Potential of Noni Juice Fermented with Lactic Acid Bacteria and Bifidobacteria. Int. j. food sci. nutr. 60:98-106.

[110] Mousavi Z, Mousavi S, Razavi S, Emam-Djomeh Z, Kiani H (2011) Fermentation of Pomegranate Juice by Probiotic Lactic Acid Bacteria. World j. microb. biot. 27:123-128.

[111] Pereiraa ALF, Maciela TC, Rodriguesa S (2011) Probiotic Cashew Apple Juice. Int. congr. eng. food. 2011: 1-6.

[112] Tsen JH, Lin YP, King VAE. (2003) Banana Puree Fermentation by Lactobacillus acidophilus Immobilized in Ca-alginate. J. gen. appl. microbiol.49:357-361.

[113] Kourkoutas Y, Xolias V, Kallis M, Bezirtzoglou E, Kanellaki M. (2005) Lactobacillus casei Cell Immobilization on Fruit Pieces for Probiotic Additive, Fermented Milk and Lactic Acid Production. Process biochem 40, 411-416.

[114] Charalampopoulos D, Pandiella S, Webb C (2002) Growth Studies of Potentially Probiotic Lactic Acid Bacteria in Cereal-based Substrates. J appl. microbiol. 92:851-859.

[115] Salovaara H, Gänzle M (2011) Lactic Acid Bacteria in Cereal-based Products. In: Lahtinen S, Salminen S, Ouwehand A, Wright A. Lactic Acid Bacteria: Microbiological and Functional Aspects. London: CRC Press. pp. 227:245.

[116] Kedia G, Wang R, Patel H, Pandiella SS (2007) Use of Mixed Cultures for the Fermentation of Cereal-based Substrates with Potential Probiotic Properties. Process biochem. 42:65-70.

[117] Gotcheva V, Hristozova E, Hrostozova T, Guo M, Roshkova Z, Angelov A (2002) Assessment of Potential Probiotic Properties of Lactic Acid Bacteria and Yeast Strains. Food biotechnol. 16: 211-225.

[118]] Kedia G, Vázquez JA (2008) Pandiella SS. Fermentability of Whole Oat Flour, PeriTec Flour and Bran by Lactobacillus plantarum. J. food eng. 89:246-249.

[119] Mårtensson O, Andersson C, Andersson K, Öste R, Holst O (2001) Formulation of an Oat-based Fermented Product and Its Comparison with Yoghurt. J. sci food agr. 81:1314-1321.

[120] Wood PJ (1997) Functional Foods for Health: Opportunities for Novel Cereal Processes and Products. Cereal 8: 233-238.

[121] Helland MH, Wicklund T, Narvhus JA (2004) Growth and Metabolism of Selected Strains of Probiotic Bacteria, in Maize Porridge with Added Malted Barley. Int. j. food microbiol. 91:305-313.

[122] Gerez C, Cuezzo S, Rollán G, Font de Valdez G (2008) Lactobacillus reuteri CRL 1100 as Starter Culture for Wheat Dough Fermentation. Food microbiol. 25:253-259.

[123] [123] Hammes W, Hertel C (1998) New Developments in Meat Starter Cultures. Meat sci. 49:S125-S138.

[124] Tyopponen S, Petaja E, Mattila-Sandholm T (2003) Bioprotectives and Probiotics for Dry Sausages. Int. j. food microbiol. 83:233-244.

[125] Axelsson L (2004) Lactic Acid Bacteria: Classification and Physiology. In: Salminen S, Wright A, Ouwehand AC, editors. Lactic Acid Bacteria: Microbiology and Functional Aspects. New York: Marcel Dekker. pp. 1-66.

[126] Leistner L (2000) Basic Aspects of Food Preservation by Hurdle Technology. Int. j. food microbiol. 55:181-186.

[127] Lücke FK (2000) Utilization of Microbes to Process and Preserve Meat. Meat sci. 56:105-115.

[128] Thapa N, Pal J, Tamang JP (2004) Microbial Diversity in Ngari, Hentak and Tungtap, Fermented Fish Products of North-East India. World j. microbiol. biotechnol. 20: 599-607.

[129] Botsoglou NA, Fletouris DJ, ebrary I (2001) Drug Residues in Foods: Pharmacology, Food Safety, and Analysis. New York: Marcel Dekker. 516 p.

[130] Langhout P (2000) New Additives for Broiler Chickens. World poultry. 16(3): 22-27.

[131] Hashemipour H, Khaksar V, Kermanshahi H (2011) Application of Probiotic on Egg Production and Egg Quality of Chukar Partridge. Afr. j. biotechnol. 10(82):19244-19248.

[132] Kawakami S, Yamad T, Nakanishi N, Cai Y (2010) Feedin of Lactic Acid Bacteria and Yeast on Growth and Diarrhea of Hostein Calves. J. Anim. Vet. Adv. 9:1112-1114.

[133] Gaggìa F, Mattarelli P, Biavati B (2010) Probiotics and Prebiotics in Animal Feeding for Safe Food Production. Int. j. Micribiol. 141:S15-S28.

[134] Balcázar JL, Blas I, Ruiz-Zarzuela I, Cunningham D, Vendrell D, Múzquiz JL (2006) The Role of Probiotics in Aquaculture. Vet. microbiol. 114:173-186.

[135] Cassán F, Maiale S, Masciarelli O, Vidal A, Luna V, Ruiz O (2009) Cadaverine Production by *Azospirillum brasilense* and Its Possible Role in Plant Growth Promotion and Osmotic Stress Mitigation. Eur. j. soil biol. 45:12-19.

[136] Long SR (2001) Genes and Signals in the Rhizobium-legume Symbiosis. Plant physiol. 125:69-72.

[137] De Vleesschauwer D, Hofte M (2007) Using *Serratia plymuthica* to Control Fungal Pathogens of Plants. CAB Rev. 2(046): 1-12.

[138] Bai Y, D'Aoust F, Smith DL, Driscoll BT (2002) Isolation of Plant-growth-promoting Bacillus Strains from Soybean Root Nodules. Can. j. microbiol. 48:230-238.

[139] Kloepper JW, Ryu CM, Zhang S (2004) Induced Systemic Resistance and Promotion of Plant Growth by *Bacillus* spp. Phytopathology. 94:1259-1266.

[140] Preston GM (2004) Plant perceptions of plant growth-promoting Pseudomonas. Philos. Trans. R. Soc Lond. B. Biol. Sci. 359:907-918.

[141] Zhao Y, Thilmony R, Bender CL, Schaller A, He SY, Howe GA (2003) Virulence Systems of *Pseudomonas Syringae* pv. Tomato Promote Bacterial Speck Disease in Tomato by Targeting the Jasmonate Signaling Pathway. Plant j. 36:485-499.

[142] Ryan RP, Monchy S, Cardinale M, Taghavi S, Crossman L, Avison MB, et al (2009) The Versatility and Adaptation of Bacteria from the Genus *Stenotrophomonas*. Nat. rev. microbial. 7:514-525.

[143] Schrey SD, Tarkka MT (2008) Friends and Foes: Streptomycetes as Modulators of Plant Disease and Symbiosis. Anton van leeuw. 94:11-19.

[144] Hartmann A, Gantner S, Schuhegger R, Steidle A, Dürr C, Schmid M, Langebartels C, Dazzo FB, Eberl L (2004) N-Acyl Homoserine Lactones of Rhizosphere Bacteria Trigger Systemic Resistance in Tomato Plants. In: Tikhonovich I, Lugtenberg B,

Provorov, editors. Biology of Molecular Plant–microbe Interactions. St. Paul, Minnoesota: IS-MPMI. 4:554-6.

[145] Unno Y, Okubo K, Wasaki J, Shinano T, Osaki M (2005) Plant Growth Promotion Abilities and Microscale Bacterial Dynamics in the Rhizosphere of Lupin Analysed by Phytate Utilization Ability. Environ. microbial. 7:396-404.

[146] Conrath U, Pieterse CM, and Mauch-Mani B (2002) Priming in Plant Pathogen Interactions. Trends plant sci. 7: 210-216.

[147] [147] van Loon LC (2007) Plant Responses to Plant Growth-promoting Rhizobacteria. Eur. j. plant pathol. 119 (3): 243-254.

[148] Matsui S (2009) Probiotics principle that can help organic farming. J. environ. sanit. eng. res .31. The Association of Environmental & Sanitary Engineering Research, Kyoto University.

[149] Antoine JM (2011) Current Challenges for Probiotics in Food In: Lahtinne S, Salminen S, Von Wright A, & Ouwehand A, editor. Lactic Acid Bacteria: Microbiological and Functional Aspects. London: CRC Press p. 213-226.

[150] Shah NP (2007) Functional Cultures and Health Benefits. Int dairy j. 17:1262-1277.

[151] Kailasapathy K, Chin JC (2000) Survival and Therapeutic Potential of Probiotic Organisms with Reference to *Lactobacillus acidophilus* and *Bifidibacerium* spp. . Immunol. cell biol. 78:80-88.

[152] Rodrigues D, Rocha-Santos TAP, Pereira CI, Gomes AM, Malcata FX, Freitas AC (2011) The Potential Effect of FOS and Inulin upon Probiotic Bacterium Performancein Curdled Milk Matrices. LWT - Food sci. technol. 44:100-108.

[153] Saarela M, Mogensen G, Fonden R, Matto J, Mattila-Sandholm T (2000) Probiotic Bacteria: Safety, Functional and Technological Properties. J. biotech. 84:197-215.

[154] [154]Saxelina M, Grenovb B, Svenssonc U, Fondénc R, Renierod R, Mattila-Sandholme T (1999) The Technology of Probiotics. Trends food sci technol. 10 (12): 387-392.

[155] Del Piano M, Morelli L, Strozzi G, Allesina S, Barba M, Deidda F, et al (2006) Probiotics: from Research to Consumer. Digest liver dis. 38:S248-S255.

[156] Ding W, Shah N (2007) Acid, Bile, and Heat Tolerance of Free and Microencapsulated Probiotic Bacteria. J. food sci. 72:M446-M450.

[157] Capela P, Hay T, Shah N (2006) Effect of Cryoprotectants, Prebiotics and Microencapsulation on Survival of Probiotic Organisms in Yoghurt and Freeze-dried Yoghurt. Food res. int. 39:203-211.

[158] Champagne CP, Girard F, Rodrigue N (1993) Production of Concentrated Suspensions of Thermophilic Lactic Acid Bacteria in Calcium-alginate Beads. Int. dairy j. 3:257-275.

[159] http://www.ganedenbc30.com/

[160] Hekmat S, Reid G (2006) Sensory Properties of Probiotic Yogurt is Comparable to Standard Yogurt. Nut. res. 26:163-166.

[161] Oliveira LB, Jurkiewicz CH (2009) Influence of Inulin and Acacia Gum on the Viability of Probiotic Bacteria in Synbiotic Fermented Milk. Braz. j. food technol. 12:138-144.

[162] Luckow T, Sheehan V, Fitzgerald G, Delahunty C (2006) Exposure, Health Information and Flavor-masking Strategies for Improving the Sensory Quality of Probiotic Juice. Appetite 47: 315-325.

[163] Stein LJ, Nagai H, Nakagawa M, Beauchamp GK (2003) Effects of Repeated Exposure and Health-related Information on Hedonic Evaluation and Acceptance of a Bitter Beverage. Appetite 40:119-129.

[164] Kahkonen P, Turoila H, Rita H (1995) How Information Enhances Acceptability of a Low-fat Spread. Food qual. pref. 7:87-94.

[165] Tuorila H, Andersson A, Martikainen A, Salovaara H (1998) Effect of Product Formula, Information, and Consumer Characteristics on the Acceptance of a New Snack Food. Food qual. pref 9:313-320.

[166] Deliza RA, Silva ALS (2003) Consumer Attitude towards Information on Non Conventional Technology. Food sci. technol 14:43-49.

[167] Rokka S, Rantamäki P (2010) Protecting Probiotic Bacteria by Microencapsulation: Challenges for Industrial Applications. Eur. food res. technol. 231:1-12.

[168] Chau CF, Wu SH, Yen GC (2007) The Development of Regulations for Food Nanotechnology. Trends food sci. technol. 18:269-280.

[169] Sozer N, Kokini JL (2009) Nanotechnology and its Applications in the Food Sector. Trends biotechnol. 27:82-89.

[170] Sekhon BS (2010) Food Nanotechnology–an Overview. Nan. sci. appl. 3:1-15.

[171] Sinha VR, Anamika V, Bhinge JR (2008) Nanocochleates: A Novel Drug Delivery Technology. Pharmainfo.net. Available: http://www.pharmainfo.net/reviews/nanocochleates-novel-drug-delivery-technology . Accessed 2012 Mar 12.

[172] O'Riordan K, Andrews D, Buckle K, Conway P (2001) Evaluation of Microencapsulation of a Bifidobacterium strain with Starch as an Approach to Prolonging Viability during Storage. J. appl. microbiol. 91:1059-1066.

[173] Lee J, Cha D, Park H (2004) Survival of Freeze-dried *Lactobacillus bulgaricus* KFRI 673 in Chitosan-coated Calcium Alginate Microparticles. J. agr food chem. 52:7300-7305.

[174] Chen KN, Chen MJ, Lin CW (2006) Optimal Combination of the Encapsulating Materials for Probiotic Microcapsules and its Experimental Verification (R1). J. food eng. 76:313-320.

[175] Chandramouli V, Kailasapathy K, Peiris P, Jones M (2004) An Improved Method of Microencapsulation and its Evaluation to Protect *Lactobacillu* spp. in Simulated Gastric Conditions. J. microbiol meth. 56:27-35.

[176] Heenan C, Adams M, Hosken R, Fleet G (2004) Survival and Sensory Acceptability of Probiotic Microorganisms in a Nonfermented Frozen Vegetarian Dessert. LWT-Food sci. technol. 37:461-466.

[177] Klaenhammer TR, Barrangou R, Buck BL, Azcarate-Peril MA & Altermann E (2005) Genomic Features of Lactic Acid Bacteria Effecting Bioprocessing and Health. FEMS microbial. rev. 29: 393-409.

[178] Ahmed FE (2003) Genetically Modified Probiotics in Foods. Trends biotechnol. 21: 491-497.

[179] Sanders ME, Heimbach JT (2005) Functional Foods in the USA: Emphasis on Probiotic Foods. In: Gibson GR, editor. Food Science and Technology Bulletin - Functional Foods, Vol 1. International Food Information Service (IFIS Publishing).

Chapter 2

Development of New Products: Probiotics and Probiotic Foods

Z. Denkova and A. Krastanov

Additional information is available at the end of the chapter

1. Introduction

Probiotics are live microorganisms that confer a beneficial effect on the host when administered in proper amounts [1, 2]. Their beneficial effects on gastrointestinal infections, the reduction of serum cholesterol, the protection of the immune system, anti-cancer properties, antimutagenic action, anti-diarrheal properties, the improvement in inflammatory bowel disease and suppression of *Helicobacter pylori* infection, Crohn's disease, restoration of the microflora in the stomach and the intestines after antibiotic treatment, etc. are proven by addition of selected strains to food products [3, 4, 5, 6].

Lactobacilli and bifidobacteria are normal components of the healthy human intestinal microflora. They are included in the composition of probiotics and probiotic foods because of their proven health effects on the body [7, 8, 9]. They are the main organisms that maintain the balance of the gastrointestinal microflora [10].

Not all strains of lactobacilli and bifidobacteria can be used as components of probiotics and probiotic foods, but only those that are of human origin, non-pathogenic, resistant to gastric acid, bile and to the antibiotics, administered in medical practice; they should also have the potential to adhere to the gut epithelial tissue and produce antimicrobial substances; they should allow the conduction of technological processes, in which high concentrations of viable cells are obtained as well as to allow industrial cultivation, encapsulation and freeze-drying and they should remain active during storage [11, 12]. This requires the mandatory selection of strains of the genera *Lactobacillus* and *Bifidobacterium* with probiotic properties. Moreover, the concentration of viable cells of microorganisms in the composition of probiotics should exceed 1 million per gram [13] in order for the preparation to exhibit a therapeutic and prophylactic effect.

Along with probiotics probiotic bacteria are most frequently included in the composition of dairy products - yogurt, cheese, etc. [14, 15]. A dairy product that delivers viable cells of

L.acidophilus, L.bulgaricus, Bifidobacterium sp. is bio-yoghurt. Adequate numbers of viable cells, namely the"therapeutic minimum" need to be consumed regularly for transfer of the "probiotic" effect to consumers. This requires, according to Rybka & Kailasapathy, 1995 [16] the consumption of 100 g per day bio-yoghurt containing more than 10^6cfu/cm^3 viable cells.

The species *L.bulgaricus* is a heterogeneous group of bacteria, including strains with probiotic properties [17]. The inclusion of such cultures in yogurt would transform this lactic acid product into a probiotic product.

Probiotic bacteria are included as components of the starter cultures for non-dairy foods [18]. For each type of non-dairy product strains that can grow in the food environment and contribute to the formation of the sensory profile are selected. So in starter cultures for raw-dried meat products probiotic bacteria that are able to grow in the meat environment are included; in soy fermented foods as components of the starter cultures lactobacilli and bifidobacteria strains which can grow and multiply in soy milk are applied; in fruit and vegetables and fruit and vegetable juices microorganisms with probiotic properties suitable for this type of food are used [19].

Some strains of lactobacilli with probiotic potential are used as components of sourdough in bread-making to extend the shelf life and to improve the quality and some technological properties of the final product [20, 21, 22, 23].

In this chapter, the new steps in obtaining probiotics and probiotic foods are discussed. The requirements for the strains of microorganisms which are implemented as components of the probiotics and probiotic foods are listed.

The chapter includes some data from the research of our research team in the field of selection of bifidobacteria and lactobacilli with probiotic properties, developing the technology for obtaining the probiotics "Enterosan", probiotic milk and beverages, probiotic starter cultures for meat foods and non-traditional fermented probiotic foods.

2. Microorganisms with probiotic properties

Enormous amount of microbial biomass inhabits the stomach and the intestines and accompanies individuals throughout their lives. Organisms that are a part of the gastrointestinal microflora, include saprophytic, pathogenic and conditionally pathogenic microorganisms, enterobacteria, lactobacilli, lactic acid cocci, bifidobacteria. They occupy a niche in the digestive tract and enter into complex relationships both among themselves and with the host - man or animal. Depending on the composition of food intake the diversity of species and the ratio between them varies significantly. Upon intake of plant foods fermenting species predominate, while in meat meal representatives of the putrefactive microorganisms take the upper hand. Microbes transform nutrients in food in different ways and excrete metabolites with diverse chemical nature. Through them the gastrointestinal microflora influences the condition and the health of the body. A part of the microflora that includes lactobacilli and bifidobacteria utilizes the substrates and forms metabolites as a result of its vital activity through which it oppresses and expels pathogenic and toxigenic bacteria from the biological niche. The degradation of nutrients from the decay performed by pathogenic and toxigenic microorganisms, which include the pathogenic genera *Clostridium* and *Bacteroides* leads to the formation of toxins and products of decay that inhibit the functioning of the organisms and cause diseases. The balance between these two groups of microorganisms determines to a considerable extent the health of the individuals. Many factors affect this balance - the quality of food, water and air, the neuro-psychological status and stress, the social and personal hygiene, the health and the use of drugs, antibiotics, etc. The age of the individuals also influences the diversity of the microflora in the stomach and intestines.

Maintaining the right balance between the species in the gastrointestinal tract is achieved through the adoption of beneficial flora (lactobacilli and bifidobacteria) in the form of concentrates of viable cells, known as probiotics, or in the composition of foods that can be enriched with them.

Probiotics are biologically active preparations containing high concentrations of beneficial natural microorganisms that allow maintaining a predominantly beneficial microflora in the gastro-intestinal tract, ensuring good health and quality of life. In the last decades, science and health care are paying serious attention to probiotics as preventive and therapeutic tools against many diseases. The first beneficial effect of their adoption is the normalization of the gastrointestinal microflora and the occurrence of recovery processes in the digestive tract. This helps to improve the health status of other organs and systems. The practical application of probiotics clearly speaks in favor of this claim. Probiotic microorganisms should be regarded as an indispensable ingredient of food. Absence, lack or destruction of part or all of the useful microflora poses serious hazards to human health. Therefore, one can neither exist without the normal probiotic microorganisms nor can replace them with something else. Neglecting this requirement is associated with serious consequences for the health and life of humans and animals. Quite often probiotics are the only key to the treatment of some diseases of gastroenterological, functional and deficiency nature.

By applying advanced technologies for fermentation, encapsulation and freeze-drying probiotic preparations (Multibionta, Enterogermina, Reuterina, Enterosan, Florastor) with proven prophilactic and healing action in children and adults against colitis, including ulcerative colitis, gastritis, enteritis, ulcerative disease, intestinal infections, disbacteriosis and some cases of dyspepsia, have been created.

Not all species and strains of lactobacilli and bifidobacteria could act as regulators of the gastrointestinal microflora, but only those who are able to survive and grow under the different conditions of the digestive tract. This requires the selection of strains of lactobacilli and bifidobacteria with probiotic properties, which are reflected in their ability:

1. To be part of the natural microflora in humans and animals.
2. To have the ability to adhere to epithelial cells or cell lines, or at least to be able to colonize the ileum temporarily [24, 25].

Adhesion can be nonspecific - related to the physicochemical factors, and specific - based on specific molecules on the surface of the probiotic cells that adhere to receptor molecules on the surface of the epithelial cells. The strains used in the production of fermented milk products are not with the best adhesion properties, while probiotic bacteria show strong adhesion that is species specific. As far as their ability to adhere is concerned lactic acid bacteria (including lactic acid bacteria used in the manufacture of milk products) show moderate to good adhesion properties when it comes to adhesion on human cell lines [26, 27, 28].

The adhesion of probiotic strains to the surface of the intestine and the subsequent colonization of the gastrointestinal tract of humans creates conditions for better retention in the intestinal tract and implementation of metabolic processes with a strong immunomodulatory effect. Adhesion provides interaction with the mucosa, supporting the contact with the intestine-associated lymphoid tissue, which in turn provides stabilization of the intestinal mucosa that performs a barrier function. The intestine-associated lymphoid tissue can interact with the cells of the probiotic strains and their components and thus has a positive effect on the immune system of the host [29].

In many species of lactic acid bacteria, including those of the genus *Lactobacillus*, the presence of surface-layer proteins [30, 31, 32] has been found. The gene for the S-layer protein has been sequenced and cloned in *Lactobacillus brevis* [33], *Lactobacillus acidophilus* [34], *Lactobacillus helveticus* [35] and *Lactobacillus crispatus* [36].

The thickness of the surface-layer (S-layer) in bacteria is typically 5 to 25 nm and it is composed of subunits arranged in a grid (lattice) with irregular, square or hexagonal symmetry [37]. In the amino acid analysis of the S-layer proteins it was found that they are rich in acidic and hydrophobic amino acids and very poor in sulfur-containing amino acids [38]. In determining the secondary structure it was found that in most S-layer proteins 40% of the amino acids form a β-sheet structure and 10-30% - α-helix [38]. Common feature of all surface-layer proteins characterized so far is their ability to crystallize spontaneously into a two-dimensional layer on the outer side of the bacterial cell wall.

In representatives of the genus *Lactobacillus* some surface located enzymes are established along with the S-layer proteins on the cell surface. The molecular weight of the S-layer proteins in lactobacilli ranges from 40 kDa to 60 kDa and they are one of the smallest known S-layer proteins [31, 36, 39, 40]. Compared with many other S-layer proteins, which are of acidic nature, those in lactobacilli are characterized by high values of their isoelectrical points [41]. The S-layer proteins in some lactobacilli give the cell surface hydrophobicity [40, 42]. Moreover, the hydrophobicity of the cell surface of the strain *Lactobacillus acidophilus* ATCC 4356 can be varied in accordance with the change of the ionic strength of the medium [43]. In a sequencing study of the S-layer proteins in *Lactobacillus acidophilus*, *Lactobacillus crispatus* and *Lactobacillus helveticus* a high degree of homology in one third of their C-terminus is demonstrated [36].

The functions of the S-layer proteins in lactobacilli are insufficiently studied. The S-layer proteins act as adhesins in many bacteria such as lactobacilli and some representatives of the genus *Bacillus*, so they determine their adhesion to epithelial cells or extracellular matrix proteins [44, 45, 46, 47].

3. To survive in the conditions of the stomach and intestines, i.e. to survive in the conditions of acidic pH in the stomach and to withstand the effects of bile [48, 49, 50].

The survival of bacteria in gastric juice depends on their ability to tolerate the low pH values of the medium. Transition time in these conditions depends on the condition of the individual and the type of the food and it ranges from 1 to 3-4 hours. The lactic acid bacteria *L.sakei, L.plantarum, L.pentosus, P.acidilactici* and *Pediococcus pentosaceus* can survive in acidic conditions [51, 52]. Therefore Klingberg et al., 2006 [51] and Pennacchia et al., 2004 [52] suggest the examination of the survival of the strains for probiotic purposes in cultural medium at pH 2.5, acidified with hydrochloric acid for 4 h. Using this criterion *Lactobacillus* strains resistant to low values of pH (pH 2) and the presence of pepsin [17] are selected.

Bacteria that survive in the conditions of the stomach then enter the duodenum, where bile salts are poured and their concentration is 0.3%. Microorganisms reduce the emulsifiable effect of bile salts by hydrolyzing them, thus reducing their solubility. Some intestinal lactobacilli, such as *L.acidophilus, L.casei* and *L.plantarum* have the ability to hydrolyze bile salts [53]. Moreover, some strains of lactic acid bacteria isolated from sausages such as *L.sakei, L.plantarum, L.pentosus* and *P.acidilactici* are resistant to 0.3% bile salts [51, 52].

The survival of probiotic bacteria in the gastrointestinal tract, their translocational and colonizational properties and the destruction of their active components are essential for the realization of their preventive role.

Different probiotic strains react differently in different parts of the gastrointestinal tract - some strains are killed very quickly in the stomach, while others pass through the entire gastrointestinal tract, retaining high concentrations of viable cells [29, 54, 55, 56, 57, 58, 59, 60].

The natural gastro-intestinal microflora, especially lactobacilli, should have the ability to hydrolyze conjugated bile acids that are present in large quantities in the intestines. Conjugated bile acids provide the emulsification, digestion and absorption of lipids more efficiently than bile acids in non-conjugated form. The hydrolysis of bile acids may be associated with the accumulation of energy in anaerobic conditions and / or the detoxication of bile acids that inhibit bacterial growth.

4. To have the ability to reproduce in the gastrointestinal tract. By primarily utilizing the substrate to oppress and expel from the biological niche the pathogenic and toxigenic microorganisms.

5. To possess antimicrobial activity against conditionally pathogenic, carcinogenic and pathogenic microorganisms, which is associated with inactivation of their enzyme systems, overcoming their adhesion, growth suppression and forcing them out of their biological niche, as a result of which gastrointestinal microflora is normalized.
6. To produce antimicrobial substances.

Probiotic strains should be able to carry out fermentation with lactic acid and bacteriocin production by utilizing the carbohydrates, thus changing the pH of the medium and suppressing the development of pathogenic and toxigenic microorganisms or acting directly on the microbial cells by producing antibacterial substances with peptide nature (bacteriocins) [61, 62].

7. To modulate the immune response.
8. To be safe for clinical and food applications.

Lactic acid bacteria applied in clinical and functional foods must be safe, especially if intended for humans.

9. To allow industrial cultivation, resulting in obtaining concentrates with high concentrations of viable cells that can be included in gel matrices (encapsulation), thus retaining their activity in the process of freeze-drying as well as in the composition of the finished products.

Donald and Brow, 1993 [13] and Wolfson, 1999 [63] conclude that in order to prevail in the balance of gastro-intestinal microbial association the number of live beneficial probiotic bacteria shoud exceed 10^9 per gram product. Achieving this value requires a better understanding of the factors of cultivation, concentration, drying and storage.

3. Lactobacilli and bifidobacteria with probiotic properties – Foundation for the probiotics "Enterosan"

Lactobacilli, bifidobacteria and lactic acid cocci are isolated from different sources (from the intestinal tract of infants naturally fermented raw-meat dried products, naturally fermented sourdough, fermented vegetables, etc.) by contemporary breeding and genetic methods, they are identified using the methods of conventional taxonomy (morphological, physiological, biochemical, cultural) and molecular genetic methods (ARDRA, pulse gel electrophoresis, RAPD).

As a result of extensive breeding work on a wide range of strains of lactobacilli and bifidobacteria, strains suitable for incorporation in starter cultures for fermented milk products, probiotics and probiotic foods and beverages that have the ability to reproduce in the model conditions of digestion, to synthesize lactic and other organic acids, bacteriocins, by inhibiting the growth of pathogens that cause toxicity, toxicoinfections and fungal infections are selected. They allow the accumulation of high concentrations of viable cells in the process of fermentation, immobilisation, freeze-drying that retain their viability in storage conditions (Table 1) [64].

Genus *Lactobacillus*	genus *Bifidobacterium*	Lactic acid cocci
L.bulgaricus BG	*B.bifidum* 1H	*Pediococcus pentosaceus*
L.bulgaricus GB	*B.bifidum* L1	*Lactococcus lactis* L4
L.bulgaricus BB	*B.infantis*	*Streptococcus thermophilus* T3
L.helveticus H	*B.breve*	
L.plantarum 226-15	*B.longum*	
L.plantarum Sw		
L.casei C		
L.acidophilus 2		
L.acidophilus A		

Table 1. Strains of lactobacilli, lactic acid cocci and bifidobacteria with probiotic properties

The human organism is a complex biological system, which requires nutrients, air, water and energy for performing the thousands of biochemical reactions, which provide its normal functioning. The food in the stomach is subjected to transformation under the action of enzyme systems and with the direct participation of microorganisms. A part of them, which are related to the genera *Lactobacillus* and *Bifidobacterium*, form the group of the beneficial microorganisms. They digest substrates and through the metabolites, produced as a result of their vital activity, they inhibit and expel from the biological niche the pathogenic, toxigenic and putrefactive microorganisms.

The assimilation of nutrients by the toxigenic and putrefactive microorganisms, which form the group of the undesired microflora, leads to the synthesis of putrefactive and toxic metabolites, which impede the functions of separate systems and the oragnism as a whole.

Pathogenic microorganisms enter the digestive tract of humans and animals and cause digestive disorders and inflammation of the intestinal mucosa, when present in high concentrations (above 10^5cfu/g).

Some of the metabolites produced by lactic acid bacteria and bifidobacteria are lactic, acetic, citric and other organic acids, through which they acidify the medium and inhibit the growth of pathogens. Another group of substances with antimicrobial action are bacteriocins, which have protein nature.

The interactions between the selected group of lactobacilli [17] and bifidobacteria and the pathogens, representatives of *Enterobacteriaceae*, causing toxicoinfections and toxicoses, as well as fungal pathogens and the cancerogenic *Helicobacter pylori* are of great interest.

Pathogenic microorganisms of human origin - *Salmonella sp., Candida albicans, Proteus vulgaris, Enterococcus faecalis, Staphylococcus aureus* subsp. *aureus, Pseudomonas aeruginosa, Klebsiella pneumoniae* subsp. *pneumoniae, Escherichia coli* with viable cell counts of the suspensions above 10^{10}cfu/cm^3 are used as test-microorganisms. The investigations are conducted using the agar diffusion method. The results from these experiments are presented in Table 2.

Bifidobacteria have inhibitory activities close to that of lactobacilli (Table 2). When cultivated together, *B. breve, B. infantis, B. longum* and *B. bifidum* L1 exhibit greater antimicrobial effect in comparison with each one of the strains separately. The titratable acidity of the liquid supernatant is comparatively higher as well. They demonstrate certain synergism, which has a positive effect on human and animal organisms. Having in mind their distribution in the gastro-intestinal tract, they are the main regulators of the microflora in the colon.

Bifidobacteria belong to the symbionts particularly important to the human and animal organism. They are some of the first inhabitants of the digestive tract of the new-born mammals. Their importance is strengthened by their regulatory role in the colon.

Bifidobacteria have active metabolism, producing other organic acids (acetic, citric, tartaric) beside lactic acid. They exhibit antimicrobial activity against pathogenic and toxigenic microorganisms. Their significant synergism with lactobacilli and the rest of their probiotic properties, as well as their important place of habitat, define the important health-promoting role of bifidobacteria.

Strain Test-microorganism	Bif.breve	Bif.longum	Bif.infantis	Bif.bifidum L1	Bifidobacterium symbiotic culture
Salmonella sp., $1,2.10^{12}$ cfu/cm³*	14	9	7	10	15
C. albicans, 5.10^{8} cfu/cm³	10	9 – 10	10	10	10
P.vulgaris, 5.10^{11} cfu/cm³	11	9	7	8	13
E. faecalis, $2,2.10^{11}$ cfu/cm³	13	11	10	9	12 – 13
S. aureus, $1,0.10^{12}$ cfu/cm³	8	10	10	-	8
P.aeruginosa, 7.10^{10} cfu/cm³	11	7	8	8	10
K. pneumoniae, $1,0.10^{11}$ cfu/cm³	20	18	19	21	20 – 21
E.coli $1,5.10^{10}$ cfu/cm³	12	10	9	11	10 – 11

* concentration of the cells of the test-microorganism in the agar medium.

Table 2. Antimicrobial properties of bifidobacteria

The antimicrobial activity of *L. acidophilus* 2, *L. bulgaricus* NBIMCC 3607, the symbiotic culture of *B. bifidum* L1, *B. longum, B. breve* on the growth of 11 strains of *H. pylori* of human origin is determined.

The symbiotic culture of bifidobacteria demonstrates the highest inhibitory effect on *H. Pylori* – the zones of inhibition are >10 mm for 50% of the strains (Table 3.)

L. acidophilus 2 and *L. bulgaricus* GB suppress the growth of half of the investigated strains of *Helicobacter pylori* (Table 3). It must be noted, that the model investigations on the influence of the tested cultures on the cells of *H. pylori* are conducted with liquid concentrates of *L. acidophilus* 2, *L. bulgaricus* GB, symbiotic culture of *B. bifidum* 1, *B. longum*, *B. breve* with viable cell counts above 10^{10} cfu/cm³ and pH of the fermentation medium 6,3. This means that the action of part of the metabolites with antimicrobial activity is eliminated.

H. pylori Mc Farland	Inhibition zone of H. pylori, mm			pH
	L. acidophilus 2	*L. bulgaricus* GB	Symbiotic culture of bifidobacteria	
MF=1	7(10)	7(17)	7(12)	6,3
MF=0.5	7	7	7	6,3
MF =0.5	7	7	7	6,3
MF =0.5	7,5	7	7	6,3
MF=0,5	7	7	15,5	6,3
MF =0.5	9,3	10	13	6,3
MF=0.5	26	20	12	6,3
MF=0.5	7	7	20	6,3
MF=2	9	11	10,2	6,3
MF=0.5	11	9,7	14	6,3
MF=0.5	7	7	8,5	6,3

Table 3. Antimicrobial activity of *L. acidophilus* 2, *L. bulgaricus* GB, the symbiotic culture of *Bif. bifidum* 1, *Bif. longum*, *Bif. breve* against *H.pylori*

4. Antibiotic resistance of bifidobacteria

Antibiotics are substances with antimicrobial action, which influence both Gram-positive and Gram-negative bacteria. They inhibit the growth of or destroy microbial cells. In order to fulfill these functions, the antimicrobial substances must penetrate the cell, conjugate with a certain cell structure, which participates in a vital processes (DNA replication and cell division) or suppress them completely.

The effect of 22 antibiotics - β-lactam (penicillin, ampicillin, cefamndole, ciprofloxacin, amoxicillin, oxacillin, piperacillin, azlocillin), aminoglicoside (streptomycin, gentamicin, kanamycin, lincomycin, clindamycin, amikacin, vancomycin, tobramycin), macrolide (rifampin, erythromycin), tetracycline (tetracycline, doxicycline), aromatic (chloramphenicol) and nalidixic acid, on the growth of the selected lactobacilli - is studied. The 22 antibiotics belong to 3 groups with different mechanism of action – inhibition of the synthesis of the cell walls (penicillin, ampicillin, cefamndole, amoxicillin, oxacillin, piperacillin, azlocillin, vancomycin), inhibition of the protein synthesis (streptomycin, gentamicin, kanamycin, lincomycin, clindamycin, amykacin, tobramycin, rifampin, erythromycin, tetracycline, doxycycline, chloramphenicol), inhibition of the synthesis of DNA and/or cell division (ciprofloxacin and nalidixic acid). The investigated concentrations are equivalent to the actual concentration in *in vivo* antibiotic therapy.

All four strains of bifidobacteria (*Bif.bifidum* L1, *Bif.breve, Bif.infantis, Bif.longum*) are resistant to the action of most of the studied antibiotics with *Bif.bifidum* expressing the best results, followed by *Bif.breve, Bif.infantis* and *Bif.longum*. They show some sensitivity towards the action of aminoglicoside antibiotics. *Bif.bifidum* L1 demonstrates dense growth when tested against 18 out of the 22 antibiotics, weak growth when examined against 3 of the 22 antibiotics and it has single colonies in the clearance zone when tested against vancomycin. *Bif.breve* shows the following results: dense growth - 9 out of 22 antibiotics, weak growth – 11 out of 22 antibiotics, no growth – 2 out of 22 antibiotics. *Bif.infantis* exibits dense growth when tested against 5 out of 22 antibiotics, weak growth – 12 out of 22 antibiotics, single colonies in the clearance zone – 3 out of 22 antibiotics, no growth – 2 out of 22 antibiotics. *Bif.longum* is characterized with dense growth when examined against 15 out of 22 antibiotics, weak growth – 6 out of 22 antibiotics, no growth – 1 out of 22 antibiotics. These results reveal the possibility for the inclusion of the strains in the complex therapy against different diseases.

The resistance of the cells of the different *Lactobacillus* [17] and *Bifidobacterium* strains to 22 of the most frequently applied in medical treatment antibiotics reveals the possibility for their application in the cases of disbacteriosis. Moreover, it is better to use strains with natural polyvalent resistance as components of probiotics for the treatment of disbacteriosis.

5. Survival of bifidobacteria in the model conditions of the digestive tract

Bifidobacteria survive in the model conditions of the digestive tract – at low pH values in the presence of enzymes (pH=2 + pepsin) and at neutral pH values in the presence of enzymes (pH=7 + pepsin) (Fig. 1). The cells of the four strains are more sensitive to pH=2 + pepsin than to pH=7 + pepsin. At pH=2 + pepsin a reduction in the number of viable cells is observed; the reduction is by over 2 to approximately 5 log cfu/g at the 24th hour from the beginning of the cultivation in comparison to the baseline concentration of viable cells in the population; *Bif.infantis* and *Bif.longum* are more sensitive to pH=2 + pepsin than *Bif.breve* and *Bif.bifidum* L1. At pH=7 + pepsin the reduction in the number of viable cells is by over 1 to approximately 3 log cfu/g at the 24th hour from the beginning of the cultivation in comparison to the baseline concentration of viable cells in the population; *Bif.infantis* and *Bif.longum* are more resistant to pH=7 + pepsin than *Bif.breve* and *Bif.bifidum* L1.

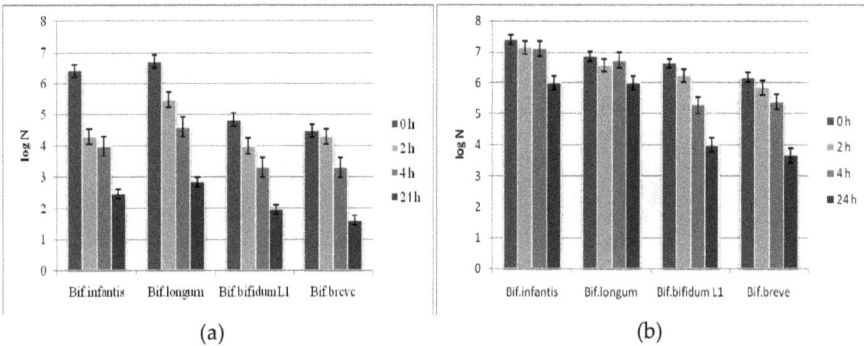

(a)   (b)

Figure 1. Reduction of the viable cells of bifidobacteria at pH=2 + pepsin (a) and at pH=7 + pepsin (b)

All bifidobacteria strains tested for their resistance to different concentrations of bile salts maintain high levels of viable cells (Fig. 2). An increase in the titre of viable cells at 0,15% bile salts is observed in Bif.infantis (Fig. 2a), Bif.bifidum L1 (Fig. 2b) and Bif.longum (Fig. 2c), while in Bif.breve (Fig. 2d) the number of viable cells at 0,15% bile salts decreases from the very beginning of the experiment. At 0,3% bile salts the number of viable cells of Bif.bifidum L1 (Fig. 2b) and Bif.longum (Fig. 2c) increases during the first 8 hours, but at the 24th hour the cell count is lower than the value at the 8th hour in both the two strains. In Bif.infantis (Fig. 2a) and Bif.breve (Fig. 2d), the concentration of viable cells starts decreasing from the beginning of the test.

On the basis of these investigations four groups of probiotics „Enterosan" are developed: probiotics for the gastro-intestinal tract, probiotics for promotion of the functions of some endocrine glands, probiotics for functional usage and probiotics for deficiency diseases [65]. They have high concentration of viable cells of probiotic bacteria (over 10^9cfu/g).

The probiotics "Enterosan" have been tested by leading experts in clinics in our country and abroad and are proven to be beneficial to the human organism - for gastrointestinal infections, rotavirus infections, disbacteriosis due to antibiotics, in chemotherapy, in osteoporosis, arthritis, multiple sclerosis, allergies, anemia, high blood pressure, etc.

The road to developing a probiotic preparation is quite long. It begins with the selection of strains of microorganisms with probiotic properties, the development of probiotic formulations and the implementation of industrial process.

There are several probiotic products on the market but the documentation is often based upon case reports, animal studies or uncontrolled small clinical trials, and only few products declare the content of microorganisms [66].

In the conducted studies on the probiotic properties of different species and strains differences not only between different types of probiotic bacteria, but also between strains within a species are established; differences that should be taken into account in the selection of strains with probiotic properties for industrial use.

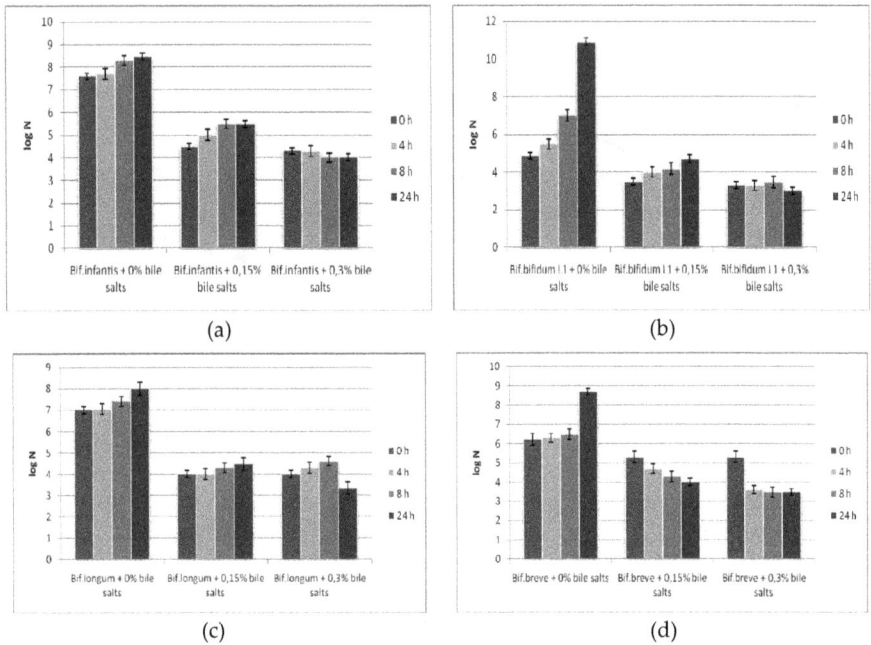

Figure 2. Change in the concentration of viable cells of *Bif.infantis* (a), *Bif.longum* (b), *Bif.bifidum* L1 (c), *Bif.breve* (d) at different concentrations of bile salts

6. Probiotic foods

6.1. Yoghurt with high concentration of viable cells of the probiotic strain *Lactobacillus delbrueckii* subsp.*bulgaricus* NBIMCC 3607

Lactic acid foods occupy a major place in the diet of our contemporaries. About 80% of the population use yoghurt for direct consumption or as a food supplement daily. A characteristic feature of this product is the addition of starters of pure cultures of *Streptococcus thermophilus* and *Lactobacillus delbrueckii* ssp.*bulgaricus* for conducting lactic acid fermentation. By using an appropriate technological process a product with characteristic taste and aroma, physicochemical and biological properties is obtained from milk as a raw material. These traditional lactic acid bacteria have a positive effect on the body, which is a result of the formed metabolites, which inhibit the putrefactive and pathogenic flora or of the improvement of the utilization of lactose [67].

Many functional foods include lactobacilli in their composition (Table 4). Lactobacilli are particularly important in the manufacture of probiotic foods [68]. Several species of the genus *Lactobacillus* are used as starters in the manufacture of yoghurt, cheese and other fermented liquid products [69, 70]. It should be noted that the properties of the strain itself are particularly important in the selection of probiotic cultures. Not all strains can be cultivated on an industrial scale because of the low reproductive capacity in the medium or because of their low survival rate in the processes of freezing and freeze-drying [71]. That is why the cultures used in the production of fermented foods must meet certain requirements (Table 5).

GENUS	SPECIES
Lactobacillus	L. acidophilus; L. delbrueckii subsp. bulgaricus; L. casei; L. crispatus; L. johnsonii; L. lactis; L. paracasei; L. fermentum; L. plantarum;L. rhamnosus; L. reuteri; L. salivarius.
Bifidobacterium	B. adolescentis; B. bifidum; B. breve; B. essensis; B. infantis; B. lactis; B. longum
Enterococcus	E. faecalis, E. Faecium
Pediococcus	P. acidilactici
Propionibacterium	P. freudenreichii
Saccharomyces	S. boulardii
Streptococcus	S. thermophilus

Table 4. Probiotic strains used in the production of fermented milk [72, 73, 74]

The selection of probiotic strains is based on microbiological criteria for food safety of the final product. This is achieved by applying non-pathogenic strains with clear health effects and proper hygiene [75].

The high concentration of viable cells and the good survival when passing through the stomach allow lactobacilli and bifidobacteria in fermented milk products to fulfill their biological role in the intestine.

Several properties of bacteria such as oxygen sensitivity, storage stability, resistance to the proteases of the digestive system, sensitivity to aldehyde or phenolic compounds produced by the metabolism of amino acids, antioxidant activity, adhesion to the intestinal mucosa are examined in *in vitro* testings [88,89]. Strains exhibit the specific properties of lactic acid bacteria in a different degree. The combination of strains with different properties allows the increase in the biological activity of fermented foods. This in turn is related to their ability to develop as symbiotic cultures.

Fermented milk products with probiotic properties are designed on the basis of the experience in the field of development of probiotics. Given that yogurt is the most popular food after bread a technology that includes the use of a starter culture with the probiotic strain *Lactobacillus delbrueckii* subsp.*bulgaricus* NBIMCC 3607, which has high reproductive capacity and meets all the requirements for probiotic cultures, has been developed. The technology is piloted for a period of over 1 year in industry. Table 6 presents the change of the acidity and the concentration of viable cells in the finished product during storage.

Industrial field	Criteria	Product	References
Suppliers of probiotic cultures	Cheap cultivation	Cultures for all groups of products	Charteris et al., 1998 [76]
	Easy concentration for obtaining high cellular density	Cultures for all groups of products	Charteris et al., 1998 [76]
Production of probiotic foods	Possibility for industrial production	Products, produced in high quantities (cheese)	Gomes and Malcata, 1999 [77]
	Compatibility with other lactic acid bacteria	All fermented products	Samona and Robinson, 1994 [78] Nighswonger et al., 1996 [79]
	Stability during storage at acidic conditions	Acidophilous milk, yoghurt, cheese	Micanel et al. 1997 [80] Gobbetti et al., 1998 [81]
	Stability during storage in non-fermented milk	Sweetened acidophilous milk	Brashears and Gilliland, 1995 [82]
	Resistance to bacteriophages	All fermented products	Richardson, 1996 [83]
	Survival in the conditions during the maturation and freezing of the ice cream	Ice-cream	Christiansen et al., 1996 [84]
	Tolerance to preservatives	Non-sterilized products	Charteris et al., 1998 [76]
	Stability during storage at temperatures under -20°C	Ice-cream, frozen products	Modler et al., 1990 [85] Christiansen et al., 1996 [84]
	Tolerance towards oxygen during growth	All fermented products	Gomes and Malcata, 1999 [77]
	Low activity at temperatures under 15°C	Cultures for all groups of products	Gomes and Malcata, 1999 [77]
	Utilization of pentanal and n-hexanal	Soy products	Scalabrini et al., 1998 [86] Murti et al., 1993 [87]
	Fermentation of raffinose and stachyose	Soy products	Scalabrini et al., 1998 [86]

Table 5. Some criteria applied in the selection of probiotic strains for fermented foods

Day	Titrable acidity, °T	Concentration of viable cells, cfu/cm^3		Proportion Str.thermophilus : L.bulgaricus	Extraneous microflora
		Str.thermophilus	L.bulgaricus		
1	104	5x10^{11}	5x10^{11}	1:1	Not found
15	106	6,5x10^{11}	6,45x10^{11}	1:1	Not found
30	108	6x10^{11}	6x10^{11}	1:1	Not found

Table 6. Physicochemical and microbiological indicators of yogurt produced using the new technology

The data show that the yoghurt produced according to this technology lasts for one month, during which the acidity is maintained within the standard requirements and the concentration of viable cells of *L.bulgaricus* NBIMCC 3607 in 1 gram of the product exceeds 1 billion by the end of the prolonged storage. Furthermore, the ratio of streptococci to lactobacilli is within the range of 1:1. A similar result can be achieved in any of the currently used technologies.

High concentrations of lactobacilli in yogurt increase its healing and preventive properties.Thus, the most popular product becomes probiotic.

6.2. Bio-yoghurt

Most of the strains of *Streptococcus thermophilus* and *Lactobacillus delbrueckii* subsp.*bulgaricus* do not retain in the intestinal tract, which limits the application of yogurt during antibiotic therapy and for other medical purposes. Therefore, probiotic bacteria are included in the composition of starter cultures for lactic acid products in addition to the traditional microorganisms *L.bulgaricus* and *Str.thermophilus*, which turns them into products with medicinal properties, known as bio-yoghurt (yogurt, dry mixes, ice cream, soft and hard cheeses, products for infant feeding).

The microflora of bio-yoghurt includes mainly *L.acidophilus, L.paracasei* ssp.*paracasei, L.paracasei* biovar *shirota, L.rhamnosus, L.reuteri, L.gasseri, Bifidobacterium infantis, Bif.breve, Bif.longum, Bif. bifidum, Bif.adolescentis* and *Bif.lactis* [90]. In addition to these species, some products contain *Bif.animalis*, which multiplies faster than other bifidobacteria, but unlike them it is not isolated from the intestinal tract of humans, although some *in vitro* studies show that some strains of *Bif.animalis* have the ability to attach to epithelial cells.

Many researchers believe that only species and strains isolated from the gastrointestinal tract of humans, provide probiotic effects on the human body. The digestive system of the fetus in the womb is sterile. It is inhabited within the first 2-3 days after birth. So right after birth the digestive system is inhabited by species and strains that form its gastro-intestinal microflora, as a result of natural selection, and they are better adapted to the conditions of the gastro-intestinal tract. Through this type of functional foods probiotic bacteria enter the body in the form of fermented milk.

Probiotic lactobacilli attach to special receptors on the epithelial wall and fill the vacant spots in the intestine. They utilize nutrients and produce lactic acid and substances with antimicrobial activity [90]. Their prophylactic role consists in changing the conditions, making them unsuitable for the development of bacteria that cause infections such as *Salmonella* sp. [90]. It has been shown that lactobacilli increase the levels of immunoglobulin Ig A and Ig G [91], thus protecting the immune system, lower cholesterol levels [59, 92], etc.

Bifidobacteria are located on the surface of the colon. In this part of the gastrointestinal tract different types of bifidobacteria utilize nutrients and produce lactic and acetic acids and antimicrobial substances (bacteriocins). The large amount of viable cells of bifidobacteria stimulate the walls of the colon to excrete the polysaccharide mucin that facilitates the passage of faeces through the colon, thereby preventing the colonization of cells of *E.coli, Candida* sp. thus protecting the body.

In recent years some yoghurt products have been reformulated to include live cells of strains of *L.acidophilus* and species of *Bifidobacterium* (known as AB-cultures) in addition to the conventional yoghurt organisms, *Str.thermophilus* and *L.bulgaricus*. Therefore bio-yoghurt is yoghurt that contains live probiotic microorganisms, the presence of which may give rise to claimed beneficial health effects [93]. In order to exert its probiotic effect, the number of viable cells of probiotic bacteria in bio-yoghurt should exceed 1 million [94] (10^8-10^9cfu/g) [10]. According to a Japanese standard the number of bifidobacteria in fresh milk must be at least 10^7 viable cells/ml. As far as the National Yoghurt Association (NYA) in the U.S. is concerned in the production of bio-yoghurt the concentration of lactic acid bacteria in the finished products must be 10^8 viable cells of lactic acid bacteria / g. Moreover, the culture must have rapid growth during fermentation as well as acid tolerance in order to maintain high microbial content during storage.

Technologies for obtaining probiotic yogurt from whole milk and lactic acid beverage with bifidobacteria from skimmed cow's milk with the participation of *Streptococcus thermophilus, Lactobacillus bulgaricus* and strains of the genus *Bifidobacterium* have been developed. The microbiological indicators of this probiotic milk are presented in Table 7.

With the inclusion of bifidobacteria in the starter culture for yoghurt a product with high concentration of active cells (more than 10^8cfu/g) with durability of 30 days is obtained (Table 7).

Day	Titrable acidity, °T	Concentration of viable cells, cfu/cm³			Proportion *Str.thermophilus* : *L.bulgaricus*	Extraneous microflora
		Str.thermophilus	*L.bulgaricus*	Bifidobacteria		
1	114	7×10^{10}	$3,5 \times 10^{10}$	7×10^9	1:2	Not found
15	120	$7,7 \times 10^{10}$	$3,75 \times 10^{10}$	$2,9 \times 10^9$	1:2	Not found
30	126	6×10^9	3×10^9	5×10^8	1:2	Not found

Table 7. Physicochemical and microbiological indicators of the probiotic yogurt with bifidobacteria during storage at $4 \pm 2°C$

A technology for obtaining fermented milk beverage with bifidobacteria has been developed and implemented. The concentration of viable cells in the product is over $10^9 cfu/cm^3$, which is consistent with the requirements for the concentration of viable probiotic cells in bio-yogurt, required to perform health beneficial effects. The beverage retains the concentration of bifidobacteria cells for 40 days when stored at $4 \pm 2^{\circ}C$ (Table 8).

Day	Concentration of viable cells, cfu/cm³		Titrable acidity, °T	Extraneous microflora
	L. delbrueckii subsp. *bulgaricus*	*Bifidobacterium* sp.		
1	$8,0 \times 10^{12}$	$7,0 \times 10^{10}$	102	Not found
10	$7,7 \times 10^{12}$	$2,9 \times 10^{10}$	104	Not found
20	$6,0 \times 10^{12}$	$5,0 \times 10^{9}$	108	Not found
30	$1,0 \times 10^{11}$	$3,0 \times 10^{9}$	110	Not found
40	$1,2 \times 10^{11}$	$2,0 \times 10^{9}$	120	Not found
90	$1,7 \times 10^{8}$	$7,0 \times 10^{8}$	125	Not found

Table 8. Physicochemical and microbiological characterization of the probiotic milk during storage at $4 \pm 2^{\circ}C$

A technology for obtaining other probiotic foods - acidophilous milk and milk, containing *Lactobacillus acidophilus* and bifidobacteria - has been developed as well, which expands the range of dairy foods with preventive role for humans, which in turn is the key to protecting public health.

Lactic acid bacteria are applied in the production of different types of cheeses. Other microorganisms that form the specific properties of cheeses are involved as well. Using molds to obtain cheeses not only radically alters the organoleptic characteristics of cheeses, but also requires changes in the production technology. Depending on the types of microorganisms in the composition of starter cultures, cheeses with starter cultures of mesophilic lactic acid bacteria, starter cultures of mesophilic and thermophilic lactic acid bacteria and propionic acid bacteria, with the participation of molds, bifidobacteria and/or *Lactobacillus acidophilus* - dietetic (functional) cheeses [90] are obtained.

In the production of certain hard cheeses with high temperature of the secondary heating propionic acid bacteria participate in the formation of the specific taste, flavor and texture of the product along with lactic acid bacteria. Propionic acid bacteria absorb part of the lactate, forming propionic and acetic acid and carbon dioxide. Therefore, as a component of these starter cultures the propionic acid bacterial species *Propionibacterium frendenreichii* subsp. *frendenreichii*, *Propionibacterium frendenreichii* subsp. *shermanii* and *Propionibacterium frendenreichii globosum* are included.

The research on the development of starter cultures for yoghurt conducted by our research team shows the importance of achieving symbiosis between the strains in the composition of the starter culture for the quality of the finished product. Few strains of *L. bulgaricus* can be used to obtain a symbiotic culture. The symbiosis between *L. bulgaricus* and *Str. thermophilus* determines the taste-aroma complex of the finished products to a great extent.

A starter culture for hard cheese with the inclusion of the strain *Propionibacterium frendenreichii* subsp. *frendenreichii* NBIMCC 328 with high antioxidant activity (catalase, peroxidase and superoxide reductase), determined by the ORAC method (Oxygen Radical Absorbance Capacity), antimicrobial ability, moderate lipolytic and proteolytic activity is created. The ability of the microorganisms to neutralize free radicals is important for milk production and health, since they enter the gastrointestinal tract with food and their growth continues after intake. Thus another source of antioxidants (bacteria capable of synthesizing antioxidants during growth) is ensured.

Probiotic bacteria are included in a starter culture for hard cheese with high temperature of second heating (50-52^{0}C), providing protection of the product in the process of maturation and storage.

At the end of the ripening process high content of beneficial microorganisms - lactic acid and propionic acid bacteria with concentration of 10^8cfu/g - remains. There are no representatives of the pathogenic microflora. Extraneous microflora is less than 100 cfu/g. Moreover, in the final hard cheese the concentration of viable cells is more than 10^8cfu/g. This opens up new paths for the usage of microorganisms with probiotic potential. The content of short-chain acids in the hard cheese with high temperature of secondary heating is determined by HPLC. The final product contains significant amount of propionate (14,9 mg/kg) and acetate (2 mg/kg).

Goat's milk improves blood composition and exhibits bactericidal properties, strengthens the immunity, accelerates the healing of bone traumas due to its significant levels of calcium, activates the work of the digestive glands and has anti-allergic properties. It also has a positive impact on diseases of the skin, joints, etc. It protects against tooth decay and helps build a healthy enamel. Gastric diseases are rapidly improved with goat's milk. In the cases of arthritis, rheumatism and all conditions in which acidic metabolic products occur predominantly such as diabetes, heart, lung, kidney, liver, etc. the health of the individual improves significantly after the inclusion of goat's milk in the diet. Goat's milk combined with soaked and peeled dates turns out to be useful combination in the case of gastric ulcer and in combination with dried figs in the case of arthritis.

Goat's milk is digested in the stomach 20 min after intake, unlike cow's milk, which requires 2 hours. Great part of the population eats goat's milk.

Yoghurts and yoghurt beverages from goat's milk with lactobacilli and bifidobacteria with probiotic properties are obtained as a result of the work of our research team (Table 9 and Table 10). They are characterized with high concentration of viable cells (above 10^8cfu/cm^3). Probiotic bacteria influence not only the functionality but also the flavor of these products.

Storage time	10 days			20 days			30 days		
	N, [cfu/cm³]		TA,	N, [cfu/cm³]		TA,	N, [cfu/cm³]		TA,
Bio-yoghurt	LAB	bifidobacteria	[°T]	LAB	bifidobacteria	[°T]	LAB	bifidobacteria	[°T]
Bif. bifidum L1	$5x10^{11}$	$3,2x10^{11}$	97	$4x10^{11}$	$8x10^{11}$	110	$6x10^{10}$	$7x10^8$	108
MZ₂ control	$2,7x10^{12}$	-	68	$3x10^{11}$	-	112	$3x10^{10}$	-	126
Lactobacillus acidophilus 2	$1,3x10^{12}$	-	94	$1,1x10^{12}$	-	105	$6x1010$	-	119
Lactobacillus acidophilus 2 + Bif. bifidum	$9x10^{12}$	$5,3x10^{11}$	82	$3,5x10^{12}$	$4,2x10^{11}$	112,5	$6x10^{11}$	$4x10^8$	120

MZ₂ – starter culture for yoghurt containing a probiotic strain of *Lactobacillus delbrueckii* ssp.*bulgaricus* and *Streptococcus thermophilus*

Table 9. Concentration of viable cells (N) and titrable acidity (TA) of goat yoghurt, produced with a probiotic starter cultures during storage

Storage time	1day			15 days			30 days		
	N, [cfu/cm³]		TA,	N, [cfu/cm³]		TA,	N, [cfu/cm³]		TA,
Beverage	LAB	bifidobacteria	[°T]	LAB	bifidobacteria	[°T]	LAB	bifidobacteria	[°T]
B. bifidum L1	$3,5x10^{12}$	$1x10^{10}$	90	$3,75x10^{11}$	$1,9x10^{10}$	98	$4x10^{11}$	$1x10^9$	102
MZ₂ control	$7x10^{11}$	-	62	$6,58x10^{11}$	-	90	$5,8x10^{10}$	-	100
Lactobacillus acidophilus 2	$5x10^{11}$	-	58	$5x10^{11}$	-	96	$3,8x10^{10}$	-	110

MZ₂ – starter culture for yoghurt containing a probiotic strain of *Lactobacillus delbrueckii* ssp.*bulgaricus* and *Streptococcus thermophilus*

Table 10. Change in concentration of viable cells (N) of probiotic lactobacilli and bifidobacteria and titrable acidity (TA) of goat yoghurt beverages during storage at temperature 4±2°C

Probiotic goat yoghurt and yoghurt beverages have high concentrations of viable cells of lactobacilli and/or bifidobacteria and can be applied as probiotic foods for 30 days.

6.3. Probiotic bacteria in the composition of the starter cultures for fermented sausages without heating

Biological preservation of ground meat is an important and topical issue for the meat industry. Its solution is associated with the search for suitable strains of microorganisms that provide protective properties and pleasant taste and flavor of the finished products. By applying this method of preservation a number of advantages can be achieved, the most important of which are extending storage, usage of softer modes of cold storage, etc. To achieve targeted fermentation and quality maturation in the production of cured meat products starter cultures of lactic acid bacteria are imported. A new trend in the production of dried meat products is the inclusion of probiotic strains in the composition of starter cultures. They provide proper conduction of the fermentation process in meat foods and significant amounts of microflora beneficial to human health.

Meat products, which are not treated thermally are suitable carriers of probiotic bacteria [95, 96]. Strains of lactic acid bacteria with probiotic properties as starter cultures for fermented sausages are given in Table 11. These species are isolated from the gastrointestinal tract. Human digestive tract is a natural biological environment for *Lactobacillus acidophillus, Lactobacillus casei* and *Bifidobacterium* sp. These microorganisms are found in various fermented foods [90, 97, 98, 99]. According to Anderssen, 1998 [97], however, lactobacilli isolated from the intestines do not grow and contribute to the implementation of fermentation of the meat substrate.

In the preparation of starter cultures for the meat industry various microbial species are included (Table 9).

Microorganisms	Species
Bacteria	
Lactic acid bacteria	*Lactobacillus acidophilus, L.alimentarius, L.casei, L.curvatus, L.plantarum, L.pentosus, L.sakei, Lactococcus lactis, Pediococcus acidilactici, P.pentosaceus*
staphylococci	*Staphylococcus xylosus, S.carnosus subsp. carnosus, S.carnosus subsp. utilis, S.equorum; Halomonadaceae, Halomonas elongata*
enterobacteria	*Aeromonas sp.*
Bifidobacterium sp.	
Actinomycetales	*Kocuria varians* *Streptomyces griseus*
Yeasts	*Debaryomyces hansenii, Candida famata*
Molds	*Penicillium nalgioevnse, Penicillium chrysogenum, Penicillium camemberti*

Table 11. Microbial species involved as components of starter cultures

A study conducted by Hammes et al., 1997 [100] clearly shows the beneficial effects of fermented meat products in the fermentation of which strains of the genus *Lactobacillus* with probiotic properties are used [100].

In studies conducted on representatives of the genus *Lactobacillus* it has been found that *Lactobacillus gasseri* JCM 1131T is suitable for meat fermentation. Moreover, *Lactobacillus gasseri* JCM 1131T and *Lactobacillus acidophilus* are the predominant species in the digestive tract of humans and *Lactobacillus gasseri* JCM 1131T has the ability to adhere to the gastrointestinal mucosa. Further research with this strain in meat environment shows some positive effects, but the culture is sensitive to the addition of NaCl and $NaNO_2$ and can only be used in meat products with low salt concentration without the addition of nitrites [101].

Lactobacillus sakei is widely used in meat industry as a species with probiotic properties, high antimicrobial activity against *Escherichia coli, Staphylococcus aureus* and *Listeria monocytogenes*, and ability to retain the sensory profile of meat products [102, 103, 104].

The strains *Lactobacillus plantarum* NBIMCC 2415 [18] and *Pediococcus pentosaceus* NBIMCC 1441 are selected. They grow well in meat environment at high concentrations of sodium chloride and low temperatures, since under such conditions the processes of salting, ripening and drying of these products are performed. They also have well expressed fermentative activity without gas release, reisitance to low pH, moderate proteolytic and lipolytic activity as well as antioxidant activity, which is associated with the formation of free amino acids, volatile fatty acids, carbonyl compounds and other substances that determine the taste and flavor of meat products, have good antimicrobial activity. The two strains are incorporated as starter cultures in a batch of sausage. *Lactobacillus plantarum* NIBMCC 2415 is imported as a monoculture with concentration of 10^8 cfu/g for the implementation of targeted lactic acid fermentation (batch I) and in a combination with *Pediococcus pentosaceus* NBIMCC 1441 (batch II). The microbiological parameters of the products are tested during the process of fermentation and drying. Experimental data are presented in Table 12 and Table 13.

Day	pH	Total Microbial Count, cfu/g	*S.aureus*, cfu/g	*Salmonella* sp., cfu/g	*E.coli*, cfu/g	*Enterococcus* sp., cfu/g	LAB, cfu/g
8	5,00	$1,1x10^3$	-	-	$3x10^3$	$1,1x10^3$	$2x10^9$
18	4,63	Under 10	-	-	-	$2,3x10^3$	$6x10^{11}$
28	5,1	Under 10	-	-	-	Under 10	$7,8x10^{10}$
40	5,5	Under 10	-	-	-	Under 10	$8x10^8$

Table 12. Microbiological parameters of the first batch of sausage in the process of fermentation and drying

Day	pH	Total Microbial Count, cfu/g	*S.aureus*, cfu/g	*Salmonella* sp., cfu/g	*E.coli*, cfu/g	*Enterococcus* sp., cfu/g	LAB, cfu/g
4	5,2	Under 10	-	-	-	Under 10^4	$8,4x10^9$
14	5,5	Under 10	-	-	-	Under 10^2	$5,4x10^{10}$
48	5,5	Under 10	-	-	-	Under 10	$3,5x10^{10}$

Table 13. Microbiological parameters of the second batch of sausage in the process of fermentation and drying

The extraneous microflora is suppressed and the total number of microorganisms is reduced as well as the number of coliforms and enterococci, which ensures safety of the product on one hand and maintaining its quality during fermentation on the other. The product also contains a high concentration of viable cells ($8x10^8$ - $3,5x10^{10}$cfu/g) of the probiotic strain *Lactobacillus plantarum* NIBMCC 2415, which turns the product into a probiotic and healthy one, and these indicators increase its durability and storage time [18].

6.4. Probiotic bacteria in the composition of bread sourdough

Bread is one of the main products in the diet of contemporary people. The quality of bread depends upon several factors. Intrinsic parameters of the flour, such as carbohydrate [105, 106], gluten [107], mineral element [108], lipid content [109, 110] and endogenous enzyme activity [111], and on the other hand extrinsic parameters referring to the breadmaking procedure, such as temperature, stages and extent of fermentation [112], water activity [113, 114], redox potential and additives [115, 116, 117], and incorporation of nutritional or rheological improvers, such as dairy ingredients [118], affect the quality of the final product. The effect of these factors can be either direct or indirect, by affecting the microflora, either this is supplied as a commercial starter or in traditional sourdough processes. These factors influence the microflora submitted in the form of a starter culture or traditional processes involving sour dough [119].

Bread is considered to be perishable food, microbial spoilage is observed quite often.The growth of molds causing huge economic losses and reduction of the safety of the bread due to the production of mycotoxins. Fungal spoilage of wheat bread is mainly due to *Penicillium* sp., which cause around 90% of wheat bread spoilage [120]. Other common bread spoilage molds belong to the genera *Aspergillus, Monilia, Mucor, Endomyces, Cladosporium, Fusarium* or Rhizopus [121]. At present a number of alternatives are applied to prevent or minimize microbial spoilage of bread, e.g. modified atmosphere packaging, irradiation, pasteurization of packaged bread and/or addition of propionic acid and its salts [121, 122].

Propionic acid has previously been shown to inhibit moulds and *Bacillus* spores, but not yeasts to a large extent, and has therefore been the traditional chemical of choice for bread preservation [123]. Legislation implemented under the European Parliament and Council Directive No. 95/2/EC requires that propionic acid may only be added to bread in a concentration not exceeding 3000 ppm [124]. However, recent studies have shown that under these conditions propionic acid is not effective against common bread spoilage organisms [125]. Additionally, a reduction of preservatives to sub-inhibitory levels might stimulate the growth of spoilage molds [126] and/or mycotoxin production [127, 128, 129]. Recent trends in the bakery industry have included the desire for high-quality foods, which are minimally processed and do not contain chemical preservatives, thus increasing the interest toward natural preservation systems [130].

Among the natural means for preservation of bread is the use of strains of lactic acid bacteria, which are imported in the form of sourdough [131, 132], providing fast and reliable stability of the dominant microflora in the production cycle. As components of the starter cultures selected strains homo- and heterofermentative lactic acid bacteria are applied. The latter utilize substrates with the formation of lactic and acetic acid, resulting in acidification of the medium (pH, total titratable acidity (TTK)) [105, 131, 133]. Acetate production by heterofermentative metabolism is of major importance for the development of flavour. The molar ratio between lactic to acetic acid in bread (fermentation quotient, FQ) is considered optimum in the range between 2.0 and 2.7 [131]. Production of suitable end-products during dough fermentation depends on the availability of soluble carbohydrates, which are attacked by the enzymes of the flour and the microbial enzyme systems [105, 134, 135, 136]. Metabolism of carbohydrates is species specific, even strain specific. It depends on the type of sugars, the co-presence of yeasts and the processing conditions [137].

Besides weak organic acids, i.e. lactic and acetic acid [138, 139, 140], LAB produce a wide range of low molecular weight substances [141], peptides [142] and proteins [143] with antifungal activity.

Sourdough is applied in the production of classic bread, sour bread, snacks, pizza and sweet baked goods. Sourdough fermentation increases the performance of the dough, improves the volume, texture, taste and nutritional value of the final product, slows down the loss of freshness and flavor and protects bread from mold and bacterial spoilage. These beneficial effects result from the appropriate balance between the metabolism of yeast strains and strains of hetero- and homofermentative lactic acid bacteria, which are the predominant microorganisms in natural sourdough. The metabolism of lactic acid bacteria is responsible for the production of organic acids and contributes, together with yeasts, to the production of aromatic components [144, 145, 146].

The activity of the lactobacilli in the composition of sourdough affects the protein fraction of flour during fermentation. This protein is particularly important for the quality of the bread, as the protein network of the bread determines its rheology, gas retention and thus the volume and texture of the bread. The substrates for the microbial conversion of amino acids in taste precursors and antifungal metabolites [147] are provided by proteolytic reactions. The levels of some peptides are reduced, which is helpful in the cases of inability to absorb cereal products by some people [148].

Bread with best quality is obtained by the simultaneous use of homo- and heterofermentative lactic acid bacteria in a certain ratio. Pure cultures of yeasts and lactic acid bacteria, imported in sufficient quantities provide fast and reliable stabilization of the dominant microbiota, normal fermentation process and actively participate in the quality of the finished bread. To observe this effect proper selection of species of lactic acid bacteria and process design, control over the purity and the activity of the cultures are required.

The strains *Lactobacillus casei* C, *Lactobacillus brevis* I, *Lactobacillus plantarum* NBIMCC 2415 and *Lactobacillus fermentum* J are isolated from naturally fermented sourdough, which defines their ability to grow in the mixture of flour and water, reaching high levels of viable cells and accumulating acid. Therefore, the growth of each of the four strains in the mixture of flour and water is examined. The change in the concentration of viable cells and the titratable acidity for 96 hours of cultivation at 30°C is traced. The proportions for the repeated kneading every 24 hours are: first day - 44% flour: 56% tap water and 5% 48-hour culture of the strain, second to fifth day: 25% starter from the previous day: 75% new mix flour / water with ratio 44% / 56%. All four strains of lactobacilli grow well in the mixture of flour and water, reaching 10^9-10^{15}cfu/g within 96 hours and the TTA of the sourdoughs increases to around 10^0N (Table 14).

Time, h	0 h		24 h		48 h		72 h		96 h	
Strain	N, [cfu/g]	TTA, [°N]	N, [cfu/g]	TTA, [°N]	N, [cfu/g]	TTA, [°N]	N, [cfu/g]	TTA, [°N]	N, [cfu/g]	TTA, [°N]
L.casei C	2×10^8	1,8	3×10^{11}	10,4	$3,8 \times 10^{11}$	12	$3,8 \times 10^{12}$	11,2	$8,1 \times 10^{14}$	10,8
L.brevis I	$7,6 \times 10^8$	1,9	3×10^{10}	13,2	4×10^{10}	13	$4,2 \times 10^{10}$	8,6	$5,6 \times 10^{10}$	8
Lactobacillus plantarum NBIMCC 2415	2×10^9	1,7	$1,4 \times 10^{11}$	11,8	9×10^{12}	11	$1,8 \times 10^{13}$	9	$1,4 \times 10^{15}$	8,8
L.fermentum J	$1,3 \times 10^8$	2	3×10^9	9,6	$5,2 \times 10^9$	10,2	$5,6 \times 10^9$	8,8	7×10^9	8

Table 14. Change in the concentration of viable cells (N) of lactobacilli and the total titrable acidity (TTA) of the medium in repeated kneading in flour/water mixture every 24 hours for 96 hours

Based on the results for the four strains of lactobacilli a starter culture for wheat bread is created by mixing them in a certain ratio. The ratio of is 2:1:1:1 = *Lactobacillus plantarum* NBIMCC 2415: *Lactobacillus casei* C: *Lactobacillus brevis* I: *Lactobacillus fermentum* J.

The accumulation of biomass and the change in TTA of the sourdoughs during the repeated kneading every 24 hours is determined. The following experiment scheme is applied: first day - 44% flour: 56% tap water and 10% of the combination; second to fifth day: 25% from the starter culture from the previous day : 75% new mix flour / water with ratio 44% / 56%. On the third day of repeated kneading yeasts are added to the sourdough (1g).

The results of the study on the starter culture for wheat bread are given in Table 15. The four strains develop with the accumulation of high concentrations of viable cells (over 10^{10} cfu / g) of lactobacilli and TTA increases to $17,3°N$.

In the sourdough molds have not been established. In addition to that, the metabolites formed by the lactic acid bacteria in the composition of the starter culture inhibit „wild" yeasts that get into sourdough through flours (Table 15). This ability is particularly important in sourdough fermentation of bread in repeated kneading for a long period of time - 6-9 months.

Time, h	0 h				48 h				96 h			
Starter culture	N [cfu/g]			TTA [°N]	N [cfu/g]			TTA [°N]	N [cfu/g]			TTA [°N]
	LAB	M	Y		LAB	M	Y		LAB	M	Y	
Wheat sterter culture	3×10^9	3×10^1	Under 10	2,5	$6,2 \times 10^{11}$	nf	Under 10	8,4	2×10^{10}	nf	Under 10	17,3

Table 15. Concentration of viable cells (N) of lactobacilli and of the Total Titrable Acidity (TTA) in the wheat starter culture and change in the microflora for 96 hours. LAB – lactic acid bacteria, M – molds, Y - yeasts, nf - not found

Along with determining the concentration of viable cells an organoleptic analysis of the starter culture is performed as well. The results show that for 48 to 72 hours of cultivation the starter culture reaches normal consistency of the sourdough and pleasant lactic acid flavor.

The starter culture is probated in industrial production - for the baking of bread 96-hour sourdough with different percentage is used; the percentage is determined by the weight of the used flour - 5%, 7% and 10%, according to the following scheme: 2 kg of flour, 1.5% NaCl, 2% yeasts, the respective percentage from the starter culture and tap water (the amount of water is determined by water absorption of the type of flour). Enhancers are added as well - 2 g/kg flour.

All the indicators of the sourdough and the bread are traced, so that the levels of incorporation of the sourdough would not adversely affect the rheological characteristics of the dough and the technologies adopted by manufacturers for the production of bread. The results of these experimental studies are presented in Table 16.

Wheat bread with the starter culture is baked as well as a control bread (without a starter culture). The data from the evaluation of the final bread with different percentages of the starter culture, including its strength and elasticity, the pieces of bread before and after baking, taste, flavor, etc. are shown in Table 16 and show acceleration of the fermentation process. The bread obtained with the starter culture is healthier, has more elasticity, the loaves of the bread are higher. The final wheat bread has softer and lighter crumb, with pleasant aroma and characteristic lactic acid odour.

Sample	1 Control (without starter culture)	2 Starter culture 5%	3 Starter culture 7%	4 Starter culture 10%
TTA of the starter culture	-	15,6	15,6	15,6
Dough		Elastic	Elastic	Elastic
Rise of the dough [min]	52	50	48	52
Amount of water [%]	53	51	50	48
Temperature of the dough [ºC]	29.1	28.4	29.5	29.4
Pieces before baking		Higher that the control		
Rise of the dough [cm]	9.0	9.0	9.2	9.2
Baking (upper crust)	Normal	Normal	Normal	Normal
Aroma of the bread	Typical wheat bread aroma	Soft lactic acid aroma	Pleasant, characteristic lactic acid aroma	Strong an sharp characteristic lactic acid aroma
TTA of the bread	1.2	1.5	1.6	1.7

Table 16. Indicators characterizing the rheology of the sourdough, the flavor and aroma of the bread, prepared with 96-hour starter cultures

The created starter culture for sourdough for wheat bread improves its technological and organoleptic characteristics. Along with this it has been found to inhibit "wild" yeasts and mold spores in flour.

6.5. Soy probiotic foods

Soy foods are essential in the diet of the people in the Far East. They are rich in protein, supplying the body with all the essential amino acids for building and maintaining the tissues [149]. They are a source of flavones and isoflavones that exhibit antioxidant activity and can reduce the damage caused by free radicals [150]. Soybeans have stachyose and raffinose, oligosaccharides that are bifidogenic factors. The body is supplied with vitamins from groups B and D, mineral elements - calcium, magnesium, iron, etc. by traditional soy foods. Anti-cancer agents - protease inhibitors, saponins, phytosterols, phenolic acids, phytic acid and isoflavones, most of which are important flavones and isoflavones, which are polyphenolic compounds and relate to the group of plant estrogens, phytoestrogens, are also present in soy foods. The general term phytoestrogens refers to substances which have the effect of female hormones, but are not steroids. It is believed that soy foods play an important role in preventing chronic diseases such as menopausal disorders, cancer, osteoporosis, atherosclerosis.

Soy milk is obtained from dried, ripened, whole soybeans. They are soaked in fresh water for 16-18 hours at room temperature. The beans are washed, drained and ground. Hot potable water is added in a blender of Osterizer. The final suspension is filtered, autoclaved at 121ºC, stored overnight at 5ºC and it is processed to obtain soy milk products.

The dense residual mass is also rich in plant protein, vitamins C and E, calcium, manganese and iron and is a soy enrichment agent.

Soy milk contains no lactose. It replaces cow's milk for all people who suffer from allergies, lactase deficiency and milk protein intolerance. It can be used to carry out lactic acid fermentation with suitable strains of lactic acid bacteria (*Lactobacillus acidophilus, Lactobacillus delbrueckii* ssp. *bulgaricus, Lactobacillus casei, Leuconostoc mesenteroides, Lactococcus lactis* ssp. *lactis, Bifidobacterium longum, Bifidobacterium bifidum*) to obtain various fermented soy foods. It is a suitable environment for the development of new probiotic supplements. Having in mind the fact that it contains oligosaccharides, the obtained concentrates are synbiotics.

Soy milk yoghurt has been studied extensively [151, 152, 153]. Fermented soy milk products may provide economic and nutritional benefits, because they can be prepared at higher protein levels at comparable or lower cost than regular fermented milk products [154]. Soy proteins have favorable amino acid balance, meeting the essential amino acid, require ments, except for methionine [155]. The researches of a number of authors [156, 157, 158] show a lot of advantages of the soy milk products in the nutrition of children and adults, suffering from allergies, diabetes, cancerous, heart and renal diseases. Soy milk products and soy milk yoghurt successfully replace fermented milk products from cow's milk [157, 158].

By selection of strains of lactobacilli (*Lactobacillus acidophilus* A) and bifidobacteria (*Bifidobacterium bifidum* L1) alone and in a combination with streptococci (*Streptococcus thermophilus* T3) soy probiotic milk and beverages, characterized by high concentration of active cells of lactobacilli and bifidobacteria (10^{11} - 10^{14}cfu/g) and moderate titratable acidity, which allows 20 days of storage under refrigerated conditions, are obtained.

It has been shown that the antioxidant activity of fermented soy foods is significantly higher in comparison with unfermented soy foods.

Wang et al., 2006 [149] explores the influence of spray-drying and freeze-drying on fermented soy milk with *L.acidophilus* and *Str.thermophilus* and bifidobacteria - *Bif. longum* and *Bif. infantis*. The authors demonstrate increased antioxidant activity in fermented soy milk and the increase is species specific. Freeze-drying of soy milk leads to lower reduction of the antioxidant activity. This opens up new opportunities to use soy milk for obtaining probiotic supplements and probiotic soy milks and beverages.

Soy cheese can be obtained from soy milk coagulated as a result of the action of lactic acid bacteria. Soy cheese is the result of fermentation with starter cultures for soy cheese and the probiotic strain *L.rhamnosus*.

Probiotic lactobacilli and bifidobacteria may be included in other non-fermented soy foods - soy mayonnaise, soy delicacies, etc.in concentration 10^6-10^7cfu/g, which provides greater durability of soy foods.

Heenan et al., 2004 [159] includes *L.acidophilus, L.rhamnosus, L.paracasei* subsp.*paracasei, Sacch.boulardii* and *Bif.lactis* in concentrations 10^6cfu/g in frozen non-fermented vegetable soy desserts made from soy beverage, sugar, butter, salt and stabilizers.

Thus, the durability of soy foods increases as well as their biological effect on the body since they deliver beneficial microflora as well. That is how the preparation of healthy foods without the application of chemical preservatives is achieved. The role of the chemical preservatives is conducted by the imported probiotic cultures.

6.6. Probiotic bacteria in the fermentation of fruit, vegetables, fruit and vegetable juices

Almost all fruits and vegetables can undergo natural fermentation as they are inhabited by many types of lactic acid bacteria. The latter vary as a function of the microflora of the raw material, the temperature and the storage conditions [160]. Currently fermented cabbage, olives, cucumbers, carrots, lettuce, peas, corn, tomatoes, onions, pickles, radishes, Brussels sprouts, etc. are being produced mainly by natural fermentation. They allow fermentation with starter cultures as well. Lactic acid bacteria including the probiotic strains that are included as components of the starter cultures for fermented fruits and vegetables have the ability to grow in the fruit matrix and the cell vitality depends on the strain, the type of the substrate, the final acidity of the product [73], their resistance to high concentrations of salt in the medium, their ability to grow at temperatures around 18ºC, to reproduce rapidly and to accumulate acids, which acidify the environment and inhibit the growth of extraneous microflora. Most of them belong to the genera *Leuconostoc* (*Leuconostoc mesenteroides*), *Lactobacillus* (*Lactobacillus brevis*, *lactobacillus plantarum*, *Lactobacillus casei*) and *Pediococcus* (*Pediococcus pentosaceus*) [161, 162] and can be used as monocultures and as combinations. During its growth in vegetable juice *Leuconostoc* helps the growth of other lactobacilli and bifidobacteria by synthesis of dextranase [163].

Different strains are characterized with different sensitivity to the pH of the juice, to the acidification as a result of the fermentation, to the metabolic products, to the environmental conditions such as temperature, etc. [164, 165]. It has been shown that the optimum temperature for the development of probiotic strains is 35-40ºC and pH varies between 4,0 and 3,6 [6]. To protect the cells from the effects of the environmental factors agar, alginate, chitosan are used [165, 166, 167]. A probiotic banana product fermented with *Lactobacillus acidophilus*, included in alginate gel structures, is obtained. The inclusion of bacteria in alginate gel and carrageenan matrices protects the cells from the damages resulting from freezing and freeze-drying [168]. Encapsulation is applied in the production of probiotics as well [169].

Many fruits and vegetables allow processing to turn into media rich in nutrients, mineral elements, vitamins and antioxidants suitable for the growth of probiotic bacteria [170]. The probiotic strain *Lactobacillus plantarum* NBIMCC 2415 grows well in such medium (tomato juice) [18]. Tomato juice is a suitable medium for the growth of *Lactobacillus acidophilus*, *Lactobacillus casei*, *Lactobacillus delbrueckii* [170], which for 48 hours of growth at 30ºC reach concentration of 10^8cfu/ml. This probiotic beverage is kept at refrigerated temperature and maintains the amount of viable cells for 4 weeks. The same author obtained probiotic cabbage juice with the same strains of lactobacilli [171].

According to Rakin et al., 2007 [172] yeast autolysate can be added to vegetable juices before lactic acid fermentation. Its addition stimulates the growth of *Lactobacillus plantarum* and *Lactobacillus delbrueckii*.

Lactobacillus acidophilus and *Lactobacillus plantarum* can grow in red beet juice, reaching up to 10^9 cfu/ml viable cells and reducing the pH from 6.3 to 4.5.

Of course during the growth of probiotic bacteria in fruit and vegetable juices it is possible to obtain a product with specific flavor and aroma. In such cases the addition of fruit juices, which remove the off flavor, is needed.

All this suggests that probiotic bacteria represent a potential for obtaining fruit and vegetable functional foods because of their ability to grow in them and their resistance to acidic environments.

7. Conclusion

Beneficial microorganisms (lactobacilli and bifidobacteria) interact with other members of the intestinal microflora. The ability of the selected strains of lactobacilli and bifidobacteria to inhibit the growth of most representatives of *Enterobacteriaceae* which cause toxemia and toxicoinfections and some molds is a criterion that the microbial strains in the composition of probiotics and probiotic foods must meet. This is particularly important for the industry because of the sustainability of their growth to the majority of antibiotics used in modern health care - while pathogenic microorganisms can develop polyvalent resistance towards antibiotics, they can not do so against probiotic bacteria. The antimicrobial effect of the beneficial microflora is due to the synthesis of lactic, acetic and other organic acids and bacteriocins (proteins associated with microbial cells).

The intact intestinal epithelium with normal intestinal microflora serves as a barrier to the migration of pathogens, antigens and other harmful substances from the intestinal contents. Thus the host is protected and normal functioning of the intestines is provided. The impaired balance of the gastrointestinal microflora leads to diarrhea, intestinal inflammation, problems with the permeability or activation of carcinogens from the intestinal contents.

The future will undoubtedly show the many benefits of the combination of compatible symbiotic bacterial strains and prebiotics in functional foods.

So far probiotics are an effective alternative to antibiotics and chemotherapy, but in the coming years they are expected to demonstrate their suitability as therapeutic and prophylactic agents for many diseases associated with disorders of the digestive system.

As far as the products themselves are concerned future studies should be directed towards the selection of strains of lactobacilli and bifidobacteria with high probiotic effect and the development of technologies for the production of improved probiotics and probiotic foods.

Author details

A. Krastanov
University of Food Technologies, Department "Biotechnology", Plovdiv, Bulgaria

Z. Denkova
University of Food Technologies, Department "Organic Chemistry and Microbiology", Plovdiv, Bulgaria

Acknowledgement

We would like to thank prof. Ivan Murgov for his help in creating the probiotics „Enterosan" and some of the probiotic products.

8. References

[1] Kalliomaki M, Salminen S, Arvilommi H, Kero P, Koskinen P, Isolauri E (2001) Probiotics in primary prevention of atopic disease: a randomised placebocontrolled trial. Lancet 357: 1076–1079.

[2] Brown A C, Valiere A (2004) Probiotics and medical nutrition therapy. Nutr. Clin. Care 7: 56–68.

[3] Agerholm-Larsen L, Raben A, Haulrik N, Hansen A S, Manders M, Astrup A (2000) Effect of 8 week intake of probiotic milk products on risk factors for cardiovascular diseases. Eur. J. Clin. Nutr. 54: 288–297.

[4] Nomoto K (2005) Review prevention of infections by probiotics. J. Biosci. Bioeng.100: 583–592.

[5] Imasse K, Tanaka A, Tokunaga K, Sugano H, Ishida H, Takahashi S (2007) *Lactobacillus reuteri* tablets suppress *Helicobacter pylori* infectionda doubleblind randomised placebo-controlled cross-over clinical study Kansenshogaku zasshi. J. Jpn. Assoc. Infect. Dis. 81: 387–393.

[6] Shah N P (2007) Functional cultures and health benefits. Int. Dairy J. 17: 1262–1277.

[7] Hirayama K, Rafter J (2000) The role of probiotic bacteria in cancer prevention. Microbes Infect. 2: 681–686.

[8] Isolauri E (2001) Probiotics in human disease. American Journal of Clinical Nutrition, 73(6): 1142S–1146.

[9] Marteau P R, de Vrese M, Cellier C J, Schrezenmeir J (2001) Protection from gastrointestinal diseases with the use of probiotics. American Journal of Clinical Nutrition 73(Suppl. 2): 430S–436S.

[10] Rybka S, Kailasapathy K (1995) The survival of culture bacteria in fresh and freeze-dried AB yoghurts. The Australian Journal of Dairy Technology 50(2): 51–57.

[11] Mitsuoka T (1999) The human gastrointestinal tract. In: Wood BJB, editor. The lactic acid bacteria. vol.1, Gaithersburg, MD, USA: Aspen Publishers Inc.: 69-114 p.

[12] Kirtzalidou E, Pramateftaki P, Kotsou M, Kyriacou A (2011) Screening for lactobacilli with probiotic properties in the infant gut microflora. Anaerobe 17: 440 - 443.

[13] Donald J, Brown D (1993) Probiotics and the intestinal ecosystem. Let's live, November, 45 – 47.

[14] Garcia-Fontan M C, Martinez S, Franco I, Carballo J (2006) Microbiological and chemical changes during the manufacture of Kefir made from cows' milk, using a commercial starter culture. Int. Dairy J. 16: 762–767.

[15] Penna A L B, Rao-Gurram S, Barbosa-Canovas GV (2007) Effect of milk treatment on acidification, physicochemical characteristics, and probiotic cell counts in low fat yogurt. Milchwissenschaft 62: 48–52.

[16] Rybka S, Kailasapathy K (1995) The survival of culture bacteria in fresh and freeze-dried AB yoghurts. The Australian Journal of Dairy Technology 50(2): 51–57.

[17] Denkova Z, Murgov I, Slavchev A (2006) Selection of lactobacilli with probiotic properties. Bulg. J. of agricultural sci. 12: 689-706.

[18] Nedelcheva P, Denkova Z, Denev P, Slavchev A, Krastanov A (2010) Probiotic strain *Lactobacillus plantarum* NBIMCC 2415 with antioxidant activity as a starter culture in the production of dried fermented meat products, Biotechnol. & Biotechnol. Eq. 24, 1: 1624-1630.

[19] Rivera – Espinosa Y, Gallardo-Navarro Y (2010) Non- dairy products. Food Microbiology 27: 1-11.

[20] Ganzle M G, Ehmann M, Hammes W (1998) Modelling in growth of *Lactobacillus sanfranciscensis* and *Candida milleriin* response to process parameters of sourdough fermentation. Applied and Enviromental microbiology 64 (7): 2616-2623.

[21] Katina K, Arendt E, Luikkonen K H, Autio K, Flander L, Poutanen K (2005) Potential sourdough for healthier cereal products. Trends in Food Science and Technology 16 (1-3): 104-112.

[22] Plessas S, Fisher A, Koureta K, Psarianos K, Nigan P, Koutinas A (2008) Application of *Kluveromyces marxianus, Lactobacillus delbrueckii* ssp. *bulgaricus* and *Lactobacillus helveticus* for sourdough bread making, Food chemistry 106: 985-990.

[23] Plessas S, Alexopoulos A, Mantzourani I, Koutinas A, Voidarou C, Stavropoulou E (2011) Application of novel starter cultures for sourdough bread production. Anaerobe 17: 486-489.

[24] Goldin B, Golbach S (1992) Probiotics for human. In R.Fuller (Ed.), Probiotics: the scientific basis. London:Chapman and Hall, 355-376 p.

[25] Ouwehand A, Salminen S, Isolauri E (2002) Probiotics: an overview of beneficial effects. Antonie Van Leeuwenhoek 82: 279-289.

[26] Lehto E M, Salminen S (1997) Adhesion of two *Lactobacillus* strains, one *Lactococcus* and one *Propionobacterium* strain to cultured human intestinal Caco-2 cell line. Biosci. Microflora 16: 13 – 17.

[27] Ouwehand A C, Tolko S, Kulmala J, Salminen S, Salminen E (2000) Adhesion of inactivated probiotic strains to intestinal mucus. Letters in Appl. Microbiology 31: 82-86.

[28] Ouwehand A, Tuomola E, Tolko S, Salminen S (2001) Assessment of adhesion properties of novel probiotic strains to humen intestinal mucus. International J.of Food Microbiology 64: 119 – 126.

[29] Saarela M, Mogensen G (2000) Probiotic bacteria: Safety, functional and technological properties. Journal of biotechnology 84: 197 – 215.

[30] Masuda K (1992) Heterogeneity of S-layer proteins of *Lactobacillus acidophilus* strains. Microbiol. Immunol. 36:297-301.

[31] Masuda K, Kawata T (1983) Distribution and chemical characterization of regular arrays in the cell walls of strains of the genus *Lactobacillus, FEMS Microbiology Letters* 20: 145–150.

[32] Yasui T, Yoda K, Kamiya T (1995) Analysis of S-layer proteins of *Lactobacillus brevis*. FEMS Microbiol. Lett. 133:181-186.

[33] Vidgrén, G, Palva I, Pakkanen R, Lounatmaa K, Palva A (1992) S-layer protein gene of *Lactobacillus brevis*: Cloning by polymerase chain reaction and determination of the nucleotide sequence. J. Bacteriol. 174:7419-7427.

[34] Boot H, Kolen C, van Noort J, Pouwels P (1993) S-layer protein of *Lactobacillus acidophilus* ATCC 4356: purification, expression in *Escherichia coli* and nucleotide sequence of the corresponding gene. J. Bacteriol.175:6089-6096.

[35] Callegari M, Riboli B, Sanders J, Cocconcelli P, Kok J, Venema G, Morelli L (1998) The S-layer gene of *Lactobacillus helveticus* CNRZ 892: cloning, sequence and heterologous expression. Microbiology 144:719-726.

[36] Sillanpää J, Martínez B, Antikainen J, Toba T, Kalkkinen N, Tankka S, Lounatmaa K, Keränen J, Höök M, Westerlund-Wikström B, Pouwels P, Korhonen T (2000) Characterization of the collagen-binding S-layer protein CbsA of *Lactobacillus crispatus*. J. Bacteriol. 182:6440-6450.

[37] Sleytr U, Beveridge T (1999) Bacterial S-layers. Trends Microbiol. 7:253-260.

[38] Sleytr U, Sára M, Pum D, Schuster B (2001) Characterization and use of crystalline bacterial cell surfacelayers. Prog. Surf. Sci. 68:231-278.

[39] Pelletier C, Bouley C, Cayuela C, Bouttier S, Bourlioux P, Bellon-Fontaine M (1997) Cell surface characteristics of *Lactobacillus casei* subsp.*casei*, *Lactobacillus paracasei* subsp. *paracasei*, and *Lactobacillus rhamnosus* strains. Applied and Environmental Microbiology 63: 1725–1731.

[40] Van der Mei H, van de Belt-Gritter B, Pouwels P, Martinez B, Busscher H (2003) Cell surface hydrophobicity is conveyed by S-layer proteins- a study in recombinant lactobacilli. Colloids Surf. B Biointerfaces. 28:127-134.

[41] Boot H, Pouwels P (1996) Expression, secretion and antigenic variation of bacterial S-layer proteins. Mol. Microbiol. 21:1117-1123.

[42] Ventura M, Jankovic I, Carey Walker D, David Pridmore R, Zink R (2002) Identification and Characterization of Novel Surface Proteins in *Lactobacillus johnsonii* and *Lactobacillus gasseri*. Applied and Environmental microbiology, Vol. 68, No. 12: 6172–6181.

[43] Vadillo-Rodríguez V, Busscher H, Norde W, de Vries J, Van der Mei H (2004) Dynamic cell surface hydrophobicity of *Lactobacillus* strains with and without surface layer proteins. J. Bacteriol. 186:6647-6650.

[44] Hynönen U, Westerlund-Wikström B, Palva A, Korhonen T (2002) Fibronectin-binding function in the SlpA surface protein of *Lactobacillus brevis*. J. Bacteriol. 184:3360-3367.

[45] Kotiranta A, Haapasalo M, Kari K, Kerosuo E, Olsen I, Sorsa T, Meurman J, Lounatmaa K (1998) Surface structure, hydrophobicity, phagocytosis, and adherence to matrix proteins of *Bacillus cereus* cells with and without the crystalline surface layer protein. Infect. Immun. 66:4895-4902.

[46] Schneitz C, Nuotio L, Lounatmaa K (1993) Adhesion of *Lactobacillus acidophilus* to avian intestinal epithelial cells mediated by the crystalline bacterial cell surface layer (S-layer). J. Appl. Bacteriol. 74:290-294.

[47] Toba T, Virkola R, Westerlund R, Bjorkman Y, Sillampaa J, Vartio T (1995) A collagen binding S-layer protein in *Lactobacillus crispatus*, *Applied and Environmental Microbiology* 61: 2467–2471.

[48] Kashtan H (1990) Manipulation of faecal pH by dietary means. Prev. Med. 19 (6): 607 – 613.

[49] Segal I (1995) Faecal short chain fatty acids in South African urban Africans and whites. Dis. Colon Rectum, 38 (7): 732 – 734.

[50] Erkkila S, Petaja E (2000) Screening of commercial meat starter cultures at low pH and in the presence of bile salts for potential probiotic use. Meat Sci. 55: 297–300.

[51] Klingberg T, Axelsson L, Naterstad K, Elsser D, Budde B (2006) Identification of potential probiotic starter cultures for Scandinavian-type fermented sausages, Int. J. of Food Microbiology 105: 419-431.

[52] Pennacchia C, Ercolini D, Blaiotta G, Pepe O, Mauriello G, Villani F (2004) Selection of *Lactobacillus* strains from fermented sausages for their potential use as probiotics. Meat Science 67: 309-317.

[53] Gilliland S, Speck M (1977) Deconjugation of bile acids by intestinal lactobacilli, Applied and Environmental Microbiology 33: 15-18.

[54] Pochart P, Mavtean P, Bouhnik Y, Goderel I, Bourlioux P, Rambrand J (1992) Survival of bififdobacteria ingested via fermented milk during their passage through the human small intestine: an in vivo study using intestinal perfusion. Am. J. Clin. Nutr. 55: 78-80.

[55] Nielsen E, Schlundt J, Gunvig A, Jacobsen B (1994) Epithelial mucus and lumen subpopulations of *Escherichia coli* in the large intestine of conventional and gnotobiotic rats. Microbial Ecol. Health Dis. 7: 263-273.

[56] Alander M, Korpela R, Saxelin M, Vilpponen-Salmela T, Mattila-Sandholen T, von Wright A (1997) Recovery of *Lactobacillus rhamnosus* GG from human colonic biopsies. Lett. Appl. Microbiol. 24: 361-364.

[57] Donohue D, Salminen S (1996) Safety assessment of probiotic bacteria. Asia Pac. J. Clin. Nutr. 5: 25-28.

[58] Donohue D, Salminen S, Marteau P (1998) Safety of probiotic bacteria. In: Salminen, S., von Wright, A(Eds.), Lactic acid bacteria. Marcel Dekker, New York, 369-384 p.

[59] Adams M R (1999) Safety of industrial lactic acid bacteria. J. Biotechnol., 68: 171-178.

[60] Nikolova D (2010) Probiotic and biotechnological characteristics of strains of the genus *Lactobacillus*, PhD thesis.

[61] Barefoot S, Klaenhammer T (1983) Detection and activity of lactacin B, a bacteriocin produced by *L.acidophilus*. Appl. Environ. Microbiol.: 1808 – 1811.

[62] Eswranandam S, Hettlarachy N, Johnson M (2004) Antimicrobial activity of citric, lactic, malic or martaric acids and nisin-incorporated soy protein film against *L. monocytogenes, E.coli* 0157:H7, and *Salmonella gaminara*. J. of Food Science, 69 (3), FMS 79.

[63] Wolfson N (1999) A probiotics primer. Nutrition Science News, 4(6): 276-280.

[64] Denkova Z, Krastanov A, Murgov I (2004) Immobilized lactic acid bacteria for application as dairy starters and probiotic preparations, J. Gen.Appl.Microbiol.50, № 2: 107-114.

[65] Denkova Z, Murgov I (2005) Probiotics "Enterosan"for protection of the health of today's man. J. Biotechnology & Biotechnical Equipment, vol.1 (19): 188-192.

[66] Ljiung A, Wasdstrom T (2005) Lactic acid bacteria as probiotics. Curr. Issues Intest. Microbiol., 7: 73-90.

[67] Hoier E (1992) Use of probiotic starter cultures in dairy products. Food Australia 44(9): 418–420.

[68] Klaenhammer T (1998) Functional activities of *Lactobacillus* probiotics: Genetic mandate. Int. Dairy J. 8: 497–506.

[69] Champagne C, Gardner N (2005) Challenges in the addition of probiotic cultures to foods. Critical Rev. Food Sci. Nutr. 45: 61-84.

[70] Drake M, Small C, Spence K, Swanson B (1996) Rapid detection and identification of *Lactobacillus* spp. in dairy products by using the polymerase chain reaction. J. Food Protection, 59: 1031–1036.

[71] Saxelin M, Salminen S (1996b) The safety of commercial products with viable *Lactobacillus* strains. Infectious Diseases Clinical Practice 5: 331 – 335.

[72] Tamime A, Robinson R (1999) Yogurt science and technology. 2nd edition. Woodhead Publishing, Cambridge and CRC Press, Boca Raton, 619 p.

[73] Shah N (2001) Functional foods from probiotics and prebiotics. Food Technol., 55(11): 46–53.

[74] Mercenier A, Pavan S, Pot B (2002) Probiotics as biotherapeutic agents: Present knowledge and future prospects. Current Pharmaceutical Design 8: 99–110.

[75] Gibson G, Fuller R (2000) Aspects of in vitro and in vivo research approaches directed toward identifying probiotics and prebiotics for human use. J. Nutr. 130: 391–395.

[76] CharterisW, Kelly P, Morelli L, Collins J (1998) Ingredient selection criteria for probiotic microorganisms in functional dairy foods. Int. J. Dairy Technol., 51(4): 123–136.

[77] Gomes A, Malcata F (1999) *Bifidobacterium* spp. and *Lactobacillus acidophilus*: Biological, biochemical, technological and therapeutical properties relevant for use as probiotics. Trends Food Sci. Technol. 10: 139–157.

[78] Samona A, Robinson R (1994) Effect of yogurt cultures on the survival of bifidobacteria in fermented milks. J. Soc.Dairy Technol. 47: 58–60.

[79] Nighswonger B, Brashears M, Gilliland S (1996) Viability of *Lactobacillus acidophilus* and *Lactobacillus casei* in fermented milk products during refrigerated storage. J. Dairy Sci. 79: 212–219.

[80] Micanel N, Haynes I, Playne M (1997) Viability of probiotic cultures in commercial Australian yogurts. Australian J. Dairy Technol. 52: 24–27.

[81] Gobbetti M, Corsetti A, Smacchi E, Zocchetti A, Angelis M (1998) Production of Crescenza cheese by incorporation of bifidobacteria. J. Dairy Sci. 81: 37–47.

[82] Brashears M, Gilliland S (1995) Survival during frozen and subsequent refrigerated storage of *Lactobacillus acidophilus* cells as influenced by the growth phase. J. Dairy Sci. 78: 2326–2335.

[83] Richardson D (1996) Probiotics and product innovation. Nutr. Food Sci. 4: 27–33

[84] Christiansen P, Edelsten D, Kristiansen J, Nielsen E (1996) Some properties of ice cream containing *Bifidobacterium bifidum* and *Lactobacillus acidophilus*. Milchwissenschaft 51: 502–504.

[85] Modler H, McKellar R, Goff H, Mackie D (1990) Using ice cream as a mechanism to incorporate bifidobacteria and fructooligosaccharides into the human diet. Cultured Dairy Products J., 25(3): 4–6, 8–9.

[86] Scalabrini P, Rossi M, Spettoli P, Matteuzzi D (1998) Characterization of Bifidobacterium strains for use in soymilk fermentation. Int. J. Food Microbiol. 39(3): 213–219.

[87] Murti T, Lamberet G, Bouillanne C, Desmazeaud M, Landon M (1993) Croissance des lactobacilles dans l'extrait de soja. Effets sur la viscosit'e, les compos'es volatils et la prot'eolyse. Sciences des Aliments 13(3): 491–500.

[88] Lin M, Yen C (1999) Antioxidative ability of lactic acid bacteria. J. Agricult. Food Chem. 47: 1460–1466.

[89] Godward G, Sultana K, Kailasapathy K, Peiris P, Arumugaswamy R, Reynolds N (2000) The importance of strain selection on the viability and survival of probiotic bacteria in dairy foods. Milchwissenschaft 55:441–445.

[90] Tamime A, Robinson R (2002) Yoghurt: Science and Technology (Eds.), CRC Press, New York, USA, 469-521 p.

[91] Salminen S, Ouwehand A, Benno Y, Lee Y (1999) Probiotics: How should they be defined? Trends Food Sci. Technol. 10: 107-110.

[92] Alerholm-Larsen L, Bell M, Astrup A (2000) The effect of probiotic milk product on plasma cholesterol: a meta –analysis of short-term intervention studies, Eur. Clin. Nutr. 54: 288-297.

[93] Lourens-Hattingh A, Viljoen B (2001) Yoghurt as probiotic carrier food, International Dairy Journal 11: 1-17.

[94] Speck M (1978) Enumeration of viable *Lactobacillus acidophilus* organisms in dairy products. Journal of Food Protection 41(2): 135–137.

[95] Hugas M, Monfort M (1997) Bacterial starter cultures for meat fermentation. Food Chemisrty 59:547-554.

[96] Incze K (1998) Dry fermented sausages, Meat Science 49: S169-S177.

[97] Anderssen L (1998) Fermented dry sausages with the admixture of probiotic cultures. 44th International Congress of Meat Science and Technology: 826-827.

[98] Arihara K, Luchansky J (1994) Dairy lactobacilli. Food Bacteriology: Microorganisms, Y.H. Hui and G.G. Khachatourians(Ed). VHC Publishers, New York 609-643 p.

[99] Goldin B, Golbach S (1992) Probiotics for human. In: Probiotics, the Saentific basis.(Ed. R. Fuller). Chapman and Hall, London 355-376 p.

[100] Hammes W (1997) Microecol.Therapy 26: 97.

[101] Arihara (1998) *Lactobacillus acidophilus* group Lactic Acid Bacteria Applied to Meat Fermentation. Journal of Food Scienc 63: 544-547.

[102] Bredholt S (2001) Industrial application of an antilisterial strain *Lactobacillus sakei* as protective culture and its effect on the sensory acceptability of cooked, sliced, vacuum-packaged meats. Int. J. Food Microbiol. 66: 191-196.

[103] Niessen H, Dainty R (1995) Comparison of the use of rRNA probes and conventional methods in identifying strains of *Lactobacillus sakei* and *Lactobacillus curvatus* isolated rom meat, Int. J. of Food Microbiology 25: 311-315.

[104] Ray B (2004) Fundamental Food Microbiology, GRC Press, Boca Raton 55–57 p.

[105] Collar C (1996) Biochemical and technological assessment of the metabolism of pure and mixed cultures of yeast and lactic acid bacteria in breadmaking applications. Food Sci Technol Int 2: 349–367.

[106] Henry R, Saini H (1989) Characterization of cereal sugars and oligosaccharides. Cereal Chem 66: 362–365.

[107] Callejo M, Gil M, Rodriguez G, Ruiz M (1999) Effect of gluten addition and storage ime on white pan bread quality: instrumental evaluation. Z Lebensm Unters Forsch A 208:27–32.

[108] Emodi A, Scialpi L (1980) Quality of bread fortified with ten micronutrients.Cereal Chem 57:1–3.

[109] Brooker B (1996) The role of fat in the stabilization of gas cells in bread dough. J Cereal Sci 24:187–198.

[110] Collar C, Armero E, Martinez J (1998) Lipid binding of formula bread doughs. Relationships with dough and bread technological performance. Z Lebensm Unters Forsch A 207: 110–121.

[111] Martinez-Anaya M (1996) Enzymes and bread flavor. J Agric Food Chem 44: 2469–2480.

[112] Spicher G, Bruemmer J (1995) Baked goods. In: Reed G, Nagodawithana TW, editors. Biotechnology. 2nd ed. VCH 243–319 p.

[113] Berland S, Launay B (1995) Rheological prperties of wheat flour doughs in steady and dynamic shear: effect of water content and some additives. Cereal Chem 72: 48–52.

[114] Czuchajowska Z, Pomeranz Y, Jeffers H (1989) Water activity and moisture content of dough and bread. Cereal Chem 66:128–132.

[115] Martinez-Anaya M, Jimenez T (1998) Physical properties of enzymesupplemented doughs and relationship with bread quality parameters. Z Lebensm Unters Forsch A 206: 134–142.

[116] Ravi R, Sai Manohar R, Haridas Rao P (2000) Influence of additives on the rheological characteristics and baking quality of wheat flours. Eur Food Res Technol 210: 202–208.

[117] Wikstrom K, Eliasson A (1998) Effects of enzymes and oxidizing agents on shear stress relaxation of wheat flour dough: additions of protease, glucose oxidase, ascorbic acid, and potassium bromate. Cereal Chem 75: 331–337.

[118] Kenny S, Wehrle K, Stanton C, Arendt E (2000) Incorporation of dairy ingredients into wheat bread: effects on dough rheology and bread quality. Eur Food Res Technol 210: 391–396.

[119] Paramithiotis S, ChouliarasY, Tsakalidou E, Kalantzopoulos G (2005) Application of selected starter cultures for the production of wheat sourdough bread using a raditional three-stage procedure, Process Biochemistry 40: 2813–2819.

[120] Legan J, Voysey P (1991) Yeast spoilage of bakery products and ingredients. Journal of Applied Bacteriology 70: 361–371.

[121] Legan J (1993) Mould spoilage of bread: the problem and some solutions. International Biodeterioration and Biodegradation 32: 33–53.

[122] Pateras I (1998) Bread spoilage and staling. In: Cauvain, S.P., Young, L.S. (Eds.), Technology of Breadmaking. Blackie Academic and Professional, London, 240–261 pp.

[123] Ponte J, Tsen C (1987) Bakery products, In: Beuchat, L. (Ed.), Food and Beverage Mycology, 2nd ed. AVI, New York, N.Y., 233–268 pp.

[124] European Union (1995) European Parliament and Council Directive No. 95/2/EC of 20February 1995 on food additives other than colours and sweeteners, p. 53. http://europa.eu.int/eur-lex/en/ consleg/pdf/1995/en_1995L0002_do_001.pdf..

[125] Lavermicocca P, Valerio F, Evidente A, Lazzaroni S, Corsetti A, Gobbetti M (2000) Purification and characterization of novel antifungal compounds from the sourdough *Lactobacillus plantarum* strain 21B. Applied and Environmental Microbiology 66: 4084–4090.

[126] Marin S, Sanchis V, Sanz D, Castel I, Ramos A, Canela R, Magan N (1999) Control of growth and fumonisin B1 production by *Fusarium verticillioides* and *Fusarium proliferatum* isolates in moist maize with propionate preservatives. Food Additives and Contaminants 16: 555–563.

[127] Yousef A, Marth E (1981) Growth and synthesis of aflatoxin by *Aspergillus parasiticus* in he presence of sorbic acid. Journal of Food Protection 44: 736–741.

[128] Gareis M, Bauer J, von Montgelas A, Gedek B (1984) Stimulation of aflatoxin-B1 and T-2-toxin production by sorbic acid. Applied and Environmental Microbiology 47: 416–418.

[129] Bullerman L (1985) Effects of potassium sorbate on growth and ochratoxin production by *Aspergillus ochraceus* and *Penicillium* species. Journal of Food Protection 48: 162–165.

[130] Ryan L, Dal Bello F, Arendt E (2008) The use of sourdough fermented by antifungal LAB to reduce the amount of calcium propionate in bread, International Journal of Food Microbiology 125: 274–278

[131] Hammes W, GaËnzle M (1998) Sourdough breads and related products. In B. J. B. Woods (Ed.), Microbiology of fermented foods, (2nd ed.) London: Blackie Academic/Professional 199–216 pp.

[132] Messens W, De Vuyst L (2002) Inhibitory substances produced by Lactobacilli isolated rom sourdoughs—a review. International Journal of Food Microbiology 72: 31–43.

[133] Corsetti A, Gobbetti M, Balestrieri F, Paoletti F, Russi L, Rossi J (1998) Sourdough lactic acid bacteria effects on bread firmness and staling. Journal of Food Science 63: 347–351.

[134] Martinez-Anaya M (1996b) Carbohydrates and nitrogen related components in wheat sourdough processes. Advances in Food Sciences 18: 185–200.

[135] Gobbetti M (1998) The sourdough microflora: interactions of lactic acid bacteria and yeasts. Trends in Food Science and Technology 9: 267–274.

[136] Robert H, Gabriel V, Lefebvre D, Rabier P, Vayssier Y, Fontagner-Faucher C (2006) Study of the behaviour of *Lactobacillus plantarum* and *Leuconostoc* starters during a complete wheat sourdough breadmaking process, LWT 39: 256–265.

[137] Gobbetti M, Corsetti A, Rossi J (1994) The sourdough microflora, evolution of soluble carbohydrates during the sourdough fermentation. Microbiologie Aliments Nutrition 12: 9–15.

[138] Rocken W (1996) Applied aspects of sourdough fermentation. Advances in Food Science 18: 212–216.

[139] Rocken W, Voysey P (1995) Sourdough fermentation in bread making. Journal of Applied Bacteriology 79: 38S–48S.

[140] Stiles M (1996) Biopreservation by lactic acid bacteria. Antonie van Leeuwenhoek 70: 331–345.

[141] Niku-Paavola M, Laitila A, Mattila-Sandholm T, Haikara A (1999) New types of antimicrobial compounds produced by *Lactobacillus plantarum*. Journal of Applied Microbiology 86: 29–35.

[142] Okkers D, Dicks L, Silvester M, Joubert J, Odendaal H (1999) Characterisation of pentocin TV35b, a bacteriocin-like peptide isolated from *Lactobacillus pentosus* with a ungistatic effect on *Candida albicans*. Journal of Applied Microbiology 87: 726–734.

[143] Magnusson J, Schnurer J (2001) *Lactobacillus coryniformis* subsp. *coryniformis* strain Si3 produces a broad-spectrum proteinaceous antifungal compound. Applied and Environmental Microbiology 67: 1–5.

[144] Damiani P, Gobbetti M, Cossignani L, Corsetti, Simonetti M, Rossi J (1996) The sourdough microflora. Characterization of hetero- and homofermentative lactic acid bacteria yeasts and their interactions on the basis of the volatile compounds produced. Lebensmittel-Wissensschaft und Technologie 29: 63–70.

[145] Martinez-Anaya M (1996a) Enzymes and bread flavor. Journal of Agricultural and Food Chemistry 44: 2469–2480.

[146] Meignen B, Onno B, Gelinas P, Infantes M, Guilois S, Cahagnier B (2001) Optimization of sourdough fermentation with *Lactobacillus brevis* and baker's yeast. Food Microbiology 18: 239–245.

[147] Thiele C, Ganzle M, Vogel R (2002) Contribution of sourdough lactobacilli, yeast, and cereal enzymes to the generation of amino acids in dough relevant for bread flavour. Cereal Chemistry 79: 45–51.

[148] Vermeulen N, Kretzer J, Machalitza H, Vogel R, Ganzle M (2006) Influence of redox-reactions catalysed by homo- and hetero-fermentative lactobacilli on gluten in wheat sourdoughs, Journal of Cereal Science 43: 137–143.

[149] Wang Y, Yu R, Yang H, Chou C (2006) Antioxidatives activities of soymilk fermented with lactic acid bacteria and bifidobacteria. Food Microbiol. 23: 128–135.

[150] Lin M, Yen C (1999) Antioxidative ability of lactic acid bacteria. J. Agric. Food Chem. 47: 1460–1466.

[151] Shirai K, Pedrasa G, Duran M, Marshall V, Moiseev S, Garibay M (1992a) Production of a yogurt-like product from plant foodstuffs and whey: Substrate preparation and ermentation. Sci.Food Agric. 59:199-204.

[152] Shirai K, Duran M, Marshall V, Moiseev S, Garibay M (1992b) Production of a yogurt-ike product from plant foodstuffs and whey: Sensory evaluation and physical attributes. Sci.Food Agric. 59: 205-210.

[153] Yadav V, Jha Y, Garg S, Mital B (1994) Effect of soy milk supplementation and additives on sensory characteristic and biochemical changes of yogut during storage. The Australian J. Dairy Technol. 49: 34-38.

[154] Karleskind K, Laye I, Halpin E and Morr C (1991) Improving acid production in soy based yoghurt by adding cheese whey proteins and mineral salts. J. Food Sci. 56: 999-1001.

[155] Snyder H, Kwon T (1987) Soybeen utilization. AVI Publication, New York.

[156] Chang C, Stone M (1990) Effect of total soymilk solids on acid production by selected Lactobacilli. J. of Food Science 55, 6: 1643-1646.

[157] Kim K, Ko Y (1987) Study of growth and acid production by lactic acid bacteria in soy milk. Korean J. Food Sci. Technol. 19,2: 151-155.

[158] Nsofor L, Nsofor O, Udegbe C, Nwoke E (1996) Evalution of pure bacterial culture rom fermented cassava as soy-yoghut starter: a research note. J. Food Research nternational 29, 5-6: 549-553.

[159] Heenan C, Adams M, Hosken R, Fleet G (2004) Survival and sensory acceptability of probiotic microorganisms in a nonfermented frozen vegetarian dessert. Lebensm. Wiss. U. Technol. 37: 461–466.

[160] Bisakowski B, Atwal A, Gardner N, Champagne C (2007) Effect of lactic acid ermentation of onions (Allium cepa) on the composition of flavonol glucosides. Int. J. Food Sci. Technol. 42: 783–789.

[161] Yan P, Xue W, Tan S, Zhang H, Chang X, (2008) Effect of inoculating lactic acid bacteria starter cultures on the nitrite concentration of fermenting Chinese paocai. Food Control 19: 50–55.

[162] Randazzo C, Restuccia C, Romano A, Caggia C (2004) Lactobacillus casei, dominant species in naturally fermented Sicilian green olives. Int. J. Food Microbiol. 90: 9–14.

[163] Sanz M, Cote G, Gibson G, Rastall R (2006) Influence of glycosidic linkages and molecular weight on the fermentation of maltose-based oligosaccharides by human gut bacteria. J. Agric. Food Chem. 54: 9779–9784.

[164] Vinderola C, Reinheimer J (2003) Lactic acid bacteria: a comparative "in vitro" study of probiotic characteristics and biological barrier resistance. Food Res. Int. 36: 895–904.

[165] Guerin D, Vuillemard J, Subirade M (2003) Protection of Bifidobacteria encapsulated in polysaccharide–protein gel beads against gastric juice and bile. J. Food Protect. 66: 2076–2084.

[166] Kailasapathy K (2002) Microencapsulation of probiotic bacteria: technology and potential application. Curr. Issues Intest. Microbiol. 3: 39–49.

[167] Kourkoutas Y, Xolias V, Kallis M, Bezirtzoglou E, Kanellaki M (2005) Lactobacillus casei cell immobilization on fruit pieces for probiotic additive, fermented milk and lactic acid production. Process. Biochem. 40: 411–416.

[168] Tsen J, Lin Y, Huang H, King V (2007) Accelerated storage testing of freeze-dried mmobilized Lactobacillus acidophilus-fermented banana media. J. Food Process. Preserv. 31: 688–701.

[169] Favaro-Trindade C, Heinemann R, Pedroso D (2011) Developments in probiotic encapsulation, CAB Reviews: Perspectives in Agriculture, Veterinary Science, Nutrition and Natural Resources 6, No 004.

[170] Yoon K, Woodams E, Hang Y (2004) Probiotication of tomato juice by lactic acid bacteria. J. Microbiol. 42: 315–318.

[171] Yoon K, Woodams E, Hang Y (2006) Production of probiotic cabbage juice by lactic acid bacteria. Bioresource Technol. 97: 1427–1430.

[172] Rakin M, Vukasinovic M, Siler-Marinkovic S, Maksimovic M (2007) Contribution of lactic acid fermentation to improved nutritive quality vegetable juices enriched with brewer's yeast autolysate. Food Chem. 100: 599–602.

Chapter 3

Nutritional Programming of Probiotics to Promote Health and Well-Being

Alice Maayan Elad and Uri Lesmes

Additional information is available at the end of the chapter

1. Introduction

The human large intesine is inhabited by a diverse and complex bacterial flora, which includes an outstanding total number of 10^{14} cells, >1000 species and a biomass of more than 1 kg [1, 2]. Thus, the gut microbiota may be conceived as a specialized 'microbial organ' within the gut, affecting human health and disease through its involvement in pathogenesis, nutrition and immunity of the host [1-3]. Recently it has also been recognized that this dynamic yet stable ecosystem plays a role in conditions such as obesity and diabetes as well as in general well-being, from infancy to ageing [1-8]. Consequently, an increasing number of studies which explore the potential of promoting health by nutrition focuses on possible ways to influence and modulate the composition and activity of the gut flora towards a healthier one [4, 9-12].

In this respect, three major dietary approaches have been studied and applied. The first approach of probiotics is to fortify the gut flora through the consumption of exogenous live microorganisms, e.g. *L. acidophilus* in dairy products. The second strategy of prebiotics seeks to selectively stimulate the growth and/or activity of one or a limited number of advantageous indigenous bacteria in the host gut flora [1, 13]. The third approach, known as synbiotics due to its synergistic nature, aims to combine the previous ones by the simultaneous administration of probiotics and prebiotics, which improves the survival and implantation of the live microbes [13].

Over the years, much attention has been drawn to indigestible carbohydrates that evade enzymatic digestion in the upper gastrointestinal tract and become available for fermentation in the colon [13]. These dietary compounds were later termed as prebiotics, a definition of which has been updated into its current form as "a selectively fermented ingredient that allows specific changes, both in the composition and/or activity in the gastrointestinal microflora that confers benefits upon host well-being and health" [14, 15].

Although a more recent development compared to probiotics, prebiotics have been at the heart of various studies and numerous commercial products since they do not share the problem of probiotic survival upon ingestion by the consumer, and they can be added to a broad range of food products (e.g. confectionary and baked foods as well as more traditional fermented milk products and fruit drinks) because the majority of prebiotics are carbohydrates [16].

Amongst the carbohydrates currently marketed as prebiotics, inulin, fructo-oligosaccharides (FOS), galacto-oligosaccharides (GOS) and lactulose are consistently supported by high quality data from *in vitro*, *in vivo* and human trials [10-12, 14, 16-19]. Specifically, human trials have established that dietary consumption of 5-20 g/day of these prebiotics stimulates the growth of *Bifidobacterium* and *Lactobacillus* and promotes the health and well-being of infants, adults, pregnant and lactating women as well as the elderly to varying extents [6, 8, 11, 20, 21].

2. Prebiotics as gut flora management tools

2.1. Established prebiotics

Overall, three major groups of compounds have been consistently established as prebiotics conferring health benefits (as detailed in Table 1): fructans, which include inulin and fructo-oligosaccharides (FOS), galacto-oligosaccharides and lactulose. Under the general term fructans one can classify three established prebiotic carbohydrates: inulin, fructo-oligosaccharides (FOS) and short chain fructo-oligosaccharides (scFOS) [16-18]. The fructans are polymers composed of D-fructose units joined by β-2-1 glycosidic linkages and terminated by an α-1-2-linked D-glucose.

Established prebiotic	Recommended efficaceous intake [g/day]	Key effects in humans	Potential adverse intake [g/day]	Suggested references
Inulin	5-15	• Stimulate bifidobacteria growth	> 15 (increase in fecal output)	[22]
Fructo-oligosaccharides	10-15	• Production of short chain fatty acids	> 15 (increase in fecal output)	[17]
Galacto-oligosaccharides	10-15		> 20 g/human body (diarrhea)	[19]
Lactulose	10	• Protection against enteric infections	> 20 (laxative)	[23]

Table 1. The main established prebiotics and their beneficial/adverse intakes.

The degree of polymerization (DP), defined by the number of monosaccharide units, is used to distinguish between inulin, FOS and scFOS. Molecules with a DP between 2-60 are referred to as inulin. Inulin is commercially produced from chicory roots, but it is present in varying extent also in onions, garlic, Jerusalem artichoke, tomato and banana [11, 16, 21]. Similarly, oligofructose, commonly referred to as FOS, is prepared from chicory in an enzymatic hydrolysis using inulinase, and defined as oligosaccharide fractions which have a maximal DP of 20 with most common commercial products having an average DP of 9. In contrast, scFOS are synthesized in an enzymatic reaction via transfer of fructosyl units from sucrose molecules to yield mixtures of fructosyl chains with a maximum DP of 5. The mixture produced is usually comprised mainly of 1-kestose (2 units of fructose linked to glucose, GF2), nystose (GF3) and 1-fructosyl nystose (GF4) [16, 17, 24].

Fructans have a long tradition as prebiotics. Since their fructose units are joined by β-linkages, they are resistant to hydrolysis by the human digestive enzymes which mainly cleave α-linkages. As a consequence, when these carbohydrates reach the colon they selectively stimulate the growth of beneficial bacteria such as bifidobacteria, which do contain specific enzymes for their degradation, i.e. β-fructosidases [16, 21, 25]. Therefore, inulin, FOS and scFOS are classified as 'nondigestible' carbohydrates, with a calorie value of 1.5-2.0 kcal/g [24]. FOS fermentation in the colon results in increased levels of short chain fatty acids (SCFA) which lower the pH in the intestinal lumen. This can provide an explanation to the reports that these fructans lead to a decrease in the number of harmful bacteria in the colon (such as *Clostridium*, *Streptococcus faecallis* and *Escherichia coli*) [21, 25].

Galacto-oligosaccharides (GOS) are galactose-containing oligosaccharide mixtures of the form Glu α-1-4[β-Gal-1-6]$_n$ where n can be between two to five. They are produced from lactose syrup using β-galactosidases, which catalyze the hydrolysis of lactose into glucose and galactose, and also the transgalactosylation reactions with lactose as acceptor of galactose units giving rise to a variety of glycosidic linkages and molecular weights [11, 16, 19, 21]. Furthermore, the use of different enzymes in the various production processes of GOS leads to variability in their purity and glycosidic linkages, with β-1-6, β-1-3 and β-1-4 being the dominant [19]. Several *in vitro* and *in vivo* experiments have demonstrated that as in inulin-type fructans, the β-glycosidic linkages in GOS render them resistant to hydrolysis by the human digestive enzymes secreted in the upper gastrointestinal tract [16, 19, 21, 26]. In light of that, manufacturers are obliged by the European regulation to clearly identify GOS-containing food products as dietary fibers, with an estimated low calorie value of 1-2 kcal/g [19].

Most of the health effects related to GOS arise from their selective fermentation by bifidobacteria and lactobacilli. In fact, it has been reported that when added to infant milk formulas, these oligosaccharides replicated the bifidogenic effect of human breast milk, not only in bacterial counts, but also with respect to the metabolic activity of the microflora in the colon [16, 27]. The growth of *Lactobacillus paracasei* and *Bifidobacterium lactis* has been shown to be preferential when grown on tri- and tetrasaccharide fractions of FOS or GOS, which supports the notion that prebiotics selectively promote the proliferation of bacteria possesing an active transport system enabling them to utilize these oligosaccharides [28-30]. In addition, it has been demonstrated that GOS compete for pathogen binding sites that coat the surface of the gastrointestinal epithelial cells [31, 32].

Finally, lactulose (β-1-4-galactosyl-fructose) is a synthetic disaccharide derived from lactose. It is commonly used as a laxative in pharmaceutical products for the treatment of constipation, in doses over 20 g/day [16, 21]. Nevertheless, human trials have shown that at lower doses, lactulose acts as a prebiotic, reaching the colon and increasing bifidobacteria counts [2, 16, 17, 23]. Although this substance is an established prebiotic, it is still heavily confined to applications as a therapeutic agent.

2.2. Novel prebiotics

The search for new and novel prebiotics is constantly driven by the increased interest in management of human health through nutrition, particularly by the modulation of gut flora. In addition, studies of established prebiotics have enabled the better understanding of mechanisms of action and properties, which provided the basis for emerging prebiotics. Among the large array of prebiotic candidates, isomalto-oligosaccharides (IMO), xylo-oligosaccharides (XOS), soy-oligosaccharides (SOS), gluco-oligosaccharides, lactosucrose and resistant starches can be classified as emerging prebiotics [17, 33-40]. Some of these compounds present advantages over established prebiotics; for example, XOS are stable across a wide range of pH, hence they are resistant to degradation in low pH juices, in contrast to inulin [21]. Besides attempts to identify and isolate naturally occurring prebiotics there are also attempts to enhance and extend the functionality of exisiting natural prebiotics through a rational design approach [41].

Promising results have been reported, including the selective growth of bifidobacteria and lactobacilli and/or the formation of beneficial metabolites, such as short chain fatty acids. However, it should be noted that these studies are still limited to *in vitro* models or small scale animal or human trials [16, 17, 40]. For example, thermally produced resistant starch has been demonstrated to possess a bifidogenic and butyrogenic effect in an *in vitro* three stage continuous fermentation system inoculated with human feces [42]. Furthermore, this study suggested that resistant starch crystalline polymorphism, resulting from different thermal treatments, could convey different prebiotic effects on the human colon flora.

3. Efficacy of prebiotics across the life span

3.1. Methods to evaluate prebiotics

Research into the efficacy of prebiotics includes a collection of methods currently in use, from pure cultures to human trials, which can be generally classified into *in vivo* and *in vitro* methods. Overall, the prebiotic effect is mainly evaluated by the presence of beneficial metabolites and measuring the growth of major bacterial groups commonly present in the human gut, in particular a selection for increased numbers of bifidobacteria and lactobacilli in comparison with undesirable bacteria such as certain clostridia and sulfate reducing bacteria [40]. Ultimately, health claims concerning prebiotic effects must rely on comprehensive well-controlled human trials. Thus, *in vivo* studies have evolved over the years to robust experimental designs which combine double blind and placebo-controlled designs with advanced microbial analyses, such as bacterial enumeration using 16s DNA probes in fluorescence *in situ* hybridization (FISH) [16]. In most human studies, the production of short chain fatty acids (SCFA) has been quantified in fecal samples, as a marker of enhanced saccharolytic fermentation in response to prebiotic treatment [13].

In spite of their high significance, *in vivo* human studies are usually limited, mainly due to financial and ethical restrictions. Therefore, animal models have been used as a possible viable alternative to the human GI tract, while allowing the researchers to perform *in vivo* experiments in tightly controlled conditions as well as access intestinal contents, tissues and organs at autopsy. Moreover, many *in vivo* experiments have used germ-free animals dosed with fecal suspensions obtained from human donors, which are considered to be a reliable model for a reconstituted human gut flora. However, data generated from animal models do not necessarily coincide with human or *in vitro* studies, as has been shown for prebiotic resistant starch type III [42].

Consequently, many *in vitro* experimental models have been developed to simulate various aspects of the human GI tract [43-45]. Seeking to closely mimic the conditions of organs along the GI tract, these models include a reactor or a series of reactors under tightly controlled settings, with the large intestine represented by an anaerobic reactor/s inoculated with fecal slurries [40]. Thus, these systems offer researchers a controlled experimental design that is relatively inexpensive, easy to set up, high throughput and raises minimal ethical issues [46].

One of the first *in vitro* GI models described in the literature was termed the simulator of the human intestinal microbial ecosystem (SHIME) [47]. This computer controlled model is composed of a five serially connected vessels simulating the conditions of the stomach, small intestine, ascending, transverse and descending colon [48, 49]. Operators can control various parameters of physiological relevance, including gastric and pancreatic secretions, pH, transit time, feed composition as well as sample different loci along the system on a regular basis [13, 46]. Another comprehensive *in vitro* GI model was developed in the Netherlands [50]. This model is actually comprised of two seperate parts: TIM-1 is a series of four computer controlled chambers simulating the upper GI, i.e. the stomach, duodenum, jejunum and ileum, while TIM-2 models the large intestine. Unlike the SHIME, this model consists of a series of linked glass vessels containing flexible walls, which allow simulation of the peristaltic movements of the GI. The hollow fiber membrane construct of the system enables to simulate absorption of water and nutrients in the lumen as well as their removal from the colon [13, 46]. Similarly, simple glass reactors have been used for in batch and three stage continuous fermentation systems to simulate the lower GI, i.e. the proximal, transverse and distal colon, and have been validated against sudden death victims [51].

Overall, *in vivo* methods and particularly human trials are essential for establishing health claims regarding prebiotic effects on human microflora. However, such methods are hindered by financial, ethical and practical reasons. *In vitro* models fail to fully mimic the GI system, particularly peristaltic movements, mucosal uptake and impact of immune components. Nevertheless, these systems offer relatively low costs, ease of use and have minimal ethical considerations, while providing researchers controllable settings for studying luminal biochemistry and microbiology.

3.2. Prebiotic efficacy in infancy and childhood

At birth, the neonate gut is considered to be sterile with rapid colonization by bacteria believed to occur in three phases: delivery, breastfeeding and weaning to solid foods [52-54]. Immediately after birth, facultative anaerobic bacteria such as *Enterobacteriaceae*, streptococci and staphylococci colonize the gut environment of the newborn, gradually consuming oxygen and producing various metabolites. Consequently, strict anaerobic bacterial population dominated by bifidobacteria, *Clostridium* and *Bacteroides* can be established [55-57]. Within the first year of life, the microflora is highly dynamic, but by the age of two years with the introduction of solid foods, the colonic microbiota is considered complete – it stabilizes and resembles that of the adult [58-60].

The interest in prebiotics as a nutritional strategy to program infant gut microbiota to favor a more advantageous population has been inspired by the beneficial effects attributed to the 200 different human milk oligosaccharides (HMO) [52-54]. Based on the observations of bifidobacteria in the feces of breastfed babies, attempts have been made to reproduce this bifidogenic aspect in infant formulas by adding commercial prebiotics, in particular FOS and GOS [8, 53]. This practical application of prebiotics was evaluated for example in double-blind, randomized and controlled studies in 90 full term infants, which demonstrated that 4 g/L or 8 g/L of FOS, GOS or their combination resulted in a significant decrease in fecal pH and a concomitant increase in bifidobacteria and lactobacilli after 28 days feeding [61, 62]. A GOS and FOS mixture at a ratio of 9:1 (GOS:FOS) has been extensively studied as a prebiotic additive to infant formulas [63], and shown to increase bifidobacteria in infant feces and lower the incidence of pathogens [64-66]. Therefore, the administration of FOS and GOS into commercial infant formulas for their prebiotic effects has spread, and researchers continue exploring additional prebiotics as possible candidates for infant formulas supplementation. Moreover, studies are also looking into the persistence of the prebiotic effects.

3.3. Prebiotic efficacy in adulthood

To date, various studies have determined fructans (inulin and FOS) induce different beneficial effects on the health and general well-being of healthy adult subjects [10, 16-18]. A daily consumption of 5-10 g of fructans has been demonstrated to exert a bifidogenic effect on healthy adults based on dose-response studies, while similar doses of GOS and lactulose have been reported in *in vitro* and human trials as stimulating a bifidogenic effect [16, 67, 68]. As to bowel habit, i.e. the frequency of bowel discharge but not fecal output, constipation and laxative effect, there is some evidence that in constipated subjects, inulin may increase bowel habit [69], whereas lactulose is prescribed at 20 g/day to increase fecal output of chronically constipated patients, however, having a bifidogenic effect on healthy adults at lower doses [68]. Moreover, numerous studies have shown that fecal output remains unchanged at a daily intake of up to 15 g fructans with a slight increase at doses of 15 g/day or higher [11]. Hence, inulin, FOS, GOS and lactulose may be defined as mild laxatives with adverse effects observed only at a consumption of over 20 g/day.

Additionally, established prebiotics have been linked to protection against enteric infections, modification of the host immune response, production of short chain fatty acids, particularly butyrate, increased mineral absorption and even the reduced risk of colon cancer [10, 11, 14, 16, 18]. Prebiotics efficacy has also been studied during pregnancy and lactation. These life periods are sometimes accompanied by irregular gastrointestinal activity, which can be improved by the consumption of dietary fibers and prebiotics [20]. Furthermore, gestational weight gain and postpartum weight retention have been suggested to be affected from prebiotics intake, since they modulate the gut microflora [5]. However, it is also important to note that the prebiotic effect has not been found to extend to neonates and infants, even when solely breast fed.

3.4. Prebiotics efficacy in ageing

At the old age, increased threshold for taste and smell as well as masticatory dysfunction can lead to a nutritionally imbalanced diet. In addition, various physiological functions deteriorate with age and may influence the absorption and/or metabolism of nutrients. Furthermore, the increased intake of drugs results in GI disturbances due to antibiotics undesired effect on indigenous bacteria in the host gut flora. Thus, changes in the GI tract, modification of diet and host immune system inevitably give rise to bacterial population alterations [70, 71]. In spite of the increasing proportion of the elderly in Western countries [72, 73], scarce data exists on the changes that occur in the intestinal microbiota during the ageing process and their possible health outcomes. Overall, an increase in facultative anaerobes and decrease in *Bacteroides* and bifidobacteria (total numbers as well as species diversity) have been reported [74].

Therefore, modulation of the colon microflora by the consumption of prebiotics is increasingly being studied as a potent, cost effective and natural way to improve the health and well-being of elderly people as well as reduce risks for various diseases [70, 71, 74]. FOS and GOS ingestion, as well as synbiotic preparations, were found to significantly increase the number of bifidobacteria at the expense of less beneficial microbiota in ageing individuals [6, 75-78]. In addition, a randomized, double-blind, controlled study with 74 subjects aged 70 and over has indicated that prebiotic addition can improve the low noise inflammatory process frequently observed in this sensitive population [79].

4. Prebiotics as therapeutics

4.1. Prebiotics therapeutic efficacy in human diseases

It is now well documented that the bacteria microflora residing in the human GI has a role not only in promoting health but also in preventing some diseases [3, 80, 81]. Prebiotics have been reported to protect against pathogenic gastrointestinal infections by promoting the growth of probiotics which help displace pathogens from the mucosa, producing antimicrobial agents and competing with pathogens on binding sites and nutrients [3]. In addition to *in vitro* data which supports this disease preventing effect of prebiotics [16, 22], a human study on 140 infants has concluded that consumption of oligofructose and cereal significantly reduced events of fever, frequency of vomiting, regurgitation and abdominal discomfort [82]. Moreover, various studies have shown that prebiotics can beneficially affect patients with antibiotic-associated diarrhea, especially when it arises from *C. difficile* [11].

Prebiotics have also been reported to reduce the risk of colon cancer as a result of gut flora modulation [11, 14, 16-18]. Specifically, they support the metabolism of carcinogenic molecules and the secretion of short chain fatty acids to the lumen by the colon microbiota [83, 84]. Furthermore, human trials have demonstrated that inulin, FOS and scFOS beneficially affect colorectal cell proliferation and genotoxicity [17], hence the potential of prebiotics in prevention and treatment of colon cancer should be further explored.

Inflammatory bowel disease (IBD), which includes ulcerative colitis (UC) and Crohn's disease (CD), has also been researched as a possible target for prebiotics [11, 16, 17]. As mucosal communities significantly change in these diseases, prebiotics may be used in order to manipulate them. For example, patients fed 15 g per day of a prebiotic mixture composed of 7.5 g inulin and 7.5 g FOS for 2 weeks prior to colonoscopy, have had more than a 10-fold increase in bifidobacterial and eubacterial numbers in the mucosa of the proximal and distal colon [85]. Similarly, in a small open-label human trial, 10 patients with active ileum-colonic CD were fed 15 g FOS daily for 3 weeks, after which a significant reduction in the Harvey Bradshaw index of disease activity was observed as well as an increase of fecal bifidobacteria numbers [11].

4.2. Prospective therapeutic targets

4.2.1. Obesity and the metabolic syndrome

Increasing evidence linking gut flora to human health and diseases have inspired further research regarding the possible link between gut flora and obesity, which has led to the notion that prebiotics could be harnessed as potential therapeutic agents or management tools to prevent and treat obesity and the metabolic syndrome [4, 5, 7, 20, 52]. The metabolic syndrome is a cluster of metabolic abnormalities, including abdominal obesity, type 2 diabetes mellitus and cardiovascular diseases [86, 87].

Various studies have shown that prebiotic intervention decreased fat storage in white adipose tissues and in the liver, decreased hepatic insulin resistance as well as systemic inflammation in several nutritional (high-fat diet-fed) and genetic (*ob/ob* mice) obese rodents [88-95]. Some beneficial effects of fructans on BMI, fat mass and insulin resistance were also shown in the limited human trials conducted so far [95-98].

However, to date, the mechanisms underlying the complex role of gut microbiota in such conditions are largely unknown [1]. It has been reported that a lower number of bifidobacteria at birth is associated with overweight later in childhood [99], and in adults, the number of bifidobacteria is slightly lower in individuals with obesity than in lean subjects [100]. The number of these bacteria is also decreased in patients with type 2 diabetes mellitus compared with nondiabetic people [101]. Hence, these results seem to suggest that bifidobacteria affects the development of obesity and its related comorbidities [52].

A remarkable increase has been observed in the number of *Bifidobacterium* spp. following inulin-type fructans supplementation to mice with diet-induced or genetically determined obesity [52]. Interestingly, the number of bifidobacteria was inversely correlated with the development of fat mass, glucose intolerance and levels of lipopolysaccharides (LPS) [102]. LPS has been found at a significantly higher level in the serum of obese individuals, which creates a metabolic endotoxemia, leading to obesity, insulin resistance and systemic inflammation [103]. Moreover, it has been reported that the overexpression of numerous host genes that are related to adiposity and inflammation was prevented by prebiotic intake [52].

A pathway involving short chain fatty acids (SCFA) has been proposed to be involved in the interplay between prebiotics, the gut flora and obesity. SCFA act as signaling molecules and are specific ligands for at least two G protein-coupled receptors, GPR41 and GPR43, which have a potential role in fat mass development [13, 104]. In addition, it has been shown that acetate and propionate can modify hepatic lipid metabolism [105]. Interestingly, a recent study has demonstrated that diet-induced obesity and insulin resistance were prevented when mice on a high-fat diet were supplemented with butyrate, which promoted energy expenditure and induced mitochondrial function [106]. Various studies have shown that a diet enriched with prebiotics leads to a greater intestinal SCFA production and thereby migitates body weight gain, fat mass development and the severity of diabetes [89, 90, 100, 107-109]. Numerous peptides secreted by the enteroendocrine cells along the GI are involved in the regulation of energy homeostasis and/or pancreatic function. Three such peptides which can modulate food intake and energy expenditure are glucagon-like peptide-1 (GLP-1), peptide YY (PYY) and ghrelin [110-113]. Thus, it has been suggested that SCFA are related to changes in the gut peptide secretion, namely increased production and secretion of GLP-1 and PYY and the reduction of ghrelin which induce metabolic effects [13, 114, 115]. Piche *et al.* were the first to report that inulin-type fructan feeding of 20 g/day significantly increased plasma GLP-1 in humans [116]. In another study, a 2-week supplementation with inulin-type fructans (16 g/day) to healthy volunteers increased GLP-1, consequently increasing satiety, lowering calorie intake and decreasing postprandial glycemia [90, 108]. Furthermore, prebiotic treatment in obese patients has been found to induce and increase PYY and decrease ghrelin levels [117]. Finally, Tarini and Wolever have demonstrated that a single dose of inulin significantly increased postprandial plasma GLP-1 and decreased plasma ghrelin [118]. This is in contrast to perceived necessity for a prolonged prebiotics administration to modulate gut microbiota and allow effect on gut endocrine function. Thus, it seems that further studies are needed to fully unravel the potential of prebiotics to offer a nutritional means to cope with the worrisome increase in human obesity and the metabolic syndrome.

5. Future challenges

5.1. Harmonization of methods to evaluate efficacy

To date, a plethora of studies have investigated the effects of prebiotics on human health and well-being, leading to the general realization prebiotics could serve as a possible method of therapeutic intervention. However, the majority of these studies cannot be compared due to the variety of methods employed. For example, results obtained by bacterial isolation techniques [39, 119] cannot be compared with data from more advanced methods for the molecular characterization of the microbiota, now considered essential to obtain a comprehensive view of the gut ecosystem. Furthermore, DNA-based techniques including the use of the 16s ribosomal RNA gene are considered as less biased, hence their results are more reliable [54]. In addition, studies focused on the effect of prebiotics on the elderly, even in healthy subjects, lack a clear definition of 'elderly', and various groups are recruited, usually on the basis of 'over 60' [120], 'over 65' [119, 121] or 'over 70' [122]. This makes is difficult to define a 'threshold age' at which the gut environment starts to be influenced from the ageing process [70]. Thus, harmonization of methods to evaluate efficacy is a prequisite step limiting the further application of prebiotics for the prevention and treatment of diseases as well as the development of novel prebiotics.

5.2. The challenge of personalization

A broad range of parameters has been known to affect the bacterial composition of the infant gut, e.g. mode of delivery, type of feeding (exclusive breastfeeding versus formula), antibiotic use and maternal infection [55-57, 123, 124]. Furthermore, various studies have indicated that the low number of certain bacteria at birth such as bifidobacteria is related to overweight later in childhood [99]. Consequently, prebiotics supplementation even in infants may be used as a preventive nutritional programming tool, which will affect the health and well-being also in adulthood. Moreover, it has been increasingly accepted that environmental factors such as nutritional habits and lifestyle may impact the gut microbiota composition, for example striking country-related differences in the effects of age on the microflora have been reported [70]. This wide variety of factors, affecting intestinal microbiota composition from infancy to elderly, drove the need for personalized nutrition, including personalized and tailored prebiotics. In addition, since prebiotics are recently considered even as therapeutic agents for the prevention and treatment of diseases, it may be beneficial to aim personalized prebiotics to people at high-risk to develop these illnesses. Thus, the challenge of personalization includes performing long-term, large-sized, well-controlled and multidisciplinary-collaborated studies which will demonstrate and establish the health promoting effects of prebiotics and enable harnessing them in the clinic or in supermarket shelves.

6. Conclusions

Prebiotics have emerged as cost-effective and efficient nutritional programming tools to beneficially and selectively promote the growth and/or activity of certain bacteria in the indigenous flora of the human GI. So far, prebiotics have been demonstrated to exert various beneficial effects during an individual's lifetime, from infancy to ageing, as well as function as therapeutic agents for the prevention and treatment of different diseases, including obesity and the metabolic syndrome.

In addition to the well-established prebiotics of FOS, GOS and lactulose, novel prebiotics are constantly being developed. State of the art techniques, *in vitro* gastrointestinal models and advanced computerization tools are leading many researchers to adopt more complete and comprehensive approaches, e.g. metabolomics and metagenomics.

Future challenges include the harmonization of methods of evaluating efficacy that will help focus research efforts and enable a more comprehensive understanding of prebiotic mechanisms of action and beneficial effects and how these can be modulated. Another important prospect is personalization, i.e. fitting tailored prebiotics to individual needs in order to nutritionally program and affect their health and well-being from infancy and into old and prosperous age.

Author details

Alice Maayan Elad and Uri Lesmes
Department of Biotechnology and Food Engineering, Technion, Israel Institute of Technology, Haifa, Israel

7. References

[1] Diamant, M., E.E. Blaak, and W.M. de Vos, Do Nutrient–Gut–Microbiota Interactions Play a Role in Human Obesity, Insulin Resistance and Type 2 Diabetes? Obesity Reviews, 2011. 12(4): p. 272-281.

[2] Venema, K., Intestinal Fermentation of Lactose and Prebiotic Lactose Derivatives, including Human Milk Oligosaccharides. International Dairy Journal, 2012. 22(2): p. 123-140.

[3] O'Hara, A.M. and F. Shanahan, The Gut Flora as a Forgotten Organ. EMBO Rep, 2006. 7(7): p. 688-693.

[4] Delzenne, N.M. and P.D. Cani, Nutritional Modulation of Gut Microbiota in the Context of Obesity and Insulin Resistance: Potential Interest of Prebiotics. International Dairy Journal, 2010. 20(4): p. 277-280.

[5] Duncan, S.H., et al., Human Colonic Microbiota Associated with Diet, Obesity and Weight Loss. International Journal of Obesity, 2008. 32(11): p. 1720-1724.

[6] Tuohy, K.M., Inulin-Type Fructans in Healthy Aging. The Journal of Nutrition, 2007. 137(11): p. 2590S-2593S.

[7] Tuohy, K.M., A. Costabile, and F. Fava, The Gut Microbiota in Obesity and Metabolic Disease - A Novel Therapeutic Target. Nutritional Therapy and Metabolism, 2009. 27(3): p. 113-133.

[8] Parracho, H., A.L. McCartney, and G.R. Gibson, Probiotics and Prebiotics in Infant Nutrition. Proceedings of the Nutrition Society, 2007. 66: p. 405-411.

[9] Fooks, L.J., R. Fuller, and G.R. Gibson, Prebiotics, Probiotics and Human Gut Microbiology. International Dairy Journal, 1999. 9(1): p. 53-61.

[10] Gibson, G.R., Prebiotics as Gut Microflora Management Tools. Journal of Clinical Gastroenterology, 2008. 42(6): p. S75-S79.

[11] Macfarlane, S., G.T. Macfarlane, and J.H. Cummings, Review Article: Prebiotics in the Gastrointestinal Tract. Alimentary Pharmacology & Therapeutics, 2006. 24(5): p. 701-714.

[12] Tuohy, K.M., et al., Using Probiotics and Prebiotics to Improve Gut Health. Drug Discovery Today, 2003. 8(15): p. 692-700.

[13] De Preter, V., et al., The Impact of Pre- and/or Probiotics on Human Colonic Metabolism: Does It Affect Human Health? Molecular Nutrition & Food Research, 2011. 55(1): p. 46-57.

[14] Gibson, G.R., From Probiotics to Prebiotics and a Healthy Digestive System. Journal of Food Science, 2004. 69(5): p. M141-M143.

[15] Schrezenmeir, J. and M. de Vrese, Probiotics, Prebiotics, and Synbiotics - — Approaching a Definition. The American Journal of Clinical Nutrition, 2001. 73(2): p. 361S-364S.

[16] Tuohy, K.M., et al., Modulation of the Human Gut Microflora Towards Improved Health Using Prebiotics – Assessment of Efficacy. Current Pharmaceutical Design, 2005. 11: p. 75-90.

[17] Rastall, R.A., Functional Oligosaccharides: Application and Manufacture. Annual Review of Food Science and Technology, 2010. 1(1): p. 305-339.

[18] Sabater-Molina, M., et al., Dietary Fructooligosaccharides and Potential Benefits on Health. Journal of Physiology and Biochemistry, 2009. 65(3): p. 315-328.

[19] Torres, D.P.M., et al., Galacto-Oligosaccharides: Production, Properties, Applications, and Significance as Prebiotics. Comprehensive Reviews in Food Science and Food Safety, 2010. 9(5): p. 438-454.

[20] Champ, M. and C. Hoebler, Functional Food for Pregnant, Lactating Women and in Perinatal Nutrition: A Role for Dietary Fibres? Current Opinion in Clinical Nutrition & Metabolic Care, 2009. 12(6): p. 565-574.

[21] Caselato de Sousa, V.M., E.F. dos Santos, and V.C. Sgarbieri, The Importance of Prebiotics in Functional Foods and Clinical Practice. Food and Nutrition Sciences, 2011. 2: p. 133-144.

[22] Bosscher, D., J. Van Loo, and A. Franck, Inulin and Oligofructose as Prebiotics in the Prevention of Intestinal Infections and Diseases. Nutrition Research Reviews, 2006. 19: p. 216-226.

[23] Panesar, P.S. and S. Kumari, Lactulose: Production, Purification and Potential Applications. Biotechnology Advances, 2011. 29(6): p. 940-948.

[24] Flamm, G., et al., Inulin and Oligofructose as Dietary Fiber: A Review of the Evidence. Critical Reviews in Food Science and Nutrition, 2001. 41(5): p. 353-362.

[25] Van den Ende, W., D. Peshev, and L. De Gara, Disease Prevention by Natural Antioxidants and Prebiotics Acting as ROS Scavengers in the Gastrointestinal Tract. Trends in Food Science & Technology, 2011. 22(12): p. 689-697.

[26] Van Loo, J., et al., Functional Food Properties of Non-Digestible Oligosaccharides: A Consensus Report from the ENDO Project (DGXII AIRII-CT94-1095). British Journal of Nutrition, 1999. 81: p. 121-132.

[27] Knol, J., et al., Colon Microflora in Infants Fed Formula with Galacto- and Fructo-Oligosaccharides: More Like Breast-Fed Infants. Journal of Pediatric Gastroenterology and Nutrition, 2005. 40(1): p. 36-42.

[28] Gopal, P.K., P.A. Sullivan, and J.B. Smart, Utilisation of Galacto-Oligosaccharides as Selective Substrates for Growth by Lactic Acid Bacteria Including Bifidobacterium lactis DR10 and Lactobacillus rhamnosus DR20. International Dairy Journal, 2001. 11(1–2): p. 19-25.

[29] Kaplan, H. and R.W. Hutkins, Fermentation of Fructooligosaccharides by Lactic Acid Bacteria and Bifidobacteria. Applied and Environmental Microbiology, 2000. 66(6): p. 2682–2684.

[30] Kaplan, H. and R.W. Hutkins, Metabolism of Fructooligosaccharides by Lactobacillus paracasei 1195. Applied and Environmental Microbiology, 2003. 69(4): p. 2217-2222.

[31] Searle, L.E.J., et al., Purified Galactooligosaccharide, Derived from a Mixture Produced by the Enzymic Activity of Bifidobacterium bifidum, Reduces Salmonella enterica Serovar Typhimurium Adhesion and Invasion In Vitro and In Vivo. Journal of Medical Microbiology, 2010. 59(12): p. 1428-1439.

[32] Shoaf, K., et al., Prebiotic Galactooligosaccharides Reduce Adherence of Enteropathogenic Escherichia coli to Tissue Culture Cells. Infection and Immunity, 2006. 74(12): p. 6920–6928.

[33] Mountzouris, K.C., et al., Modeling of Oligodextran Production in an Ultrafiltration Stirred-Cell Membrane Reactor. Enzyme and Microbial Technology, 1999. 24(1–2): p. 75-85.

[34] Rycroft, C.E., et al., A Comparative In Vitro Evaluation of the Fermentation Properties of Prebiotic Oligosaccharides. Journal of Applied Microbiology, 2001. 91(5): p. 878-887.

[35] Kaneko, T., et al., Effects of Isomaltooligosaccharides with Different Degrees of Polymerization on Human Fecal Bifidobacteria. Bioscience, Biotechnology, and Biochemistry, 1994. 58(12): p. 2288-2290.

[36] Saito, Y., T. Takano, and I. Rowland, Effects of Soybean Oligosaccharides on the Human Gut Microflora in In Vitro Culture. Microbial Ecology in Health and Disease, 1992. 5(2): p. 105-110.

[37] Sharp, R., S. Fishbain, and G.T. Macfarlane, Effect of Short-Chain Carbohydrates on Human Intestinal Bifidobacteria and Escherichia coli In Vitro. Journal of Medical Microbiology, 2001. 50(2): p. 152-160.

[38] Hopkins, M.J., J.H. Cummings, and G.T. Macfarlane, Inter-Species Differences in Maximum Specific Growth Rates and Cell Yields of Bifidobacteria Cultured on Oligosaccharides and Other Simple Carbohydrate Sources. Journal of Applied Microbiology, 1998. 85(2): p. 381-386.

[39] Hopkins, M.J. and G.T. Macfarlane, Changes in Predominant Bacterial Populations in Human Faeces with Age and with Clostridium difficile Infection. Journal of Medical Microbiology, 2002. 51(5): p. 448-454.

[40] Fuentes-Zaragoza, E., et al., Resistant Starch as Prebiotic: A Review. Starch - Starke, 2011. 63(7): p. 406-415.

[41] Hernandez-Hernandez, O., et al., Characterization of Galactooligosaccharides Derived from Lactulose. Journal of Chromatography A, 2011. 1218(42): p. 7691-7696.

[42] Lesmes, U., et al., Effects of Resistant Starch Type III Polymorphs on Human Colon Microbiota and Short Chain Fatty Acids in Human Gut Models. Journal of Agricultural and Food Chemistry, 2008. 56(13): p. 5415-5421.

[43] Hur, S.J., et al., In Vitro Human Digestion Models for Food Applications. Food Chemistry, 2011. 125(1): p. 1-12.

[44] Kong, F. and R.P. Singh, A Human Gastric Simulator (HGS) to Study Food Digestion in Human Stomach. Journal of Food Science, 2010. 75(9): p. E627-E635.

[45] Macfarlane, G.T. and S. Macfarlane, Models For Intestinal Fermentation: Association between Food Components, Delivery Systems, Bioavailability and Functional Interactions in the Gut. Current Opinion in Biotechnology, 2007. 18(2): p. 156-162.

[46] Benshitrit, R.C., et al., Development of Oral Food-Grade Delivery Systems: Current Knowledge and Future Challenges. Food & Function, 2012. 3(1): p. 10-21.

[47] Molly, K., et al., Validation of the Simulator of the Human Intestinal Microbial Ecosystem (SHIME) Reactor Using Microorganism-associated Activities. Microbial Ecology in Health and Disease, 1994. 7(4): p. 191-200.

[48] De Boever, P., B. Deplancke, and W. Verstraete, Fermentation by Gut Microbiota Cultured in a Simulator of the Human Intestinal Microbial Ecosystem Is Improved by Supplementing a Soygerm Powder. The Journal of Nutrition, 2000. 130(10): p. 2599-2606.

[49] Gmeiner, M., et al., Influence of a Synbiotic Mixture consisting of Lactobacillus acidophilus 74-2 and a Fructooligosaccharide Preparation on the Microbial Ecology Sustained in a Simulation of the Human Intestinal Microbial Ecosystem (SHIME Reactor). Applied Microbiology and Biotechnology, 2000. 53(2): p. 219-223.

[50] Minekus, M., et al., A Multicompartmental Dynamic Computer-Controlled Model Simulating the Stomach and Small Intestine. Atla Alternatives To Laboratory Animals, 1995. 23(2): p. 197-209.

[51] Macfarlane, G.T., S. Macfarlane, and G.R. Gibson, Validation of a Three-Stage Compound Continuous Culture System for Investigating the Effect of Retention Time on the Ecology and Metabolism of Bacteria in the Human Colon. Microbial Ecology, 1998. 35(2): p. 180-187.

[52] Delzenne, N.M., et al., Targeting Gut Microbiota in Obesity: Effects of Prebiotics and Probiotics. Nature Reviews Endocrinology, 2011. 7(11): p. 639-646.

[53] Chichlowski, M., et al., The Influence of Milk Oligosaccharides on Microbiota of Infants: Opportunities for Formulas. Annual Review of Food Science and Technology, 2011. 2(1): p. 331-351.

[54] Marques, T.M., et al., Programming Infant Gut Microbiota: Influence of Dietary and Environmental Factors. Current Opinion in Biotechnology, 2010. 21(2): p. 149-156.

[55] Morelli, L., Postnatal Development of Intestinal Microflora as Influenced by Infant Nutrition. The Journal of Nutrition, 2008. 138(9): p. 1791S-1795S.

[56] Adlerberth, I. and A.E. Wold, Establishment of the Gut Microbiota in Western Infants. Acta Pædiatrica, 2009. 98(2): p. 229-238.

[57] Penders, J., et al., Factors Influencing the Composition of the Intestinal Microbiota in Early Infancy. Pediatrics, 2006. 118(2): p. 511-521.

[58] Palmer, C., et al., Development of the Human Infant Intestinal Microbiota. PLoS Biol, 2007. 5(7): p. e177.

[59] Harmsen, H.J.M., et al., Analysis of Intestinal Flora Development in Breast-Fed and Formula-Fed Infants by Using Molecular Identification and Detection Methods Journal of Pediatric Gastroenterology & Nutrition, 2000. 30(1): p. 61-67.

[60] Rubaltelli, F.F., et al., Intestinal Flora in Breast- and Bottle-Fed Infants. Journal of Pediatric Gastroenterology & Nutrition, 1998. 26(3): p. 186–191.

[61] Moro, G., et al., Dosage-Related Bifidogenic Effects of Galacto- and Fructooligosaccharides in Formula-Fed Term Infants. Journal of Pediatric Gastroenterology and Nutrition, 2002. 34(3): p. 291-295.

[62] Moro, G.E., et al., Effects of a New Mixture of Prebiotics on Faecal Flora and Stools in Term Infants. Acta Pædiatrica, 2003. 92: p. 77-79.

[63] Fanaro, S., et al., Galacto-Oligosaccharides and Long-Chain Fructo-Oligosaccharides as Prebiotics in Infant Formulas: A Review. Acta Paediatrca Supplement, 2005. 94(449): p. 22–26.

[64] Boehm, G., et al., Supplementation of a Bovine Milk Formula with an Oligosaccharide Mixture Increases Counts of Faecal Bifidobacteria in Preterm Infants. Archives of Disease in Childhood - Fetal and Neonatal Edition, 2002. 86(3): p. F178-F181.

[65] Haarman, M. and J. Knol, Quantitative Real-Time PCR Assays To Identify and Quantify Fecal Bifidobacterium Species in Infants Receiving a Prebiotic Infant Formula. Applied and Environmental Microbiology, 2005. 71(5): p. 2318-2324.

[66] Knol, J., et al., Increase of Faecal Bifidobacteria due to Dietary Oligosaccharides Induces a Reduction of Clinically Relevant Pathogen Germs in the Faeces of Formula-Fed Preterm Infants. Acta Paediatrca Supplement, 2005. 94(449): p. 31-33.

[67] Bouhnik, Y., et al., Administration of Transgalacto-Oligosaccharides Increases Fecal Bifidobacteria and Modifies Colonic Fermentation Metabolism in Healthy Humans. The Journal of Nutrition, 1997. 127(3): p. 444-448.

[68] Salminen, S. and E. Salminen, Lactulose, Lactic Acid Bacteria, Intestinal Microecology and Mucosal Protection. Scandinavian Journal of Gastroenterolgy Supplement, 1997. 222: p. 45-48.

[69] Den Hond, E., B. Geypens, and Y. Ghoos, Effect of High Performance Chicory Inulin on Constipation. Nutrition Research, 2000. 20(5): p. 731-736.

[70] Biagi, E., et al., Ageing of the Human Metaorganism: The Microbial Counterpart. AGE, 2012. 34(1): p. 247-267.

[71] Tiihonen, K., A.C. Ouwehand, and N. Rautonen, Human Intestinal Microbiota and Healthy Ageing. Ageing Research Reviews, 2010. 9(2): p. 107-116.

[72] Cohen, J.E., Human Population: The Next Half Century. Science, 2003. 302(5648): p. 1172-1175.

[73] Christensen, K., et al., Ageing Populations: The Challenges Ahead. The Lancet, 2009. 374(9696): p. 1196-1208.

[74] Woodmansey, E.J., Intestinal Bacteria and Ageing. Journal of Applied Microbiology, 2007. 102(5): p. 1178-1186.

[75] Guigoz, Y., et al., Effects of Oligosaccharide on the Faecal Flora and Non-Specific Immune System in Elderly People. Nutrition research, 2002. 22(1): p. 13-25.

[76] Bartosch, S., et al., Microbiological Effects of Consuming a Synbiotic Containing Bifidobacterium bifidum, Bifidobacterium lactis, and Oligofructose in Elderly Persons, Determined by Real-Time Polymerase Chain Reaction and Counting of Viable Bacteria. Clinical Infectious Diseases, 2005. 40(1): p. 28-37.

[77] Bouhnik, Y., et al., Four-Week Short Chain Fructo-Oligosaccharides Ingestion Leads to Increasing Fecal Bifidobacteria and Cholesterol Excretion in Healthy Elderly Volunteers. Nutrition Journal, 2007. 6(1): p. 42.

[78] Vulevic, J., et al., Modulation of the Fecal Microflora Profile and Immune Function by a Novel Trans-Galactooligosaccharide Mixture (B-GOS) in Healthy Elderly Volunteers. The American Journal of Clinical Nutrition, 2008. 88(5): p. 1438-1446.

[79] Schiffrin, E.J., et al., Systemic Inflammatory Markers in Older Persons: The Effect of Oral Nutritional Supplementation with Prebiotics. Journal of Nutrition Health & Aging, 2007. 11(6): p. 475-479.

[80] Fava, F., et al., The Gut Microbiota and Lipid Metabolism: Implications for Human Health and Coronary Heart Disease. Current Medicinal Chemistry, 2006. 13(25): p. 3005-3021.

[81] Guarner, F. and J.-R. Malagelada, Gut Flora in Health and Disease. The Lancet, 2003. 361(9356): p. 512-519.

[82] Saavedra, J.M. and A. Tschernia, Human Studies with Probiotics and Prebiotics: Clinical Implications. British Journal of Nutrition, 2002. 87: p. S241-S246.

[83] Louis, P. and H.J. Flint, Diversity, Metabolism and Microbial Ecology of Butyrate-Producing Bacteria from the Human Large Intestine. FEMS Microbiology Letters, 2009. 294(1): p. 1-8.

[84] McGarr, S.E., J.M. Ridlon, and P.B. Hylemon, Diet, Anaerobic Bacterial Metabolism, and Colon Cancer: A Review of the Literature. Journal of Clinical Gastroenterology, 2005. 39(2): p. 98-109.

[85] Langlands, S.J., et al., Prebiotic Carbohydrates Modify the Mucosa Associated Microflora of the Human Large Bowel. Gut, 2004. 53(11): p. 1610-1616.

[86] Hotamisligil, G.S., Inflammation and Endoplasmic Reticulum Stress in Obesity and Diabetes. International Journal of Obesity, 2008. 32(S7): p. S52-S54.

[87] Shoelson, S.E. and A.B. Goldfine, Getting Away from Glucose: Fanning the Flames of Obesity-Induced Inflammation. Nature Medicine, 2009. 15(4): p. 373-374.

[88] Cani, P.D. and N.M. Delzenne, Interplay Between Obesity and Associated Metabolic Disorders: New Insights into the Gut Microbiota. Current Opinion in Pharmacology, 2009. 9(6): p. 737-743.

[89] Cani, P.D., et al., Improvement of Glucose Tolerance and Hepatic Insulin Sensitivity by Oligofructose Requires a Functional Glucagon-Like Peptide 1 Receptor. Diabetes, 2006. 55(5): p. 1484-1490.

[90] Cani, P.D., et al., Oligofructose Promotes Satiety in Rats Fed a High-Fat Diet: Involvement of Glucagon-like Peptide-1. Obesity Research, 2005. 13(6): p. 1000-1007.

[91] Cani, P.D., et al., Changes in Gut Microbiota Control Inflammation in Obese Mice through a Mechanism involving GLP-2-Driven Improvement of Gut Permeability. Gut, 2009. 58: p. 1091–1128.

[92] Daubioul, C., et al., Dietary Fructans, but Not Cellulose, Decrease Triglyceride Accumulation in the Liver of Obese Zucker fa/fa Rats. The Journal of Nutrition, 2002. 132(5): p. 967-973.

[93] Daubioul, C.A., et al., Dietary Oligofructose Lessens Hepatic Steatosis, but Does Not Prevent Hypertriglyceridemia in Obese Zucker Rats. The Journal of Nutrition, 2000. 130(5): p. 1314-1319.

[94] Delmee, E., et al., Relation between Colonic Proglucagon Expression and Metabolic Response to Oligofructose in High Fat Diet-Fed Mice. Life Sciences, 2006. 79(10): p. 1007-1013.

[95] Roberfroid, M., et al., Prebiotic Effects: Metabolic and Health Benefits. British Journal of Nutrition, 2010. 104: p. S1-S63

[96] Abrams, S.A., et al., Effect of Prebiotic Supplementation and Calcium Intake on Body Mass Index. The Journal of Pediatrics, 2007. 151(3): p. 293-298.

[97] Maurer, A.D., et al., Changes in Satiety Hormones and Expression of Genes Involved in Glucose and Lipid Metabolism in Rats Weaned Onto Diets High in Fibre or Protein Reflect Susceptibility to Increased Fat Mass in Adulthood. The Journal of Physiology, 2009. 587(3): p. 679-691.

[98] Maurer, A., et al., Consumption of Diets High in Prebiotic Fiber or Protein During Growth Influences the Response to a High Fat and Sucrose Diet in Adulthood in Rats. Nutrition & Metabolism, 2010. 7(1): p. 77.

[99] Kalliomaki, M., et al., Early Differences in Fecal Microbiota Composition in Children May Predict Overweight. The American Journal of Clinical Nutrition, 2008. 87(3): p. 534-538.

[100] Cani, P.D., C. Dewever, and N.M. Delzenne, Inulin-Type Fructans Modulate Gastrointestinal Peptides Involved in Appetite Regulation (Glucagon-Like Peptide-1 and Ghrelin) in Rats. British Journal of Nutrition, 2004. 92(3): p. 521-526.

[101] Wu, X., et al., Molecular Characterisation of the Faecal Microbiota in Patients with Type II Diabetes. Current Microbiology, 2010. 61(1): p. 69-78.

[102] Delzenne, N.M. and C.M. Williams, Prebiotics and Lipid Metabolism. Cuurent Opinion in Lipidology, 2002. 13(1): p. 61-67.

[103] Cani, P.D., et al., Metabolic Endotoxemia Initiates Obesity and Insulin Resistance. Diabetes, 2007. 56(7): p. 1761-1772.

[104] Cani, P.D. and N.M. Delzenne, The Gut Microbiome as Therapeutic Target. Pharmacology & Therapeutics, 2011. 130(2): p. 202-212.

[105] Wong, J.M.W., et al., Colonic Health: Fermentation and Short Chain Fatty Acids. Journal of Clinical Gastroenterology, 2006. 40(3): p. 235-243.

[106] Gao, Z., et al., Butyrate Improves Insulin Sensitivity and Increases Energy Expenditure in Mice. Diabetes, 2009. 58(7): p. 1509-1517.

[107] Cani, P.D., et al., Oligofructose Promotes Satiety in Healthy Human: A Pilot Study. European Journal of Clinical Nutrition, 2005. 60(5): p. 567-572.

[108] Cani, P.D., et al., Gut Microbiota Fermentation of Prebiotics Increases Satietogenic and Incretin Gut Peptide Production with Consequences for Appetite Sensation and Glucose Response After a Meal. The American Journal of Clinical Nutrition, 2009. 90(5): p. 1236-1243.

[109] Whelan, K., et al., Appetite During Consumption of Enteral Formula as a Sole Source of Nutrition: The Effect of Supplementing Pea-Fibre and Fructo-Oligosaccharides. British Journal of Nutrition, 2006. 96(2): p. 350-356.

[110] Chaudhri, O.B., B.C.T. Field, and S.R. Bloom, Gastrointestinal Satiety Signals. International Journal of Obesity, 2008. 32(S7): p. S28-S31.

[111] Cowley, M.A., et al., The Distribution and Mechanism of Action of Ghrelin in the CNS Demonstrates a Novel Hypothalamic Circuit Regulating Energy Homeostasis. Neuron, 2003. 37(4): p. 649-661.

[112] Druce, M.R., C.J. Small, and S.R. Bloom, Minireview: Gut Peptides Regulating Satiety. Endocrinology, 2004. 145(6): p. 2660-2665.

[113] Wynne, K., et al., Appetite Control. Journal of Endocrinology, 2005. 184(2): p. 291-318.

[114] Freeland, K.R., C. Wilson, and T.M. Wolever, Adaptation of Colonic Fermentation and Glucagon-Like Peptide-1 Secretion with Increased Wheat Fibre Intake for 1 Year in Hyperinsulinaemic Human Subjects. British Journal of Nutrition, 2010. 103(1): p. 82-90.

[115] Freeland, K.R. and T.M. Wolever, Acute Effects of Intravenous and Rectal Acetate on Glucagon-Like Peptide-1, Peptide YY, Ghrelin, Adiponectin and Tumour Necrosis Factor-Alpha. British Journal of Nutrition, 2010. 103(3): p. 460-466.

[116] Piche, T., et al., Colonic Fermentation Influences Lower Esophageal Sphincter Function in Gastroesophageal Reflux Disease. Gastroenterology, 2003. 124(4): p. 894-902.

[117] Parnell, J.A. and R.A. Reimer, Weight Loss During Oligofructose Supplementation is Associated with Decreased Ghrelin and Increased Peptide YY in Overweight and Obese Adults. The American Journal of Clinical Nutrition, 2009. 89(6): p. 1751-1759.

[118] Tarini, J. and T.M.S. Wolever, The Fermentable Fibre Inulin Increases Postprandial Serum Short-Chain Fatty Acids and Reduces Free-Fatty Acids and Ghrelin in Healthy Subjects. Applied Physiology, Nutrition, and Metabolism, 2010. 35(1): p. 9-16.

[119] Woodmansey, E.J., et al., Comparison of Compositions and Metabolic Activities of Fecal Microbiotas in Young Adults and in Antibiotic-Treated and Non-Antibiotic-Treated Elderly Subjects. Applied and Environmental Microbiology, 2004. 70(10): p. 6113-6122.

[120] Mueller, S., et al., Differences in Fecal Microbiota in Different European Study Populations in Relation to Age, Gender, and Country: A Cross-Sectional Study. Applied and Environmental Microbiology, 2006. 72(2): p. 1027-1033.

[121] Claesson, M.J., et al., Comparative Analysis of Pyrosequencing and a Phylogenetic Microarray for Exploring Microbial Community Structures in the Human Distal Intestine. PLoS ONE, 2009. 4(8): p. e6669.

[122] Mariat, D., et al., The Firmicutes/Bacteroidetes ratio of the human microbiota changes with age. BMC Microbiology, 2009. 9(1): p. 123.

[123] Reinhardt, C., C.S. Reigstad, and F. Backhed, Intestinal Microbiota During Infancy and Its Implications for Obesity. Journal of Pediatric Gastroenterology and Nutrition, 2009. 48(3): p. 249-256

[124] Biasucci, G., et al., Cesarean Delivery May Affect the Early Biodiversity of Intestinal Bacteria. The Journal of Nutrition, 2008. 138(9): p. 1796S-1800S.

Chapter 4

Conjugated Linoleic and Linolenic Acid Production by Bacteria: Development of Functional Foods

Carina Paola Van Nieuwenhove, Victoria Terán and Silvia Nelina González

Additional information is available at the end of the chapter

1. Introduction

Over the years, the biological significance of conjugated fatty acids has been demonstrated. Among them, there are two that are present naturally in milk and dairy products, from ruminant origin which have been intensively studied in recent times: conjugated linoleic acid and conjugated linolenic acid.

Conjugated linoleic acid (CLA) refers to a mixture of positional and geometric isomers of linoleic acid (c9,c12-C18:2, LA) with a conjugated double bond. It is a natural compound mainly found in ruminant products such as meat, milk and other dairy food that represent the main source of CLA for humans. Of the two biologically important isomers, c9,t11 is the most prevalent one comprising around 80 to 90% of total CLA in ruminant products, and t10,c12 is present in lower amounts as 3-5% of total CLA [1].

CLA is formed as an intermediate product of the biohydrogenation (BH) process that occurs in rumen, as multi-step mechanism carried out by different microorganisms on unsaturated fatty acids to produce stearic acid (C18:0). Also , it can be produced by desaturation of trans vaccenic acid (t11-C18:1, TVA), process that occurs in different tissues such as mammary gland,.

Conjugated linolenic acid (CLNA) are representing by different conjugated isomers of the linolenic acid (c9, c12, c15-C18:3, LNA). It is also resulting of the ruminal microbial metabolism on fatty acids present in foods, but they are also found in some plant seed oils, like pomegranate seed oil rich in punicic acid (c9,t11, c13-CLNA) [2-3] and tung seed oil where α-eleostearic acid (c9,t11,t13-CLNA) content is about 70% [2-3].

Both conjugated fatty acids has undoubted effects on health, with important biological functions demonstrated in animal models, making them a target of intensive study.

Over the years, CLA has received great attention due to their beneficial properties on health. There exist near 28 different CLA isomers produced by natural and industrial process during fatty acid hydrogenation [4], but the most important according to their biological effects are c9, t11 and t10,c12 forms. However, CLA isomer in milk fat according to importance are c9,t11 (around 80%) followed by t7,c9, which is quantitatively the second most important reaching level so high as 3 to 16 % of total CLA [5]. Factors affecting CLA content in milk, such as the food of ruminants [6-7], the animal breeding type and the stage of lactation [8] were widely reported.

Many studies demonstrated the action of CLA as anti-carcinogenic [9], anti-diabetic [10] and immune-modulator [11] compound. Although there is no agreement regarding its function on fat metabolism, some authors revealed that its consumption also decreases the fat deposition [12].

In addition, CLA produced trough chemical isomerization of LA is offer as dietary supplement in many countries. However, unexpected isomers are produced by this process. To consider CLA as a nutraceutical or medicinal compound, a selective isomer production must be done.

On the other hand, CLNA showed anti-carcinogenesis effects *in vitro* and *in vivo* models [9, 13-14] and other isomers were reported as hypolipidemic compound in human liver derived HepG2 cells [15]. Moreover, it was demonstrated that CLNA exhibits stronger cytotoxic effect on tumoral cells than CLA isomers [16].

Since the most important sources of both conjugated fatty acids for human consumption are milk and dairy products, and due to the microbial production of these compounds, several attempts are being developed to increase its content in food using natural process for it production. In the field of human and animal health, it is interesting to understand the potential beneficial role of selection of bacteria with the ability to form conjugated fatty acids to be then included in foods. Thus, the processed products could be considered as functional foods and sometimes as probiotics, as we detailed below.

2. Ruminal production of conjugated linoleic and linolenic acid

Fatty acids are present in forages and concentrate feeds, mainly as esterified form, mostly present as phospholipids and glycolipids in forrages and triglycerides in plant seeds, comonly used in concentrates.

The two most abundant fatty acids from animal diet are linoleic and linolenic acids. Both are incorporated through diet and once they reach the rumen, are extensively modified by microbial enzymes, such as lipases. These enzymes produce as results LA and LNA as free form for further reactions of isomerization and hydrogenation.

The biohydrogenation of both fatty acids occur in a similar manner, but differ in the intermediate products, as shown in *Figure 1*.

Hydrogenation of linoleic acid produces as first intermediate c9, t11-CLA isomer, by a process where the double bond at carbon-12 position is transferred to carbon-11, carried out by linoleate isomerase (EC 5.3.1.5, LAI). The second step, is the rapid conversion to t11-C18:1 (trans vaccenic acid, TVA) by a reduction mechanism and further hydrogenated to stearic acid (C18:0) [17].

The other CLA isomer resulting of rumen metabolism is t10, c12, which is produced by different microorganism such as *Butyrivibrio fibrisolvens* [18] and *Megasphaera eldsenii* YJ-4 [19]. But the hidrogenation of this isomer not produced TVA but c6, t10-C18:2 which is further converted to C18:0. According to authors, some bacteria can produce hydroxiacids previously to its conversion to CLA isomers [20-21].

As we mentioned above, the other fatty acid of importance in ruminant feeding is linolenic acid, which is also converted to C18:0 by microbial action. In this pathway, LNA is isomerized at *cis*-12 position forming as first intermediate product c9,t11,c15 isomer, named conjugated linolenic acid (CLNA). This compound is further reduced to t11,c15-C18:2 and after that converted to three different products: t11-C18:1; c15-C18:1 and t15-C18:1. As shown in *Figure 1*, only t11-C18:1 is reduced up to C18:0.

Note that metabolic pathway of both LA and LNA fatty acids produce TVA as result of a reduction process, forming conjugated fatty acids as intermediate products. All conjugated fatty acids are absorbed by intestine cells, reason why they are further present in milk and meat fat [22-23].

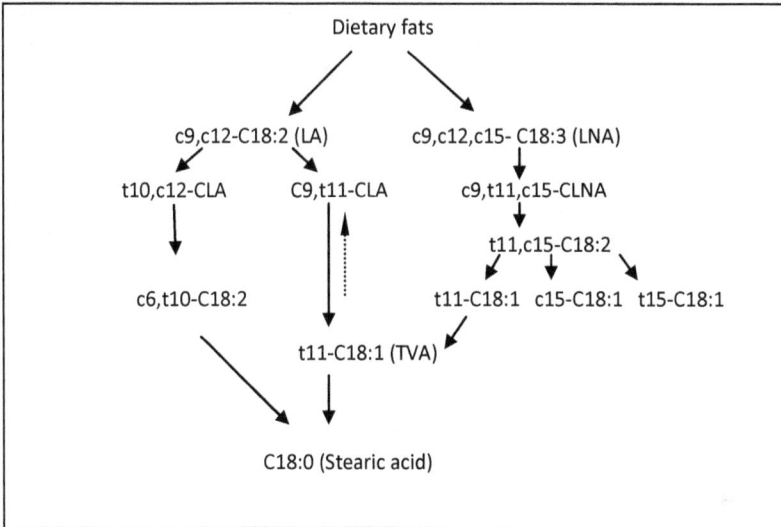

Figure 1. Biohydrogenation process of linoleic and linolenic fatty acid in rumen (adapted from Harfoot and Hazlewood [17]) and endogenous synthesis of CLA in mammary gland (dotted arrow).

Of the rumen microorganism, bacteria are largely responsible for biohydrogenation of unsaturated fatty acids and protozoa seem to be of only minor importance [17].

Kemp and Lander [24] divided bacteria into two groups according to reactions and end products of biohydrogenation. Group A includes those bacteria able to hydrogenate linoleic acid and α-linolenic acid producing t11- C18:1 as an end product. On the other hand, Group B bacteria including those able to use t11-C18:1 as one of the main substrates to produce stearic acid as end product. A listing of the bacteria species of both groups is provided in the review by Harfoot and Hazlewood [17].

Instead of ruminal biohydrogenation, there is another CLA synthesis pathway carried out through the Δ9-desaturase enzyme activity on trans-vaccenic acid (t11-C18:1-TVA) in different tissues, especially in the mammary gland [25]. This endogenous synthesis of CLA is the responsible for most of CLA level found in milk fat, being according to findings around a 64 % [25] to > 80% [26].

But other pathway of CLNA isomers synthesis, in addition to ruminal production, was not yet evidenced. For that reason, its content in ruminant milk apparently comes exclusively from BH of linolenic acid and diet.

As results of microorganism metabolism, many isomers originated in rumen are present in milk. Due to biological properties of both conjugated fatty acids researchers are looking to develop natural foods enriched in CLA and CLNA and thus increase daily intake by humans.

As it was previously mentioned, ruminant milk and meat are the most abundant sources of CLA for humans. Different studies have demonstrated that CLA content of ruminant milk and meat products varies between 4-6 mg/g fat [27-29]. From this value, near the 80 to 90% corresponds to the c9,t11 isomer [30-31]. However, the concentration of CLA can vary widely, where differences are largely related to diet. So, milk fatty acid profile can be modified according to animal feeding.

In the last years, different supplements such as vegetal oils, animal fat, natural pasture and seeds were used to improve fatty acid profile of milk, to attempt higher levels of CLA [32-33] or CLNA [22, 34].

Respect to CLA synthesis in non-ruminant animal, an increase on CLA content in tissues was evidenced in studies using rats [35] and mice [23] after TVA supplementation.

In humans, an endogenous synthesis of CLA was also shown by Adolf et al. [36]. But tisular human production in human tissues is so low, that the concentration found in tissues are directly related to food consumption.

Although ruminant foods are the richest source of CLA for humans, it is also found in monogastric animal products, such as swine [37], chicken [30], turkey [30], fish and rabbit [38] meat but in much lower levels. Among south-american camelids, CLA was determined in llama's (Lama glama) milk [39]. Vegetable oils contain little CLA and according to some authors no CLA content were evidenced in vegetal oils. Typical values of CLA in non-ruminant foods are given in *Table 1*.

Product	Total CLA (mg/ 100 g of fat)	Author
Meat Turkey	0.25	Chin *et al.* [30]
Fish	0.01-0.09	Fristche and Steinhart [105]
Swine	0.3-0.9	Ross *et al.*[37]
Rabbit	0.11	Fristche and Steinhart [105]
Chicken	0.09-0.2	Chin *et al.* [30]
Eggs yolk	N.D	Raes *et al.* [106]
	N.D	Gultemiriam *et al.* [107]
Milk Human	0.1	Park *et al.* [108]
Horse	0.05-0.12	Jahreis *et al.* [8]
Sow	0.19-0.27	Jahreis *et al.* [8]
Llama *(Lama glama)*	0.7	Schoos *et al.* [39]
Vegetable oils	<0.01	Fristche and Steinhart [105]

ND: not determined

Table 1. CLA content in non-ruminant foods

So as CLA, different CLNA isomers occur naturally, some of which could be formed by ruminal biohydrogenation and further incorporated into milk and meat fat.

Only a few studies were done respect to CLNA content in ruminant products and according to data informed, the only isomer present in cow milk is c9,t11,c15 form [40] while in muscle is also present c9,t13,c15 isomer [40].

CLNA content in milk is around of 0.3-0.39 mg/g fat [23, 40]. At the present, the effect of diet on CLNA concentration in milk was only reported by one work, where cows not fed with extruded linseed (control) have no CLNA in milk, but linseed supplementation in diet increased both CLA and CLNA content, reaching the latest fatty acid a value of 0.15% of total fatty acids [22]. In this study, CLNA was also present only as c9, t11, c15 isomer.

CLNA content in non-ruminant products were determined in different seed oils, being the most abundant source of these fatty acid isomers *(Table 2)*. Moreover, tung, pomegranate and catalpa oils showed high level of CLNA but in different isomer ratio. On this way, punicic acid (c9, t11, c15-CLNA) is contained about 72% in pomegranate seed oil [3]. In bitter gourd oil and tung seed oil the main isomer present correspond to α-eleostearic acid (c9,t11,t13-CLNA) in about 60% and 70%, respectively [3, 41]. Catalpa seed oil contains CLNA at a level of 31 %, found as catalpic acid (t9, t11, c12-CLNA) isomer.

Product	CLNA (%)	Author
Pomegranate oil	75	Suzuki *et al.* [3]
	86	Yücel *et al.* [2]
Catalpa oil	27.5	Yücel *et al.*[2]
	31	Suzuki *et al.* [3]
Bitter gourd oil	60	Yücel *et al.* [2]; Suzuki *et al.* [3]
Tung oil	70	Suzuki *et al.* [3]
Cow milk	0.3-0.39	Loor *et al.* [23]
		Plourde *et al.* [40]

Table 2. CLNA content in cow milk and seed oils

3. CLA recommended human intake

CLA concentration in dairy products widely varied according to data reported (0.55–9.12 mg/g fat), but even though are lower than required to achieve a biological effect in humans.

Biological properties after CLA administration is depending on isomer and doses administered and the period of study. Those, studies on animal models reported anti-atherosclerosis effect after 0.1-1% of total CLA per day to rabbits [42]. Moreover, anti-carcinogenic effect was determined by authors using levels from 0.5% to 4% into the diet [43-44].

Although the action mechanism is not well understood, CLA was reported as antioxidant compound in animals and *in vitro* models [15].

Just as there are variations in experimental models about effective doses of CLA, depending on animal model and the biological effect evaluated, the recommended dose from human daily intake also widely varied.

In general, by extrapolation of results found in animals, the recommended CLA daily intake is around 0.35 to 1 g/day [15]. Some authors estimated a daily dose of 650 mg [45], but other studies considered that higher doses (3.0 to 4.2 g/day) are adequate to reduce body fat mass [46-47].

However, at the present the real consumption in different countries is lower than recommended dose. Studies on German population estimated a daily CLA intake of 0.35 to 0.43 g for men and women, respectively [38]. In other countries, CLA daily intake was informed so lower as 120 to 140 mg per day [27].

A few epidemiological studies were done in humans, and evidence show that no all isomers are absorbed to a similar extent. According to result is difficult to predict the impact of CLA consumption on humans and the preventive effect of isomers.

Thus, a short-term (4 to 12 weeks) human studies showed that 2.2 g/d, administered as a mixture of c9,t11 and t10,c12 isomers, produces a decrease on inflammatory markers [48]. A higher dose (3 g/d) were used by Moloney *et al.* [49] who found an increase on HDL levels and a decrease on the ratio of LDL cholesterol to HDL cholesterol, but did not show positive effect on insulin levels in diabetics patients.

Smedman *et al.* [50] reported a reduction of body fat in humans after consumption of 4.2 g/d of a mixture of CLA isomer (c9,t11 and t10,c12) during 12 weeks.

Even though there are many positive findings about CLA supplementation by animals, some negative aspects were informed by other authors, such as the induction of fatty liver and spleen and resistance to insulin [51].

Studies concerning to increase CLA content in foods receives great attention since bacterial inclusion improves CLA levels in some fermented dairy products or could generate CLA at intestinal level after a probiotic administration. In this way, studies on bacterial CLA or CLNA production are relevant in this field, and are detailed in this chapter.

4. Bacterial CLA and CLNA production

The ruminal anaerobe *Butyrivibrio fibrisolvens* was the first bacteria were CLA production was evidenced [18]. After years, it was revealed that not only ruminal bacteria were able to form CLA. So, microorganisms isolated from dairy products, human and animal intestine were demonstrated as CLA-producing bacteria, including lactic acid bacteria (LAB) and bifidobacteria. At the present, *Lactobacillus reuteri, Lactobacillus rhamnosus, Lactobacillus plantarum; Lactobacillus brevis, Lactobacillus acidophilus; Lactococcus lactis, Propionibaterium freudenrehichii, Bifidobacterium sp, Streptococcus*, among others, were able to form CLA [52-54].

Some years ago, it was reported the formation of another isomers of conjugated fatty acid from α and γ-linolenic in *Lactobacillus plantarum*, named as CLNA [21]. Even though this conjugated fatty acid production was reported since 2003, it was only recently informed for bifidobacterium strains [55-56].

Conjugation of linoleic and linolenic acid were proposed as a detoxification mechanism to avoid the growth inhibition effect of fatty acid on bacteria [57-58].

CLA/CLNA production varied among strains being influenced by substrate concentration, culture media, temperature and time of fermentation, among other factors. The isomer formed is also strain-dependent, showing some microorganism the production of only one isomer while others produce two or more CLA/CLNA forms.

As an example of the influence of culture condition, Ogawa et al. (2001)[59] informed CLA production by *L. acidophilus* cultured in microaerophilia conditions, but when bacteria were cultured in aerophilia conditions not CLA formation was determined.

Nowadays, different processes are being carried out to increase CLA production by strains. So, Lin et al (2005) [60] immobilized cells of Lactobacilli strains in two matrix (chitosan and poliacrilamide). In this study, *L. delbruekii* ssp. *bulgaricus* and *L. acidophilus* showed higher CLA production than not immobilized cells. Washed cell instead of growth cultures is another way to produce high CLA levels ([20, 59, 61].

Further studies informed that the uses of enzyme extract of *L. acidophilus* at 50ºC and pH 5 produce more than eight CLA isomers, being around 48% as c,t/t,c form [62].

The transformation of linoleic and linolenic acid to the conjugated form is carried out by linoleate isomerase (LAI) enzyme, which is bound to the bacterial membrane [63]. This enzyme will be treated in other section of this chapter.

At the present, the *in vitro* bioproduction of conjugated fatty acids has been shown in lactic acid bacteria (LAB), propionibacteria and bifidobacteria strains.

A different mechanism of CLA production via 10-OH-C18:1 seems to be the most common pathway in human intestine bacteria according to McIntosh *et al.* (2009) [64], who evidenced this metabolic pathway in *Roseburia*, *Ruminococcus* and other intestinal strains.

5. Lactic acid bacteria (LAB)

CLA production by LAB strains were informed during years. The mechanism, isomer and optimum condition for CLA formation makes these the most variable group on the literature.

Some strains as *L. plantarum* AKU 1009a were informed as CLA-producing bacteria via a two-step reaction: first the hydration of linoleic acid to 10-hydroxy-18:1, followed by dehydration of the resulting hydroxy acid to CLA. In this strain, CLA was formed as c9,t11 (CLA1) and t10,c12 (CLA2) isomers [21].

Xu *et al.* [65] also informed CLA production as c9,t11 and t10,c12 isomer of CLA, at different ratio, in LAB and propionibacteria strains cultured in a fat milk model supplemented with hydrolized soy oil for 24 to 48 h. Among these, *L. acidophilus*, *L. casei*, *L. plantarum*, *E. faecium*, *L. rhamnosus*, *Pediococcus (Ped.) acidilactici* and yogurt cultures (mixture of *L. delbruekii* ssp. *bulgaricus* and *Str. salivarius* ssp. *thermophilus*, 1:1 ratio) were reported as CLA-producing bacteria in the mentioned condition. Increasing time from 24 to 48 h did not increase CLA content, except in *Ped. acidilactici* and *L. rhamnosus* strains. The main isomer found was c9,t11 followed by t10,c12 after 24 h of incubation, except in *E. faecium* were t10,c12 were not determined.

The ability to produce CLA in Lactobacilli strains from human origin was also informed by Lee *et al* [66]. In this study, *L. rhamnosus, L. paracasei* and *L. pentosus* also showed different CLA isomer ratio production. So, *L. rhamnosus* and *L. pentosus* were able to transform LA to c9, t11 and t10,c12- CLA, while *L. paracasei* only produce the c9,t11 isomer.

Other study revealed six LAB able to form CLA after 24 h of incubation, varying percentage of LA conversion between 17% and 36%. Here, *L. casei, L. rhamnosus,* and *Strep. thermophilus* showed the highest LA conversion in MRS broth, and increased two- or threefold in milk than MRS broth [53]. *Strep. thermophilus* has importance by it uses as starter culture during fermentation process of dairy products.

Some authors informed a positive correlation between CLA production and tolerance to LA [53, 67] using different substrate concentration. However, the efficiency of CLA production in some LAB and *bifidobacterium* decreases at higher levels of free LA in the medium [53].

Other studies using LAB showed CLA production mainly as c9,t11 form (60-65 %), followed by t10,c12 (30-32%) and other minor isomers like t9,t11 and t10,t12 (2-5%) in *L. acidophilus, L. plantarum* and *Lact. lactis* cultured in MRS broth and skim milk during 24 h. [68].

In a recent work, a low CLA production was informed by strains of *L. sakei* and *L. curvatus* (1.6 % and 4.2 %, respectively), commonly present in meat fermentation as starter cultures or natural microorganism [56, 69].

The reaction sequence of isomerization of LA seems to involve different steps according to bacterial strain.

Respect to CLNA production, *L. plantarum* AKU 1009a was able to transform ricinoleic acid to CLA (CLA1 and CLA2) [20]. Further studies demonstrated that this lactobacilli strain has the capacity of use α- and γ-linoleic acids as substrate to generate the corresponding conjugated trienoic acids [21] named CALA and CGLA, respectively. Authors reported a CALA production rate of 40% under two isomer forms: c9, t11, c15-C18:3 (CALA 1, 67% of total CALA) and t9,t11,c15-C18:3 (CALA 2, 33% of total CALA). A higher CGLA production rate was determined in this study (68%) as a mixture of two isomer: c6, c9, t11-C18:3 (CGLA 1, 40 % of total CGLA) and c6, t9, t11-C18:3 (CGLA 2, 60% of total CGLA).

Recently, determination of CLNA production by other LAB strains were informed [69]. Among these, a high production levels were determined in *L. sakei* and *L. curvatus*, reaching a percentage of conversion of 22.4 % and 60.1 %, respectively. Authors evidenced that the isomerization process of LA to CLA and LNA to CLNA is different according to LAB strain, so as isomer resulting after culturing. Some microorganisms were able to form both conjugated fatty acids, but predominantly convert LNA to CLNA, while others not were able to form CLA but effectively converted LNA to CLNA. Results are given in *Table 3*.

Strain	c9,t11	t10,c12	Other isomer	LA conversion (%)	Author
L. curvatus	+	+	-	1.6%	Gorissen *et al.* [69]
L. plantarum	+	+	-	4.6%	Gorissen *et al.* [69]
	+	-	+	N.D	Kishino *et al.* [20]
	+	+	-	N.D	Ogawa *et al.* [109]
	+	+	-	N.D	Rodríguez-alcalá *et al.* [68]
	+	+	-	N.D	Xu *et al.* [65]
L. sakei	+	+	-	4.2	Gorissen *et al.* [69]
L. reuteri	+	+		26	Lee *et al.* [110]
L. rhamnosus	+	+	-		Lee *et al.* [66]
	+	+	-		Ogawa *et al.* [109]
	+	-	-	34	Van Nieuwenhove *et al.* [53]
L. paracasei	+	-	-	N.D	Lee *et al.* [66]
L. pentosus	+	+	-	N.D	Lee *et al.* [66]
	+	+	-		Ogawa *et al.* [109]

Strep. thermophilus	+	-	-	33	Van Nieuwenhove et al. [53]
L. brevis	+	+	-	N.D	Ogawa et al. [109]
L.curvatus	+	+	-	1.6	Gorissen et al. [69]
L. acidophilus	+	-	-	20	Van Nieuwenhove et al. [53]
	+	+	-	N.D	Ogawa et al. [109]
	+	+	-	N.D	Xu et al. [65]
L. reuteri	N.I	N.I	N.I	26	Lee et al. [110]
Lact. lactis	+	+	-	N.D	Rodríguez- Alcalá et al. [68]

+: positive production. -: no production. N.D: not determined. N.I: not informed

Table 3. CLA production by LAB strains cultured in presence of free LA

6. Propionibacteria

Propionibacteria are commonly present in milk and dairy products and some species play an important role in the creation of cheeses, such as emmental cheese. Propionibacteria represents another important group of bacteria where the capacity of LA isomerization *in vitro* was demonstrated, being relevant since it could be included in fermented products as cheeses. So, *P. freudenrehichii* was able to produce CLA mainly as c9,t11 form according to different studies [58, 65, 70-71] although other author reported eight different isomers of CLA produced by enzyme extract in this bacteria [72].

CLA production in a fat milk model supplemented with hydrolyzed soy oil for 24 to 48 h was demonstrated in two *P. freudenreichii ssp shermanii* and *P. freudenreichii* ssp *freudenreichii* [65]. Higher levels of CLA were determined in skim milk than MRS broth.

The ability of *P. acnes*, isolated from sheep, to form CLA only as t10, c12 form was also evidenced [73].

The results clearly demonstrate that propioniacteria strains show a great variability on CLA production, according to many factors as origin, species, substrate and culture conditions.

To the best of our knowledge, CLNA production by propionibacteria strains was recently evidenced by Henessy et al. [74]. In this work, bacteria were culture in presence of different fatty acid used as substrate to evaluate it further conversion into the conjugated form. Thus, LA, α and γ-LNA, stearidonic (c6, c9, c15-C18:4) and other polyunsaturated fatty acids were individually incorporated to culture medium. Strains of *P. freudenreiichii* ssp *shermanii* and *P. freudenreihichii* ssp *freudenreichii* were able to conjugate different PUFA, showing different percentage of conversion of each particular fatty acid. Thus, *P. freudenreiichii* ssp *shermanii* 9093 reached a rate conversion of 50.5; 53.5 and 3.09 for LA, α-LNA and stearidonic acid, respectively. On the other hand, *P. freudenreihichii* ssp *freudenreichii* Propioni-6 reached a conversion rate of 44.65; 8.94; and 3.58 for the same fatty acids. The isomerization process on γ-LNA was not evidenced for these bacteria. The increase of substrate concentration caused a decrease on the percentage of bioconversion (as is shown in *Table 4*).

Strain	c9,t11,c15	t9,t11,c15	CLA (%)	CLNA (%)	Author
L. curvatus LMG 13553	+	+	1.6%	22.4	Gorissen et al. [69]
L. plantarum ATCC 8014	+	+	4.6%	26.8	Gorissen et al. [69]
L. sakei LMG 13558	+	+	4.2	60.1	Gorissen et al. [69]
CG1	+	+	ND	28.4	
B. bifidum LMG 10645	+	+	40.7	78.4	Gorissen et al. [55]
B. breve LMG 11040	+	+	44	65.5	Gorissen et al. [55]
B. breve LMG 11084	+	+	53.5	72.0	Gorissen et al. [55]
B. breve LMG 11613	+	+	19.5	55.6	Gorissen et al. [55]
B. breve LMG 13194	+	+	24.2	63.3	Gorissen et al. [55]
B. pseudolongum ssp pseudolongum LMG 11595	+	+	42.2	62.7	Gorissen et al. [55]
B. breve NCIMB 8807*	+	+	66	68	Hennessy et al. [74]
B. breve DPC6330*	+	+	67	83	Hennessy et al. [74]
B. longum DPC6315*	-	-	12	0.0	Hennessy et al. [74]
P. freudenreichii ssp. freudenreichii Propioni-6 **	+	+	44.6	8.9	Hennessy et al. [74]
P. freudenreichii ssp. shermanii 9093**	+	+	50.5	53.5	Hennessy et al. [74]

*: production of conjugated isomers of γ-LNA and stearidonic acid were also reported. **: production of conjugated stearidonic acid was also informed. ND: not determined

Table 4. CLNA isomers production by bacteria cultured in presence of α-LNA

7. Bifidobacterium strains

Bifidobacteria are found as normal inhabitants of the human gut and is among the first colonizers of the sterile gastrointestinal tracks of newborns [75]. Due to their health's benefits on humans, it uses as probiotic strains is indubitable [76]. As results after years of investigations, many functional foods have been developed with the addition of bifidobacteria to the food matrix [77-79].

For this reason, it is not surprising that many studies on the ability of these bacteria to produce CLA have been carried out for a long time.

Bifidobacteria species able to produce CLA was reported at first time by Coakley et al. [57], who informed a considerable interspecies variation. So, *Bifidobacterium breve* and *B. dentium* were the most efficient CLA producers among the range of evaluated strains. The highest percentage of LA conversion was determined for *B. breve*, reaching a value of 65% (c9, t11-CLA). In this study, strains also varied considerably with respect to their tolerance to linoleic acid concentration in the medium.

Other authors showed that strains of *Bifidobacterium breve* and *B. pseudocatenulatum* isolated from human feces, were able to form CLA in a rate conversion of 69% and 78%, respectively [80].

Moreover, CLA production in *B. bifidum* cultured in skim milk, using as substrate hydrolyzed soy oil was reported by Xu *et al.* [65], where authors detected CLA production after 24-48 h only as c9,t11 isomer, and traces of the t10,c12 form.

In a recently study the ability to form CLA in two strains of *B. animalis* were reported [68]. Authors found CLA production from free LA and safflower oil added to MRS broth and skim milk. Strains were able to transform LA to CLA after 24-48 h of incubation. In order to abundance, the most important isomer produced was c9, t11 isomer, followed by t10, c12.

Bifidobacterium breve LMC520 can actively convert linoleic acid to c9,t11-CLA, which is the major isomer derived from microbial conversion according to results from Park *et al.* [81].

The study with the highest number of bifidobacteria were carried out by Gorissen *et al.* [55], which performed a screening of 36 different Bifidobacteria strains to investigate their ability to produce CLA and/or CLNA. As substrate they used free LA and α- LNA, revealing that only six strains were able to convert it to different conjugated fatty acid isomers. Strains were identified as a *Bifidobacterium bifidum*, *Bifidobacterium pseudolongum* and four *B. breve* strains, named *B. breve* LMG 11084, *B. breve* LMG 11613, *B. breve* LMG 13194, *B. bifidum* LMG 10645 and *B. pseudolongum* subsp. *pseudolongum* LMG 11595. Moreover, all strains have been shown to be more efficient in converting LNA to CLNA than LA to CLA, in percentages from 55.6% to 78.4% and 19.5% to 53.5%, respectively. In addition, the CLNA isomers that were mainly found were in order c9, t11, c15-CLNA followed by t9, t11, c15-CLNA isomer.

Hennessy *et al.* [74] also informed about isomerization process of different fatty acids by bifidobacteria strains. Moreover, different PUFA such as stearidonic, araquidonic and docosapentanoic and docosahexanoic acid were supplemented to the culture. A general patron of isomerization was determined on *B. breve* and *B. longum* strains, being able to transform LA, α and γ-LNA and stearidonic acid to it conjugated form. As was observed in propionibacteria, the percentage of conversion varied among strains, showing around 12 to 67% of LA conversion, mainly into c9, t11 and t10,c12 isomer. α- LNA was converted among 0 to 83% among strains, and lower rate conversion was determined for γ-LNA (0.5- 37%). The conjugation of stearidonic acid varied from 3.8 to 27%. *B. breve* DPC6330 was the most effective conjugated fatty acid producer, showing a bioconversion rate of 70% for LA, 90% of α-LNA, 17% for γ-LNA and 28% for stearidonic acid.

As well as different ability to isomerize fatty acids was determined in LAB and propionibacteria, bifidobacteria also exhibit a wide range of bioconversion rate. Many factors affect the mechanism of the fatty acids isomerization, such as culture conditions and substrate concentration. The production of different isomers ratio was reported for all evaluated strains.

To the best of our knowledge, this is the only work reporting the conjugation of stearidonic acid by bacteria. Results are given in *Table 4*.

8. Alternative substrate to CLA production

Although free fatty acids is the most commonly substrate employed by authors to analyze CLA or CLNA production by strains, alternative substrates are being evaluated. Many studies using vegetable oils (hydrolyzed or not hydrolyzed) and mono or dilinoleins as exogenous source of fatty acids were determined to be further incorporated to food matrix. Therefore, bacteria must have the ability to hydrolyze the triglycerides and liberate linoleic acid or linolenic acid for further conversion. Only hydrolyzed oils can offer the fatty acid as free form.

While vegetable oils are the richest source of linoleic and linolenic acid, data about the utilization of monolinolein by *B. breve* were informed. This strain, from human origin, was able to generate CLA at higher bioconversion rate than free LA or dilinolein was added to the medium [82].

CLA production in milk system models was described by many authors using vegetal oils as substrate for further isomerization. At the present, soy, sunflower, canola, castor and safflower oils were used as source of linoleic acid [20, 61, 68, 83].

Kishino *et al.*[20] determined CLA production in *L. plantarum* using castor oil and ricinoleic acid as substrate, showing the same end product than using free LA. Moreover, the production of the previously reported hydroxyacids as intermediate compounds, were also evidenced in the assay.

CLA formation by LAB and *Bifidobacterium* strain using safflower oil as LA source added to skim milk at 1 mg/ml was reported by other authors [68], where they informed that some bacteria produced higher CLA using safflower oil than free linoleic acid in skim milk broth after 24 h of incubation. Among these group of microorganism was *B. animalis, L. acidophilus* and *Lact. lactis*.

Among bacteria isolated from rumen, *L. brevis* was reported as CLA-producing strain in presence of sunflower oil [84].

However, there was informed no CLA production after the addition of soy oil to skim milk in *P. freudenreihchii; L. casei; L. acidophillus, L. plantarum; P. acidilactici, B. bifidum, L. rhamnosus* and *E. faecium* [65]. But once hydrolyzed soy oil was supplemented to the medium as substrate, CLA production from 0.6 to 2.2 mg/g fat was determined in all selected strains.

According to results, the utilization of vegetable oils by bacteria as source of fatty acid for it further isomerization is also depending on metabolism of strains.

9. LAI enzyme

As we previously mentioned, linoleate isomerase is an enzyme present in some bacteria, which is bound to the membrane. In the most of bacteria, CLA production is primarily located in the extracellular phase [71] but it can be also found in the cellular membrane as an structural lipid [80]. Moreover, both LA and CLA incorporated to the membrane represent less than 1.7% of the total amount of CLA formed [80].

CLNA isomers are also found primarily in the cell-free supernatants compared to the cell pellet [55]. Authors reported that around 7% of LNA and 5% of CLNA corresponding to the cellular pellet in bacteria cultured in presence of LNA.

For this reason, the analysis methods of fatty acids of cultures did not involve the remotion of bacterial cells. Moreover, total fatty acids content is necessary to determine the complete bioavailability of those compounds once bacteria are included in a food matrix or is considered as probiotic strain.

At the present, LAI has been isolated from bacteria such as *L. delbrueckii* subsp. *bulgaricus*, *But. fibrisolvens*, *L. acidophilus* and *P. freudenreichii* subsp. *shermanii* showing some differences.

LAI from *But. fibrisolvens* A-38 was isolated by Park *et al* [85], determining the molecular weight and partial amino acid sequence of the enzyme. According to findings, this LAI consist of a single polypeptide with a molecular weight of 19 kDa.

Other authors isolated and characterized the LAI from *L. reuteri* MRS8 [86], showing a molecular weight of more than 100 kDa. In this study, the optimal activity of the enzyme was in the pH range of 4.7 to 5.4.

A genotypic identification of LAI gene from ten strains able to form CLA and/or CLNA was recently performed [69]. This work presented the homologies of LAI sequence in a dendrogram comparing to other LAI sequence from known LAB.

Moreover, the molecular weight forms LAI from *L. reuteri*, *P. acnes* and *C. sporogenes* were 68 kDa, 45 kDa and 55 kDa, respectively [87-88].

10. Functional foods and probiotics

The development of healthier food is looking for taking in account their benefits for humans. Among these, dairy products represent a good alternative to manufacture functional and/or probiotic foods. Functional food includes processed food or foods fortified with health-promoting additives. By other hand, probiotics are live microorganisms which when administered in adequate amounts confer a health benefit to the host. Several bacteria are informed as probiotic strains during years, where several positive effects on health have been supported [89].

At the present, conjugated fatty acids have attracted considerable attention because of their potentially beneficial biologic effects. Important properties were attributed to CLA and CLNA, and scientific evidence has been demonstrated both in humans and animal models, including anti-tumor, anti-obese, anti-atherogenic and anti-diabetic activities.

Microbiota present in intestine plays an important physiological rol to the host, modulating some metabolic functions, conferring resistance to microorganism infection and increasing immune response, among other functions.

The bioconversion of LA to CLA and LNA to CLNA by bacteria at intestinal level, result a novel and interesting topic to be developed with the objective to obtain probiotic foods with microorganism able to produce it or functional foods with high levels of CLA and /or CLNA.

The uses of CLA or CLNA-producing bacteria as probiotics have received great attention for nutrition, since many studies evidenced their benefits for the promotion of human health.

It has been demonstrated that isomer of CLA has different function and according to reports t10, c12 is more potent than c9,t11 CLA to prevent cancer cell proliferation [90]. This isomer is also associated to a decrease on body fat in animals [91-92] and humans [93-94].

Previous studies informed that CLA content in cheeses varied according to strain used as starter or adjunct culture [95] and to the ripening time [96]. Therefore, the inclusion of bacteria able to form it during the fermentation process has been received great attention by researchers.

At the present, different functional foods (yogurt, cheese, fermented milk) were manufactured with CLA-producing bacteria, obtaining a final product with a high CLA content. cheeses manufactured with CLA-producing bacteria were developed using sunflower oil as exogenous source of LA, reporting a modification of fatty acids profile in mice tissues after it administration [83]. Mice fed functional cheeses showed a protective effect on viability of intestinal cells after a treatment of 1,2-dimethylhydrazine drug, used as oxidant compound.

Nowadays, CLA production by probiotic bacteria has received special interest in the research field, being well established that bacteria isolated from intestine or fecal samples can form it. However, *in vitro* production was intensely informed, while a few studies have established an *in vivo* CLA production after ingestion of bacteria. Authors revealed that according to administered strain, a high t10, c12 isomer [66, 98] or c9,t11 isomer [99] content in animal tissues occurs.

Linoleic acid excretion in humans is estimate at 340 mg/day [100], being this fatty acid available to further isomerization process by intestinal microbiota. Nevertheless, this local CLA production was only reported after probiotic treatment, but if CLA amount produced is enough to exert a preventive effect require better understanding.

Strains daily administered as probiotic, in a short-term study, produced an increase on CLA systemic content [66]. Authors showed that consumption of *L. rhamnosus* PL60 (10^7-10^9 CFU/day) during 8 weeks increased t10, c12 isomer content in plasma and tissues of diet-induced obese mice. Animals receiving PL60 showed a significant reduction of fat adipose tissue (epididymal and perineal). No liver steatosis were observed in this study, being the most adverse effect informed to t10, c12-CLA. The increasing amount of CLA in tissues after oral treatment with *L. rhamnosus* was explained as an intestinal production once bacterium has been colonized the intestine. Lower leptin levels in PL60 group were also informed. Obese mice selection as animal model was supported by t10, c12-CLA as the main isomer formed by this probiotic strain.

Another work supporting the generation of CLA at intestine using animal models have also reported by same researchers and in this study, they use as probiotic strain *L. plantarum* PL62 in obese mice, at daily dose of 10^7-10^9 CFU/mice. The presence of PL62 was determined in fecal samples after the first week of its intake, and after 5 weeks of feeding a weight reduction in mice receiving PL62 was determined. Similar results were observed after two experimental doses. Respect to CLA, as in the previous study, the main isomer formed by bacterium was t10,c12-CLA [98].

So, both human bacteria *L. rhamnosus* PL60 and *L. plantarum* PL62 were demonstrated to be able to form *in vivo* CLA [66, 98].

But. fibrisolvens from goat rumen was able to rapidly convert LA to CLA and LNA to CLNA, showing similar rate conversion for both fatty acids [101]. In this work, selective strain was administered to mice using a daily dose of 10^{11} CFU/mouse, during 4 weeks. After the trial period, a higher CLA amount in feces was determined. CLA content in tissues was also increased after probiotic treatment. Although a high dose of bacteria was employed, no adverse effect was determined. The aim of this study was to develop a probiotic for animals to generate a continuous CLA production and absorption.

The administration of a mix of bacteria able to form CLA as c9, t11 and t10, c12, called VSL3 was used as probiotic for mice administration [102]. The combination of all strains (*L. casei*, *L. plantarum, L. acidophilus, L. delbrueckii subsp bulgaricus, B. infantis, B. breve, B. longum, Strep. salivarius subsp. thermophilus*) did not increase CLA production compared with individual strains. Probiotic was prepared as lyophilized form and mice were fed 30 μL of probiotic (0.03 g VSL3 in 10 ml water) for 3 days. Feces were collected at day 0 and 3, and were incubated with LA. Results shown that murine feces with LA after administering VSL3 yielded 100-fold more CLA than feces collected prior to VSL3 feeding. This work also reported that the incorporation of probiotic into conditioned medium produced a reduction of viability and induced apoptosis of HT- 29 and Caco-2 cells.

Another important work using bacteria able to produce CLA as probiotics for animal models was showed by Wall et al. [99]. The administration of *B. breve* NCIMB 702258 to mice and pigs, combined with dietary linoleic acid, showed changes on fatty acid composition of liver and adipose tissues. Higher levels of c9, t11 in liver tissues were determined for both animals receiving *B. breve*, and were also associated with reductions of the pro-inflammatory cytokines level.

Recently, an study to investigate if recombinant lactobacillus expressing LAI (from *P. acnes*, producing t10, c12 isomer) administered to mice produce changes on fatty acids profile was carried out [103]. Authors found that after a daily administration of *L. paracasei* NFBC 338 (10^9 UFC/mouse) during 8 weeks, and 4-fold increase of t10, c12 content in adipose tissue was produced comparing with control mice group. Moreover, in liver a 2.5-fold higher level of the same isomer was reported in treatment group. To the best of our knowledge, this is the only work about using genetically modified strains with the ability to produce t10, c12-CLA, administered as probiotic in mice.

There is few data respect to probiotic administration and *in vivo* CLA production in humans. Lee and Lee [104] reported the effect of PL60 consumption by humans. Here, volunteers consumed PL60 as freeze-dried at a dose of 1g/day (10^{12} CFU/g) during 3 weeks. After one week of uptake, PL60 was recovered from feces, as was previously determined in mice. Respect to CLA content in tissues, both c9,t11 and t10,c12 isomers were higher respect to day 0 of treatment (baseline). Leptin levels were also lower at the end of the study.

11. Conclusion

Although one of the most effective method to increase CLA uptake by humans consist of increase CLA levels in milk and dairy products by modification of animal diet or the inclusion of bacteria able to form it during manufacture process, in the last years the *in vivo* CLA production appears as an alternative way to make it.

Since CLA was recognized as an important biolipid with health benefic properties, there was an increasing interest on this field. However, there is another conjugated fatty acid recently included in studies: conjugated linolenic acid (CLNA). This fatty acid is also generating great attention since anti-atherogenic properties were attributed to them. Some bacteria could produce CLNA using as substrate linolenic acid. CLNA isomers in foods and its biological effects in animal models were lesser understanding than CLA, being the mechanism of it production by bacteria recently investigated. So, in the literature there is not yet recommended dose for this compound for humans.

Development of functional foods enriched on conjugated fatty acids is being extensively studied by researchers, since benefits of health properties were related to humans. The physiological role of conjugated fatty acids like CLA or CLNA is well documented on the literature.

The ability of some species of lactic acid bacteria, propionibacteria and bifidobacteria to *in vitro* conjugate the LA and/or LNA has been established over the years. Manufacture of functional food enriched in conjugated fatty acids by using it as starter or adjunct culture is a promising topic to be developed.

The variation on CLA and CLNA production among bacteria depends on many factors such as intrinsic characteristic of each particular strain, conditions of experimental design and methodology for isomer determination, among others. For this reason, studies must be carefully done before the inclusion of strain during food manufacture.

Few authors have demonstrated the action of bacteria intake on *in vivo* CLA production using experimental animal models and human, but results are promising in this field.

Instead of some technological developments have been performed, many points remain undiscovered at this issue. Some aspects of technological processed foods must be considered, such as CLA-enriched products are also high in fat, being difficult to recommend a single daily dose of CLA after food intake. As we earlier mentioned, not all isomers are incorporated at the same way into tissues fat.

Respect to microorganisms able to form conjugated fatty acids, it is not unreasonable to assume a production of these bioactive compounds at intestinal level, since fatty acid substrate are present in human diet.

Further studies are necessary to understand the kinetic mechanism of it particular production. Questions such as if LAI enzyme is the responsible for both LA and LNA conversion need to be clarified so as the factors determining the isomer production by each strain.

Indeed, taking in account the lack of information respect to some epidemiological and technological aspects of conjugated fatty acids, further studies are required to fully understand the utility of CLA and CLNA in disease prevention. The development of products as probiotic or functional foods to ensure the bioavailability of both compounds for humans is a valuable strategy to be considered.

List of abbreviations

But.: *Butyrivibrio*
B.: *Bifidobacterium*
C.: *Clostridium*
c: cis
CALA: conjugated of alpha linolenic acid
CFU: colony forming unit
CGLA: conjugated of gamma linolenic acid
CLA: Conjugated linoleic acid
CLNA: Conjugated linolenic acid
E.: *Enterococcus*
L.: *Lactobacillus*
LA: linoleic acid (c9,c12-C18:2)
LAB: lactic acid bacteria
Lac.: *Lactococcus*
LAI: linoleate isomerase
LNA: linolenic acid (c9,c12,c15-C18:3)
P.: *Propionibacteria*
Ped.: *Pediococcus*
Strep.: *Streptococcus*
t: trans
TVA: trans vaccenic acid (t11-C18:1)

Author details

Carina Paola Van Nieuwenhove
CERELA-CONICET, S. M. de Tucumán, Argentina
Facultad de Ciencias Naturales e IML- Universidad Nacional de Tucumán,
S. M. de Tucumán, Argentina

Victoria Terán
CERELA-CONICET, S. M. de Tucumán, Argentina

Silvia Nelina González
CERELA-CONICET, S. M. de Tucumán, Argentina
Facultad de Bioquímica, Química y Farmacia- Universidad Nacional de Tucumán,
S. M. de Tucumán, Argentina

Acknowledgments

This work was supported by grants of Consejo Nacional de Investigaciones Científicas y Técnicas and Consejo de Investigaciones de la Universidad Nacional de Tucumán (PIP 0343 and CIUNT 26/D-429).

12. References

[1] Parodi PW. Conjugated linolenic acid in food. Advances in conjugated linolenic acid research. AOCS Press, Champaign, IL. 2003;2:101-21.

[2] Yücel O. Determination of conjugated linoleic acid content of selected oil seeds grown in Turkey. Journal of the American Oil Chemists Society. 2005;82(12):893-7.

[3] Suzuki R, Noguchi R, Ota T, Abe M, Miyashita K, Kawada T. Cytotoxic effect of conjugated trienoic fatty acids on mouse tumor and human monocytic leukemia cells. Lipids. 2001 May;36(5):477-82.

[4] Bhattacharya A, Banu J, Rahman M, Causey J, Fernandes G. Biological effects of conjugated linoleic acids in health and disease. The Journal of Nutritional Biochemistry. 2006 Dec;17(12):789-810.

[5] Yurawecz MP, Roach JA, Sehat N, Mossoba MM, Kramer JK, Fritsche J, et al. A new conjugated linoleic acid isomer, 7 trans, 9 cis-octadecadienoic acid, in cow milk, cheese, beef and human milk and adipose tissue. Lipids. 1998 Aug;33(8):803-9.

[6] Dhiman TR, Anand GR, Satter LD, Pariza MW. Conjugated linoleic acid content of milk from cows fed different diets. Journal of Dairy Science. 1999 Oct;82(10):2146-56.

[7] Sarrazin P, Mustafa AF, Chouinard PY, Raghavan G, Sotocinal S. Performance of dairy cows fed roasted sunflower seed. Journal of the Science of Food and Agriculture. 2004(84):1179-85.

[8] Jahreis G, Fristche J, Möckel P, Schöne F, Möller U, Steinhart H. The potential anticarcinogenic conjugated linoleic acid, cis-9,trans-11 C18:2, in milk of different species: Cow, goat, ewe, spw, mare, woman. Nutrition Research. October 1999;19(10):1541-9.

[9] Ip C, Chin SF, Scimeca JA, Pariza MW. Mammary cancer prevention by conjugated dienoic derivative of linoleic acid. Cancer Research. 1991 Nov 15;51(22):6118-24.

[10] Houseknecht KL, Vanden Heuvel JP, Moya-Camarena SY, Portocarrero CP, Peck LW, Nickel KP, et al. Dietary conjugated linoleic acid normalizes impaired glucose tolerance in the Zucker diabetic fatty fa/fa rat. Biochemical and Biophysical Research Communications. 1998 Mar 27;244(3):678-82.

[11] Hayek MG, Han SN, Wu D, Watkins BA, Meydani M, Dorsey JL, et al. Dietary conjugated linoleic acid influences the immune response of young and old C57BL/6NCrlBR mice. Journal of Nutrition. 1999 Jan;129(1):32-8.

[12] Chouinard PY, Corneau L, Barbano DM, Metzger LE, Bauman DE. Conjugated linoleic acids alter milk fatty acid composition and inhibit milk fat secretion in dairy cows. Journal of Nutrition. 1999 Aug;129(8):1579-84.

[13] Kelly GS. Conjugated linoleic acid: a review. Alternative Medicine Reviews. 2001 Aug;6(4):367-82.

[14] Ip MM, Masso-Welch PA, Shoemaker SF, Shea-Eaton WK, Ip C. Conjugated linoleic acid inhibits proliferation and induces apoptosis of normal rat mammary epithelial cells in primary culture. Experimental Cell Research. 1999 Jul 10;250(1):22-34.

[15] MacDonald HB. Conjugated linoleic acid and disease prevention: a review of current knowledge. Journal of American College of Nutrition. 2000 Apr;19 (2 Suppl):111S-8S.

[16] Igarashi M, Miyazawa T. Newly recognized cytotoxic effect of conjugated trienoic fatty acids on cultured human tumor cells. Cancer Letters. 2000 Feb 1;148(2):173-9.

[17] Harfoot CG, Hazlewood GP. Lipid metabolism in the rumen. In the rumen microbial ecosystem Elsevier Science Publishers, London, UK. 1988:285-322.

[18] Kepler CR, Hirons KP, McNeill JJ, Tove SB. Intermediates and products of the biohydrogenation of linoleic acid by Butyrinvibrio fibrisolvens. The Journal of Biological Chemistry. 1966 Mar 25;241(6):1350-4.

[19] Kim YJ, Liu RH, Bond DR, Russell JB. Effect of linoleic acid concentration on conjugated linoleic acid production by Butyrivibrio fibrisolvens A38. Applied and Environmental Microbiology. 2000 Dec;66(12):5226-30.

[20] Kishino S, Ogawa J, Ando A, Omura Y, Shimizu S. Ricinoleic acid and castor oil as substrates for conjugated linoleic acid production by washed cells of Lactobacillus plantarum. Bioscience, Biotechnology and Biochemistry. 2002 Oct;66(10):2283-6.

[21] Kishino S, Ogawa J, Ando A, Shimizu S. Conjugated α-linolenic acidproduction from α-linolenic acid by Lactbacillus plantarum AKU1009a. European Journal of Lipid Science and Technology. 2003(105):572–7.

[22] Akraim F, Nicot MC, Juaneda P, Enjalbert F. Conjugated linolenic acid (CLnA), conjugated linoleic acid (CLA) and other biohydrogenation intermediates in plasma and milk fat of cows fed raw or extruded linseed. Animal. 2007 Jul;1(6):835-43.

[23] Loor JJ, Lin X, Herbein JH. Dietary trans-vaccenic acid (trans11-18:1) increases concentration of cis9,transll-conjugated linoleic acid (rumenic acid) in tissues of lactating mice and suckling pups. Reproduction Nutrition Development. 2002 Mar-Apr;42(2):85-99.

[24] Kemp P, Lander DJ. Hydrogenation in vitro of alpha linolenic acid to stearic acid by mixed cultures of pure strains of rumen bacteria. Journal of General Microbiology. 1984(130):527-33.

[25] Griinari JM, Corl BA, Lacy SH, Chouinard PY, Nurmela KV, Bauman DE. Conjugated linoleic acid is synthesized endogenously in lactating dairy cows by Delta(9)-desaturase. Journal of Nutrition. 2000 Sep;130(9):2285-91.

[26] Lock AL, Garnsworthy PC. Independent effects of dietary linoleic and linolenic fatty acids on the conjugated linoleic acid content of cows milk. Animal Science. 2002(74):163-76.

[27] Dhiman TR, Nam SH, Ure AL. Factors affecting conjugated linoleic acid content in milk and meat. Critical Reviews in Food Science and Nutrition. 2005;45(6):463-82.

[28] Jiang J, Bjorck L, Fondén R. Conjugated linoleic acid in Swedish dairy products with special reference to the manufacture of hard cheeses. International Dairy Journal. 1997;(241):863-7.

[29] Schmid A, Collomb M, Sieber R, Bee G. Conjugated linoleic acid in meat and meat products: A review. Meat Science. 2006 May;73(1):29-41.

[30] Chin SF, Liu W, Storkson JM, Ha YL, Pariza MW. Dietary sources of conjugated dienoic isomers of linoleic acid, a newly recognized class of anticarcinogens. Journal of Food Composition and Analysis. 1992;5(3):185-97.

[31] Parodi PW. Conjugated octadecadienoic acids of milk fat. Journal of Dairy Science. 1977(60):1550-3.

[32] Luna P, Fontecha J, Juarez M, Angel de la Fuente M. Changes in the milk and cheese fat composition of ewes fed commercial supplements containing linseed with special reference to the CLA content and isomer composition. Lipids. 2005 May;40(5):445-54.

[33] Khanal RC, Olson KC. Factors affecting conjugated linoleic acid(CLA) content in milk, meat and egg: A review. Pakistan Journal of Nutrition. 2004(3):82-98.

[34] Destaillats F, Trottier JP, Galvez JM, Angers P. Analysis of alpha-linolenic acid biohydrogenation intermediates in milk fat with emphasis on conjugated linolenic acids. Journal of Dairy Science. 2005 Sep;88(9):3231-9.

[35] Corl BA, Barbano DM, Bauman DE, Ip C. cis-9, trans-11 CLA derived endogenously from trans-11 18:1 reduces cancer risk in rats. Journal of Nutrition. 2003 Sep;133(9):2893-900.

[36] Adlof RO, Duval S, Emken EA. Biosynthesis of conjugated linoleic acid in humans. Lipids. 2000 Feb;35(2):131-5.

[37] Ross GR, Van Nieuwenhove CP, Gonzalez SN. Fatty Acid Profile of Pig Meat after Probiotic Administration. Journal of Agriculture and Food Chemistry. 2012 Apr 16.

[38] Fritsche J, Steinhart H. Amounts of conjugated linoleic acid (CLA) in German foods and evaluation of daily intake. European Food Research and Technology. 1998;206(2):77-82.

[39] Schoos V, Medina M, Saad S, Van Nieuwenhove CP. Chemical and microbiological characteristics of Llama's (Lama glama) milk from Argentina. Milchwissenschaft. 2008;63(4):398-401.

[40] Plourde M, Destaillats F, Chouinard PY, Angers P. Conjugated alpha-linolenic acid isomers in bovine milk and muscle. Journal of Dairy Science. 2007 Nov;90(11):5269-75.

[41] Kohno H, Suzuki R, Noguchi R, Hosokawa M, Miyashita K, Tanaka T. Dietary conjugated linolenic acid inhibits azoxymethane-induced colonic aberrant crypt foci in rats. Japanese Journal of Cancer Research. 2002 Feb;93(2):133-42.

[42] Lee KN, Kritchevsky D, Pariza MW. Conjugated linoleic acid and atherosclerosis in rabbits. Atherosclerosis. 1994 Jul;108(1):19-25.

[43] Ip C, Carter CA, Ip MM. Requirements of essencial fatty acid for mammary tumorigenesis in the rat. Cancer Research. 1985(45):1997-2001.

[44] Park HS, Ryu JH, Ha YL, Park JH. Dietary conjugated linoleic acid (CLA) induces apoptosis of colonic mucosa in 1,2-dimethylhydrazine-treated rats: a possible mechanism of the anticarcinogenic effect by CLA. British of Journal Nutrition. 2001 Nov;86(5):549-55.

[45] Van Wijlen RPJ, Colombani PC. Grass-based ruminant production methods and human bioconversion of vaccenic acid with estimations of maximal dietary intake of conjugated linoleic acids. International Dairy Journal. 2010(20):433-48.

[46] Whigham LD, Watras AC, Schoeller DA. Efficacy of conjugated linoleic acid for reducing fat mass: a meta-analysis in humans. Am J Clin Nutr. 2007 May;85(5):1203-11.

[47] Ha YL, Grimm NK, Pariza MW. Newly recognized anticarcinogenic fatty acids: Identification and quantification in natural and processed cheeses. Journal of Agricultural and Food Chemistry. 1989;37(1):75-81.

[48] Mullen A, Moloney F, Nugent AP, Doyle L, Cashman KD, Roche HM. Conjugated linoleic acid supplementation reduces peripheral blood mononuclear cell interleukin-2 production in healthy middle-aged males. The Journal of Nutritional Biochemistry. 2007 Oct;18(10):658-66.

[49] Moloney F, Yeow TP, Mullen A, Nolan JJ, Roche HM. Conjugated linoleic acid supplementation, insulin sensitivity, and lipoprotein metabolism in patients with type 2 diabetes mellitus. The American Journal of Clinical Nutrition. 2004 Oct;80(4):887-95.

[50] Smedman A, Vessby B. Conjugated linoleic acid supplementation in humans--metabolic effects. Lipids. 2001 Aug;36(8):773-81.

[51] Wang Y, Jones PJ. Dietary conjugated linoleic acid and body composition. Am J Clin Nutr. 2004 Jun;79(6 Suppl):1153S-8S.

[52] Kim YJ, Liu RH. Increase of conjugated linoleic acid content in milk by fermentation with lactic acid bacteria. Journal of Food Science. 2002;67(5):1731-7.

[53] Van Nieuwenhove CP, Oliszewski R, Gonzalez SN, Perez Chaia AB. Conjugated linoleic acid conversion by dairy bacteria cultured in MRS broth and buffalo milk. Lett Appl Microbiol. 2007 May;44(5):467-74.

[54] Chung SH, Kim IH, Park HG, Kang HS, Yoon CS, Jeong HY, et al. Synthesis of conjugated linoleic acid by human-derived Bifidobacterium breve LMC 017: utilization as a functional starter culture for milk fermentation. Journal of Agriculture and Food Chemistry. 2008 May 14;56(9):3311-6.

[55] Gorissen L, Raes K, Weckx S, Dannenberger D, Leroy F, De Vuyst L, et al. Production of conjugated linoleic acid and conjugated linolenic acid isomers by Bifidobacterium species. Applied Microbiology and Biotechnology. 2010 Aug;87(6):2257-66.

[56] Gorissen L, Leroy F, Raes K, De Vuyst L, De Smet S. Conjugated linoleic acid and conjugated linolenic acid production by bifidobacteria. Communications in Agriculture and Applied Biological Sciences. 2011;76(1):7-10.

[57] Coakley M, Ross RP, Nordgren M, Fitzgerald G, Devery R, Stanton C. Conjugated linoleic acid biosynthesis by human-derived Bifidobacterium species. Journal of Applied Microbiology. 2003;94(1):138-45.

[58] Jiang J, Bjorck L, Fonden R. Production of conjugated linoleic acid by dairy starter cultures. Journal of Applied Microbiology. 1998 Jul;85(1):95-102.

[59] Ogawa J, Matsumura K, Kishino S, Omura Y, Shimizu S. Conjugated linoleic acid accumulation via 10-hydroxy-12-octadecaenoic acid during microaerobic transformation of linoleic acid by Lactobacillus acidophilus. Applied and Environmental Microbiology. 2001 Mar;67(3):1246-52.

[60] Lin TY, Hung TH, Cheng TSJ. Conjugated linoleic acid production by immobilized cells of Lactobacillus acidophilus. Food Chemistry. 2005;(92):23-8.

[61] Kishino S, Ogawa J, Omura Y, Matsumura K, Shimizu S. Conjugated linoleic acid production from linoleic acid by lactic acid bacteria. JAOCS, Journal of the American Oil Chemists' Society. 2002;79(2):159-63.

[62] Lin TY, Lin CW, Wang YJ. Production of conjugated linoleic acid by enzyme extract of Lactobacillus acidophilus CCRC 14079. Food Chemistry. 2003;83:27-31.

[63] Bauman DE, Baumgard LH, Corl BA, Griinari JM. Biosynthesis of conjugated linoleic acid in ruminants. Proceedings of the American Scociety of Animal Science. 1999.

[64] McIntosh FM, Shingfield KJ, Devillard E, Russell WR, Wallace RJ. Mechanism of conjugated linoleic acid and vaccenic acid formation in human faecal suspensions and pure cultures of intestinal bacteria. Microbiology. 2009;155(1):285-94.

[65] Xu S, Boylston T, Glatz B. Effect of lipid source on probiotic bacteria and conjugated linoleic acid formation in milk model systems. Journal of the American Oil Chemists Society. 2004(81):589-95.

[66] Lee HY, Park JH, Seok SH, Baek MW, Kim DJ, Lee KE, et al. Human originated bacteria, Lactobacillus rhamnosus PL60, produce conjugated linoleic acid and show anti-obesity effects in diet-induced obese mice. Biochimica et Biophysica Acta. 2006 Jul;1761(7):736-44.

[67] Xu H, Lee HY, Hwang B, Nam JH, Kang HY, Ahn J. Kinetics of microbial hydrogenation of free linoleic acid to conjugated linoleic acids. J Appl Microbiol. 2008 Dec;105(6):2239-47.

[68] Rodríguez-Alcalá LM, Braga T, Xavier Malcata F, Gomes A, Fontecha J. Quantitative and qualitative determination of CLA produced by Bifidobacterium and lactic acid bacteria by combining spectrophotometric and Ag +-HPLC techniques. Food Chemistry. 2011;125(4):1373-8.

[69] Gorissen L, Weckx S, Vlaeminck B, Raes K, De Vuyst L, De Smet S, et al. Linoleate isomerase activity occurs in lactic acid bacteria strains and is affected by pH and temperature. Journal of Applied Microbiology. 2011 Sep;111(3):593-606.

[70] Rainio A, Vahvaselka M, Laakso S. Cell-adhered conjugated linoleic acid regulates isomerization of linoleic acid by resting cells of Propionibacterium freudenreichii. Applied Microbiology and Biotechnology. 2002 Dec;60(4):481-4.

[71] Rainio A, Vahvaselkä M, Suomalainen T, Laakso S. Production of conjugated linoleic acid by Propionibacterium freudenreichii ssp. shermanii. Lait. 2002;82(1):91-101.

[72] Lin TY, Lin CW, Wang YJ. Linoleic Acid Isomerase Activity in Enzyme Extracts from Lactobacillus acidophilus and Propionibacterium freudenreichii subsp. shermanii. Journal of Food Science. 2002;(67):1502-5.

[73] Wallace RJ, Chaudhary LC, McKain N, McEwen BS, Richardson AJ, Vercoe PE, et al. Clostridium proteoclasticum: A ruminal bacterium taht forms stearic acid from linoleic acid. FEMS Microbiology Letters. 2006;265:195-201.

[74] Hennessy AA, Barrett E, Paul Ross R, Fitzgerald GF, Devery R, Stanton C. The production of conjugated alpha-linolenic, gamma-linolenic and stearidonic acids by strains of bifidobacteria and propionibacteria. Lipids. 2012 Mar;47(3):313-27.

[75] Favier CF, Vaughan EE, De Vos WM, Akkermans AD. Molecular monitoring of succession of bacterial communities in human neonates. Appl Environ Microbiol. 2002 Jan;68(1):219-26.

[76] Picard C, Fioramonti J, Francois A, Robinson T, Neant F, Matuchansky C. Review article: bifidobacteria as probiotic agents -- physiological effects and clinical benefits. Alimentary Pharmacology and Therapeutics. 2005 Sep 15;22(6):495-512.

[77] Saarela M, Virkajärvi I, Alakomi H-L, Sigvart-Mattila P, Mättö J. Stability and functionality of freeze-dried probiotic Bifidobacterium cells during storage in juice and milk. International Dairy Journal. [doi: 10.1016/j.idairyj.2005.12.007. 2006;16(12):1477-82.

[78] Vinderola G, de los Reyes-Gavilán C, Reinheimer J. Probiotics and prebiotics in fermented dairy products. In Contemporary Food Engineering. 2009:601-34

[79] Vinderola G, Binetti A, Burns P, Reinheimer J. Cell viability and functionality of probiotic bacteria in dairy products. Frontiers in Microbiology. 2011;2:70.

[80] Oh DK, Hong GH, Lee Y, Min S, Sin HS, Cho SK. Production of conjugated linoleic acid by isolated Bifidobacterium strains. World J Microbiol Biotechnol. 2003(19):907-12.

[81] Park HG, Cho SD, Kim JH, Lee H, Chung SH, Kim SB, et al. Characterization of conjugated linoleic acid production by Bifidobacterium breve LMC 520. Journal of Agriculture and Food Chemistry. 2009 Aug 26;57(16):7571-5.

[82] Choi NJ, Park HG, Kim YJ, Kim IH, Kang HS, Yoon CS, et al. Utilization of monolinolein as a substrate for conjugated linoleic acid production by Bifidobacterium breve LMC 520 of human neonatal origin. Journal of Agriculture and Food Chemistry. 2008 Nov 26;56(22):10908-12.

[83] Van Nieuwenhove CP, Gauffin Cano P, Pérez-Chaia AB, González SN. Effect of functional buffalo cheese on fatty acid profile and oxidative status of liver and intestine of mice. Journal of Medicinal Food. 2011 Apr;14(4):420-7.

[84] Puniya AK, Chaitanya S, Tyagi AK, De S, Singh K. Conjugated linoleic acid producing potential of lactobacilli isolated from the rumen of cattle. Journal of Industrial Microbiology and Biotechnology. 2008 Nov;35(11):1223-8.

[85] Park SJ, Park KA, Park CW, Park WS, Kim JO, Ha YL. Purification and aminoacids sequence of the linoleate isomerase from Butyrivbrio fibrisolvens A-38 Journal of Food Science and Nutrition. 1996;1:244-51.

[86] Irmak S, Dunford NT, Gilliland SE, Banskalieva V, Eisenmenger M. Biocatalysis of linoleic acid to conjugated linoleic acid. Lipids. 2006 Aug;41(8):771-6.

[87] Deng MD, Grund AD, Schneider KJ, Langley KM, Wassink SL, Peng SS, et al. Linoleic acid isomerase from Propionibacterium acnes: purification, characterization, molecular cloning, and heterologous expression. Applied Biochemistry and Biotechnology. 2007 Dec;143(3):199-211.

[88] Rosson RA, Deng MD, Grund AD, Peng SS. PCT WO0100846. 2001.

[89] Ross GR, Gauffin Cano P, Gusils León CH, Medina RB, González SN, Van Nieuwenhove CP. Lactic acid bacteria activities to promote health benefits. Multidisciplinary approaches on food science and nutrition for the 21st century. Research signpost ed. 2011:155-74.

[90] Cho HJ, Kim WK, Jung JI, Kim EJ, Lim SS, Kwon DY, et al. Trans-10,cis-12, not cis-9,trans-11, conjugated linoleic acid decreases ErbB3 expression in HT-29 human colon cancer cells. World Journal of Gastroenterology. 2005 Sep 7;11(33):5142-50.

[91] Park Y, Albright KJ, Liu W, Storkson JM, Cook ME, Pariza MW. Effect of conjugated linoleic acid on body composition in mice. Lipids. 1997 Aug;32(8):853-8.

[92] Yamasaki M, Ikeda A, Oji M, Tanaka Y, Hirao A, Kasai M, et al. Modulation of body fat and serum leptin levels by dietary conjugated linoleic acid in Sprague-Dawley rats fed various fat-level diets. Nutrition. 2003 Jan;19(1):30-5.

[93] Mougios V, Matsakas A, Petridou A, Ring S, Sagredos A, Melissopoulou A, et al. Effect of supplementation with conjugated linoleic acid on human serum lipids and body fat. The Journal of Nutritional Biochemistry. 2001 Oct;12(10):585-94.

[94] Thom E, Wadstein J, Gudmundsen O. Conjugated linoleic acid reduces body fat in healthy exercising humans. Journal of International Medical Research. 2001 Sep-Oct;29(5):392-6.

[95] Lin TY, Lin CW, Lee CH. Conjugated Linoleic Acid Concentration as Affected by Lactic Cultures and Added Linoleic Acid. Food Chemistry. 1999;(67):1-5.

[96] Shantha NC, Ram LN, O Leary J, Hicks CL, Decker EA. Conjugated linoleic acid concentrations in dairy products as affected by processing and storage. Journal of Food Science. 1995(60):695-7.

[97] Colakoglu H, Gursoy O. Effect of lactic adjunct cultures on conjugated linoleic acid (CLA) concentration of yogurt drink. Journal of Food, Agriculture and Environment. 2011;9(1):60-4.

[98] Lee K, Paek K, Lee HY, Park JH, Lee Y. Antiobesity effect of trans-10,cis-12-conjugated linoleic acid-producing Lactobacillus plantarum PL62 on diet-induced obese mice. Journal of Applied Microbiology. 2007 Oct;103(4):1140-6.

[99] Wall R, Ross RP, Shanahan F, O'Mahony L, O'Mahony C, Coakley M, et al. Metabolic activity of the enteric microbiota influences the fatty acid composition of murine and porcine liver and adipose tissues. American Journal of Clinical Nutrition. 2009 May;89(5):1393-401.

[100] Edionwe AO, Kies C. Comparison of palm and mixtures of refined palm and soybean oils on serum lipids and fecal fat and fatty acid excretions of adult humans. Plant Foods for Human Nutrition. 2001;56(2):157-65.

[101] Fukuda S, Suzuki Y, Murai M, Asanuma N, Hino T. Isolation of a novel strain of Butyrivibrio fibrisolvens that isomerizes linoleic acid to conjugated linoleic acid without hydrogenation, and its utilization as a probiotic for animals. Journal of Applied Microbiology. 2006 Apr;100(4):787-94.

[102] Ewaschuk JB, Walker JW, Diaz H, Madsen KL. Bioproduction of conjugated linoleic acid by probiotic bacteria occurs in vitro and in vivo in mice. Journal of Nutrition. 2006 Jun;136(6):1483-7.

[103] Rosberg-Cody E, Stanton C, O'Mahony L, Wall R, Shanahan F, Quigley EM, et al. Recombinant lactobacilli expressing linoleic acid isomerase can modulate the fatty acid composition of host adipose tissue in mice. Microbiology. 2011 Feb;157(Pt 2):609-15.

[104] Lee K, Lee Y. Production of c9, t11- and t10, c12- conjugated linoleic acids in humans by Lactobacillus rhamnosus PL60. Journal of Microbiology and Biotechnology. 2009 Oct;19(12):1617-9.

[105] Fritsche J, Steinhart H. Analysis, occurence and physiological properties of trans fatty acids(TFA) with particular emphasis on conjugated linoleic acid isomers (CLA). A review. Fet/Lipid. 1998(100):190-210.

[106] Raes K, Balcaen A, Claeys E, De Smet S, Demeyer D. Effect of duration of feeding diets rich in n-3 PUFA to Belgian Blue double-muscled young bulls, on the incorporation of long-chain n-3 and n-6 PUFA in the phospholipids and triglycerides of the longissimus thoracis. Proceedings of the 48th ICoMST. Rome, Italy. 2002;2:724-5.

[107] Gultemiriam L, Van Nieuwenhove CP, Pérez Chaia A, Apella MC. Physical and chemical characterization of eggs from Araucana hens of free range fed in Argentina. Journal of the Argentine Chemical Society. 2009;97(2):19-30.

[108] Park Y, Storkson JM, Albright KJ, Liu W, Pariza MW. Evidence that the trans-10,cis-12 isomer of conjugated linoleic acid induces body composition changes in mice. Lipids. 1999 Mar;34(3):235-41.

[109] Ogawa J, Kishino S, Ando A, Sugimoto S, Mihara K, Shimizu S. Production of conjugated fatty acids by lactic acid bacteria. Journal of Bioscience and Bioengineering. 2005 Oct;100(4):355-64.

[110] Lee SO, Kim CS, Cho SK, Choi HJ, Ji GE, Oh DK. Bioconversion of linoleic acid into conjugated linoleic acid during fermentation and by washed cells of Lactobacillus reuteri. Biotechnology Letters. 2003 Jun;25(12):935-8.

Chapter 5

Probiotics in Dairy Fermented Products

Emiliane Andrade Araújo, Ana Clarissa dos Santos Pires,
Maximiliano Soares Pinto, Gwénaël Jan and Antônio Fernandes de Carvalho

Additional information is available at the end of the chapter

1. Introduction

Since ancient times, food has been considered essential and indispensable to human life. Numerous studies clearly show that an individual's quality of life is linked to daily diet and lifestyle (Moura, 2005).

Interest in the role of probiotics for human health began as early as 1908 when Metchnikoff associated the intake of fermented milk with prolonged life (Lourens-Hattingh and Vilijoen, 2001b). However, the relationship between intestinal microbiota and good health and nutrition has only recently been investigated. Therefore, it was not until the 1960's that health benefit claims began appearing on foods labels.

In recent years, there has been an increasing interest in probiotic foods, which has stimulated innovation and fueled the development of new products around the world. Probiotic bacteria have increasingly been incorporated into foods in order to improve gut health by maintaining the microbial gastrointestinal balance. The most popular probiotic foods are produced in the dairy industry because fermented dairy products have been shown to be the most efficient delivery vehicle for live probiotics to date.

In this chapter, we will discuss the application of probiotic microorganisms in fermented dairy products, particularly cheeses. In addition, we will also discuss the benefits of probiotic fermented foods on human health.

2. Probiotic concepts

The word "probiotic" comes from Greek and means "for life" (Fuller, 1989). Over the years, the term "probiotic" has been given several definitions. "Probiotic" is used to refer to cultures of live microorganisms which, when administered to humans or animals, improve properties of indigenous microbiota (Margoles and Garcia, 2003). In the food industry, the term is described as "live microbial food ingredients that are beneficial to health" (Clancy, 2003).

It is important to mention that for a microorganism to be considered probiotic, (Figure 1), it must survive passage through the stomach and maintain its viability and metabolic activity in the intestine (Hyun and Shin, 1998). Native inhabitants of the human or animal gastrointestinal tract, such as lactobacilli and bifidobacteria, are considered to be probiotic, but often display low stress tolerance, which reduces their viability in probiotic applications. Microorganisms traditionally grown in fermented foods, such as lactic acid bacteria, propionibacteria and yeasts, are also considered for these applications..

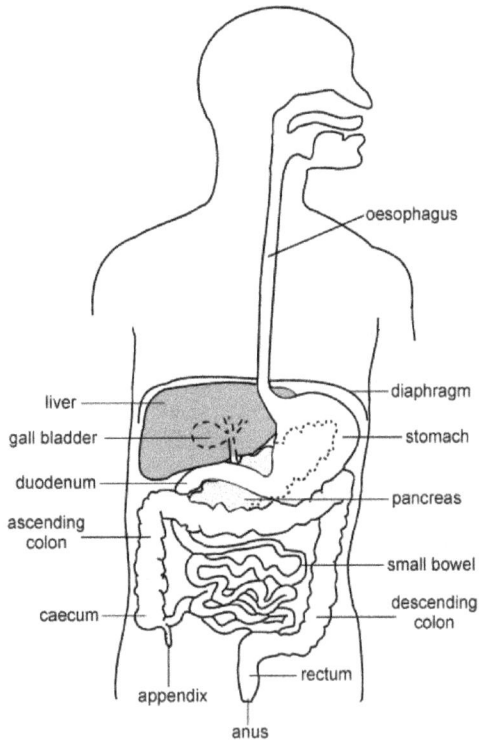

Figure 1. Schematic representation of gastrointestinal tract

It is essential that commercialized probiotic products which make health claims meet the minimum criterion of one million viable probiotic cells per milliliter of product at the expiration date. Accordingly, the minimum dosage of probiotic cells per day for any beneficial effect on the consumer is considered to be $10^8 - 10^9$ probiotic CFU ml^{-1} or CFU g^{-1}, which corresponds to an intake of 100 g product containing $10^6 - 10^7$ CFU ml^{-1} or CFU g^{-1} per day (Lorens-Hattingh and Viljoen, 2001a).

2.1. Selection of probiotic microorganisms

The human intestinal tract constitutes a complex ecosystem of microorganisms. The bacterial population in the large intestine is very high and can reach maximum counts of 10^{12} CFU g^{-1}. In the small intestine, the bacterial content is considerably lower at only 10^4–10^8 CFU g^{-1}. In the stomach only 10^1-10^2 CFU g^{-1} are found due to the low pH of the environment (Lorens-Hattingh and Viljoen, 2001b).

It is known that microbiota in the human intestine changes during human development. The intestine of newborn babies is fully sterile, however immediately after birth, colonization of many kinds of bacteria begins. On the first and second days after birth, coliforms, enterococci, clostridia and lactobacilli have been shown to be present present in infants' feces. Within three to four days, bifidobacteria begins colonization and becomes predominant around the fifth day. Simultaneously, coliform counts decrease. Breast-fed babies show 1 log-count more of bifidobacteria in feces than bottle-fed babies. Enterobacteriaceae, streptococci, and other putrefactive bacteria counts are higher in bottle-fed babies, suggesting that breast-fed babies are more resistant to gastrointestinal infections than the bottle-fed infants (Lorens-Hattingh and Viljoen, 2001b).

In addition to the microbiota changes that occur during human aging, the microbiota in the gastrointestinal system can also change because of the food and health conditions of an individual. For example, use of antibiotics can damage the equilibrium of intestinal microbiota, reducing counts of bifidobacteria and lactobacilli and increasing clostridia. The ensuing imbalance can cause diarrhea in elderly and immunocompromised people.

To help improve the balance of intestinal microbiota, probiotic microorganisms can be added to the human diet in order to stimulate the growth of preferred microorganisms, crowd out potentially harmful bacteria, and reinforce the body's natural defense mechanisms.

The selection of probiotic microorganisms is based on safety, functional and technological aspects, as reported by (Saarela et al., 2000). These are summarized in Figure 2.

Certain probiotic bacteria have been extensively studied and are already on the market, as shown in Table 1.

Before probiotic strains can be delivered to consumers, they must first be able to be manufactured under industrial conditions. They must then survive and retain their functionality during storage as frozen or freeze-dried cultures, as well as in the food products into which they are finally formulated. Moreover, they must be able to be incorporated into foods without producing off-flavors or textures (Saarela et al., 2000).

Functional food requirements must take into consideration the following aspects in relation to the probiotics: The preparation should remain viable for large-scale production; it should remain stable and viable during storage and use; it should be able to survive in the intestinal ecosystem (Prado et al., 2008).

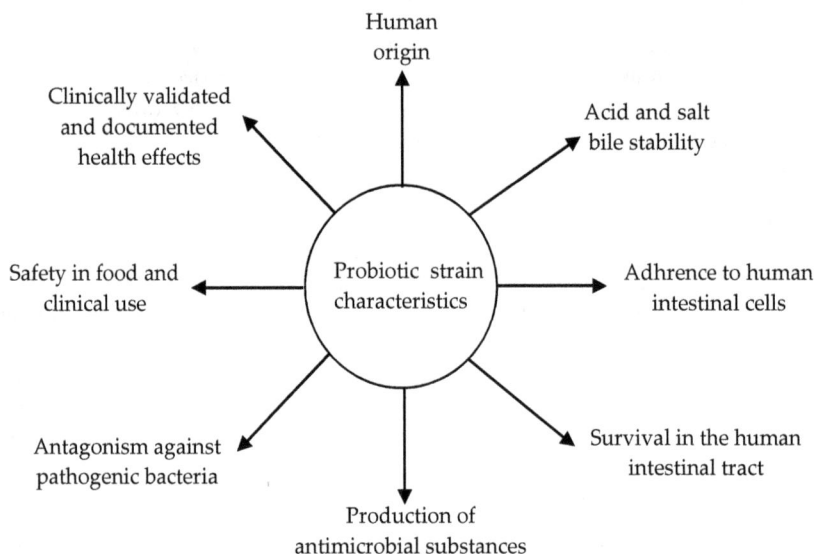

Figure 2. Theoretical basis for selection of probiotic microorganism selection (adapted from Saarela et al., 2000).

Strains	Origin
Lactobacillus casei Shirota	Yakult, Japan
Lactobacillus reuteri MM53	BioGaia, Sweden
Bifidobacterium lactis HN019	Danisco, France
Lactobacillus rhamnosus GG	Valio, Finland
Lactobacillus acidophilus NCFM	Nestle, Switzerland
Lactobacillus casei DN-173 010	Danone, France
Lactobacillus casei CRl-431	Chr. Hansen, USA
Bifidobacterium animalis BB12	Chr. Hansen, Denmark
Bifidobacterium animalis DN173010	Danone, France

Source: Prado et al., 2008

Table 1. Probiotic bacteria marketed worldwide

3. Beneficial effects of probiotics

The role of balanced nutrition for health maintenance has attracted the attention of the scientific community, which in turn has produced numerous studies in order to prove the performance of certain foods in reducing the risk of Some diseases. There has also been considerable growing interest in encouraging research into new natural components (Thamer and Penna, 2006).

In a healthy host, a balance exists among members of the gut microbiota, such that potential pathogenic and non-pathogenic organisms can be found in apparent harmony. In the case of bacterial infection, this balance can become disturbed, leading to often dramatic changes in the composition.

For most bacterial infections, nonspecific antibiotics are used, killing both non-pathogenic members of gut microbiota as well as pathogenic members. This can lead to a substantial delay in the restoration of healthy gut microbiota (Reid et al, 2011). The restoration of the gut microbiota balance is believed to be important because maintaining a healthy and balanced gut microbiota throughout life is thought to help preserve health and favor longevity.

The most comprehensive analysis of human microbiota to date examined 27 distinct sites in the body and revealed the presence of 22 bacterial phyla, with most sequences (92.3%) related to just four phyla: Actinobacteria (36.6%), Firmicutes (34.3%), Proteobacteria (11.9%) and Bacteroidetes (9.5%) (Costelo, 2008).

The metabolic capacity of gut bacteria is extremely diverse. This diversity is influenced by the large number of bacterial genera and species. Lactic acid species are present, as well as peptide-degrading bacteria, amino acids, and other methanogenic bacteria components of the gut microbiota which grow with the intermediate products of fermentation such as hydrogen, lactate, succinate and ethanol (Topping and Clifton, 2001).

In host's diet residue (matter undigested by its digestive system including resistant starch, fibers, proteins and peptides) substrates for primary fermentation can be found. Other important available substrates derive from mucin glycoproteins, exfoliated epithelial cells and pancreatic Secretions (MacFarlane et al., 1992).

Hydrolysis and carbohydrate metabolism in the large intestine is influenced by a variety of physical, chemical, biological and environmental parameters. Probably the nature and quantity of available substrate that has greater meaning, making the diet easier and the main mechanism by which to influence the profile of fermentation. Other factors affecting the colonization and growth of bacteria in the intestine are intestinal pH, which inhibits the production of metabolites (acids and peroxides) and specific inhibitory substances (bacteriocins), bile salts and molecules and cells which constitute the immune system (Rastall et al., 2000) .

Knowledge of intestinal gut microbiota and their interactions led to the development of food strategies aimed at the stimulation and maintenance of normal bacteria present in the gut (Gibson and Fuller, 2000).

According to Wohlgemuth (2010), strategies for studying mechanisms of probiotic action involve in-vitro models, or conventional or gnotobiotic animal models, plus development of a simplified human intestinal gut microbiota. Wohlgemuth's article proposes certain requirements that a model should ideally fulfill:

- Selected bacterial species should represent numerically dominant organisms of the human gut microbiota.
- By and large, the metabolic activity of this community should mimic that of normal human gut microbiota.
- The genome sequence of all members of the microbial community should be known.
- The members of this consortium should form a stable community in rodents. It should be possible to maintain this community under gnotobiotic conditions from generation to generation.
- The composition of the microbial community should be modifiable when required.

It is possible to increase the number of health-promoting microorganisms in gut microbiota through the introduction of probiotics in the diet. The probiotics will selectively modify the composition of the gut microbiota, providing the probiotic microorganisms demonstrate a competitive advantage over other bacteria in the ecosystem (Crittenden, 1999). Probiotic therapeutic properties are listed in Table 2.

Probiotic therapeutic properties
Influence on host gut microbiota and pathogenic bacteria
Improvement of specific enzymatic activities
Production of antibacterial substances
Competitive exclusion of pathogenic bacteria
Induction of defensin production
Improvement of intestinal barrier function
Modulation of host immune functions
Modulation of intestinal carcinogenesis
Modulation of cholesterol uptake

Wohlgemuth et al. (2010); Reddy and Rivenson (1993); Chen et al. (1984); Zhu et al., Cancer letters (2011); Jones et al., Br J Nutr (2012)

Table 2. Therapeutic Properties of Probiotics

There is a growing body of evidence that ingested beneficial bacteria, called probiotics, can beneficially modulate chronic intestinal inflammation, diarrhea, constipation, vaginitis, irritable bowel syndrome, atopic dermatis, food allergies and liver disease (Wallace et al., 2011, Nutrition reviews).

Probably the most promising area is the alleviation of symptoms linked to inflammatory bowel diseases (IBD), a growing health concern. As an example, the probiotic preparation VSL#3 induced remission in children (n=18) with mild to moderate ulcerative colitis (UC) (Huynh et al., 2009, Inflamm. Bowel Dis.) Accordingly, VSL#3 was tested in a 1-year, placebo-controlled, double-blind clinical study on UC children (n=29). Remission was achieved in 36.4% of children receiving IBD therapy and placebo, but in 92.8% of children receiving IBD therapy and VSL#3 (Milele et al., 2009, Am J Gastroeterol.) Similar promising results were obtained with the probiotic *Escherichia coli* Nissle 1917 strain (Kruis et al., 2004, Gut ; Do et al., Ann Pharmacother, 2010). However, a review of available data indicates that more clinical studies are needed to confirm the beneficial effects of these products in UC and in inactive pouch patients (Jonkers et al., 2012, Drugs). This review also states that there is no evidence to support the use of probiotics in Crohn's disease.

Other studies confirm these findings. Miele et al. (2009) reported that all of 29 patients studied responded to inflammatory bowel disease therapy. Remission was achieved in 92.8% of patients treated with mixed probiotics and 36.4% of patients treated with placebo. Overall, 21.4 % patients treated with a mix of probiotics and 73.3 % patients treated with placebo relapsed within 1 year of follow-up.

Urinary tract infections (UTIs) are a common and frequently recurrent infection among women. Depletion of vaginal lactobacilli is associated with UTI risk, which suggests that repletion of the bacteria may be beneficial. Young women with a history of recurrent UTI were randomized to receive either a probiotic or placebo daily. Recurrent UTI occurred in 15% of women receiving probiotic compared with 27% of women receiving placebo (Stapleton et al., 2011).

Probiotics have considerable potential for preventive and therapeutic applications in gastrointestinal disorders. However, it is important to note that many probiotic health claims have not yet been substantiated through experimental evidence. In addition, the efficacy demonstrated for a single given bacterial strain cannot be extrapolated to other probiotic organisms. Moreover, the mechanisms underlying probiotic action have not yet been fully elucidated. A better understanding of these mechanisms will be able to shed light on the disparate clinical data and provide new tools to help the prevention or treatment of health disorders (Wohlgemuth et al., 2010; Yan et al., 2011).

4. Application of probiotic bacteria in dairy foods

There is evidence that food matrices play an important role in the beneficial health effects of probiotics on the host (Espirito Santo et al., 2011).

Fermented foods, particularly dairy foods, are commonly used as probiotic carriers. Fermented beverages provide an important contribution to the human diet in many countries because fermentation is an inexpensive technology which preserves food, improves its nutritional value and enhances its sensory properties (Gadaga et al., 1999). However, the increasing demand for new probiotic products has encouraged the development of other matrices to deliver probiotics, such as ice cream, infant milk power and fruit juice.

Davidson et al. (2000) evaluated the viability of probiotic strains in low-fat ice cream. They used cultures containing *Streptococcus salivarius* ssp. *thermophilus* and *Lactobacillus delbrueckii* ssp. *Bulgaricus*, *Bifidobacterium longum* and *Lactobacillus acidophilus*, and verified that culture bacteria did not decrease in the yogurt during frozen storage. Also, the presence of probiotic bacteria did not alter the sensory characteristics of the ice cream. The ice cream matrix may offer a good vehicle for probiotic cultures due to its composition, which includes milk proteins, fat and lactose, as well as other compounds. Moreover, its frozen state contributes to its efficiency. However, a probiotic ice cream product should have relatively high pH values - 5.5 to 6.5, in order to favor an increased survival of lactic cultures during storage. The lower acidity also results in increased consumer acceptance, especially among consumers who prefer milder Products. (Cruz et al., 2009b).

Growth of a probiotic yeast, *Saccharomyces boulardii*, in association with the bio-yogurt microflora, which is done by incorporating the yeast into commercial bio-yogurt, has been suggested as a way to stimulate growth of probiotic organisms and to assure their survival during storage. Lorens-Hattingh and Viljoen (2001a) studied the ability of probiotic yeast to grow and survive in dairy products, namely bio-yogurt, UHT yogurt and UHT milk. *S. boulardii* was incorporated into these dairy products and stored at 4 ℃ over a 4-week period. It was observed that the probiotic yeast species, *S. boulardii*, had the ability to grow in bio-yogurt and reach maximum counts exceeding 10^7 CFU g^{-1}. The number of yeast populations was substantially higher in the fruit-based yogurt, mainly due to the presence of sucrose and fructose derived from the fruit. Despite the inability of *S. boulardii* to utilize lactose, the yeast species utilized available organic acids, galactose and glucose derived from bacterial metabolism of the milk sugar lactose present in the dairy products.

The viability of strains of *L. acidophilus* and *Bifidobacterium animalis* ssp. *lactis* in stirred yoghurts with fruit preparations of mango, mixed berry, passion fruit and strawberry was evaluated during shelf-life (Godward et al., 2000; Kailasapathy et al., 2008). The authors observed that regardless of concentrations, the addition of any of the fruit preparations had no effect on the counts of the two probiotics tested.

Fermented milks supplemented with lemon and orange fibers increased the counts of *L. acidophilus* and *L. casei* during cold storage compared to the control set. This was not the case for *B. bifidum*, possibly owing to the well-known sensitivity of bifidobacteria species to an acidic environment (Sendra et al., 2008).

5. Probiotic cheeses

Probiotic foods are currently primarily found in fermented milk drinks and yogurt, both of which have limited shelf life compared to cheeses. Incorporation of probiotic cultures in cheeses offers the potential not only to improve health but also product quality. It also opens the way to increasing the range of probiotic products on the market. The manufacture of most cheeses involves combining four ingredients: milk, rennet, microorganisms and salt These are processed using a number of common steps such as gel formation, whey expulsion, acid production and salt addition. Variations in ingredient blends and subsequent processing have led to the evolution of all cheese varieties.

Cheeses are dairy products which have a strong potential for delivering probiotic microorganisms into the human intestine, due to their specific chemical and physical characteristics. Cheeses have higher pH levels, lower titratable acidity, higher buffering capacity, more solid consistency, relatively higher fat content, higher nutrient availability and lower oxygen content than yogurts. These qualities protect probiotic bacteria during storage and passage through the gastrointestinal tract (Karimi et al., 2011; Ong et al., 2006).

As mentioned above, the physicochemical properties of food influence probiotic bacteria survival in the digestive tract, due to the low pH in the stomach, typically between 2.5 and 3.5 (Holzapfel et al., 1998), and the anti-microbial activity of pepsin that serve as effective barriers against the entrance of bacteria into the intestinal tract. Values of pH between 1 and 5 are commonly employed in determining the *in vitro* acid tolerance of *Lactobacillus* and *Bifidobacterium* spp. (Charteris et al., 1998). Bile salt concentrations between 0.15% and 0.3% have been recommended as appropriate for selection of probiotic bacteria for human consumption (Yang and Adams, 2004).

A variety of microorganisms, typically food-grade lactic acid bacteria (LAB), have been evaluated for their probiotic potential and have been applied as adjunct cultures in various food products or therapeutic preparations (Rodgers, 2008). *Lactobacillus* and *Bifidobacterium* species may be found in many foods; some are frequently regarded as probiotics due to their capacity to improve certain biological functions in the host. Complex interactions occur among resident microbiota, epithelial and immune cells and probiotics. These interactions play a major role in the development and maintenance of the beneficial activities for healthy humans (Medici el al., 2004).

According to Karimi et al. (2012), recommendations for the minimum viable counts of each probiotic strain in gram or millilitre of probiotic products vary when it comes to providing health benefits related to probiotic organisms. For example, the minimum viable levels of 10^5 cfu g^{-1} have been recommended (Shah, 1995); while 10^6 cfu g^{-1} (Karimi and Amiri-Rigi, 2010; Talwalkar and Kailasapathy, 2004) and 10^7 cfu g^{-1} (Samona and Robinson, 1994) have been suggested for probiotics in different products. However, populations of 10^6-10^7 CFU/g in the final product have been shown to be more acceptable as efficient levels of probiotic cultures in processed foods (Talwalkar, Miller, Kailasapathy and Nguyen, 2004), with numbers attaining 10^8 - 10^9 CFU when provided by a daily consumption of 100 g or 100 mL of probiotic food, and hence benefiting human health (Jayamanne & Adams, 2006). It is important to emphasize that the incorporation of probiotic cultures into cheeses would produce functional foods only if the cultures remained viable in recommended numbers during maturation and shelf life of the products.

One of the preconditions for a bacterial strain to be called probiotic is the strain's ability to survive in the gastrointestinal environment, although the importance of viability for the beneficial effects of probiotics has not been well defined since inactivated and dead cells can also have immunological and health-promoting effects (Ghadimi et al., 2008; Lopez et al., 2008). Moreover, there are significant technological challenges associated with the introduction and maintenance of high numbers of probiotic microorganisms in foods that depend on the form of the probiotic inoculant, and with the viability and maintenance of probiotic characteristics in the food product up to the time of consumption. Spray drying has been used as a preservation method for microbial cultures. Gardiner et al. (2002) produced spray-dried probiotic milk powder containing the probiotic *Lactobacillus paracasei* NFBC 338. The powder contained 1×10^9 CFU.g^{-1} *L. paracasei* which was used as adjunct inoculums during probiotic Cheddar cheese manufacture. After three months of ripening, the count was 7.7×10^7 CFU.g^{-1}, without any adverse effects on the cheese. The researchers' data shows that probiotic spray-dried powder may be a useful means for adding probiotic strains to dairy products.

In order to use probiotic bacteria in the manufacture of cheese products, the process may have to be modified and adapted to the requirements of the strains employed. Overall, probiotic strains should be technologically compatible with the food manufacturing process involved. With regard to the development of probiotic cheeses, this means that such strains should be cultivable to high cell density for inoculation into the cheese vat, or that the strains are capable of proliferating during the manufacturing and/or ripening process (Ross et al., 2002). In general, a probiotic cheese should have the same attributes as a conventional cheese: the incorporation of probiotic bacteria should not imply a loss of quality of the product. In this context, the level of proteolysis and lipolysis must be the same or even better than for cheese which does not have functional food appeal (Cruz et al., 2009a).

Proteolysis plays a critical role in determining typical sensory characteristics and represents a significant quality indicator for certain cheeses. Proteolysis is caused by enzymes found in milk (plasmin), rennet (pepsin and chymosin) and microbial enzymes released by starter cultures. The activities of these enzymes hydrolyze the fractions of caseins, which leads to the formation of peptides. These peptides may be further hydrolyzed with proteolytic enzymes originating from microbiota such as starter bacteria, non-starter lactic acid bacteria (NSLAB) and probiotic adjuncts to the cheeses, into smaller peptides and free amino acids, which are important for flavor development in some cheeses (Ong et al., 2007; Cliffe et al., 1993; Lynch et al., 1999).

Three batches of Cheddar cheeses (Batch 1, with only starter lactococci; Batch 2, with lactococci and *Lactobacillus acidophilus* 4962, *Lb. casei* 279, *Bifidobacterium longum* 1941; Batch 3, with lactococci and *Lb. acidophilus* LAFTIs L10, *Lb. paracasei* LAFTI L26, *B. lactis* LAFTI B94) were manufactured in triplicate to study the survival and influence of probiotic bacteria on proteolytic patterns and production of organic acid during a ripening period of 6 months at 4 °C. All probiotic adjuncts survived the manufacturing process and maintained their viability of 7.5 log10 cfu g^{-1} at the end of the ripening term. The number of lactococci decreased by one to two log cycles, but their counts were not significantly different (P> 0.05) in either the control or the probiotic cheeses. No significant differences were observed in composition (fat, protein, moisture, salt content), although acetic acid concentration was higher in the probiotic cheeses. Proteolysis assessment during ripening showed no significant differences (P> 0.05) in the level of water-soluble nitrogen (primary proteolysis), but the levels of secondary proteolysis indicated by the concentration of free amino acids were significantly higher (P> 0.05) in probiotic cheeses. These data thus suggested that Cheddar cheese is an effective vehicle for the delivery of probiotic organisms (Ong et al., 2006).

Phillips et al. (2006) have also studied probiotic Cheddar cheese. They manufactured six batches of Cheddar cheese containing different combinations of commercially-available probiotic cultures. Duplicate cheeses contained organisms from each supplier, *Bifidobacterium* spp., *Lactobacillus acidophilus* and either *Lactobacillus casei*, *Lactobacillus paracasei*, or *Lactobacillus rhamnosus*. Using selective media, the different strains were assessed for viability during Cheddar cheese maturation over 32 weeks. *Bifidobacterium* sp. remained at high numbers with the three strains present in cheese at 4×10^7, 1.4×10^8, and 5×10^8 CFU/g respectively after 32 weeks. Similarly, the *L. casei* (2×10^7 CFU/g), *L. paracasei* (1.6×10^7 CFU/g), and *L. rhamnosus* (9×10^8 CFU/g) strains survived well. However, the *L. acidophilus* strains performed poorly. Both decreased in a similar manner and were recorded at 3.6×10^3 CFU/g and 4.9×10^3 CFU/g after 32 weeks.

Numerous scientific papers have been published on the development of fresh cheeses containing recognized and potentially probiotic cultures. They have described suitable viable counts as well as a positive influence on texture and sensorial properties of the cheeses. Cottage cheese in particular shows an adequate profile for the incorporation of probiotic cells and/or prebiotic substances. In addition, cottage cheese is a healthy alternative to many other cheeses by virtue of its low fat content.

Araújo et al. (2010) developed a symbiotic cottage cheese containing *Lactobacillus delbrueckii* UFV H2b20 and inulin, and evaluated the survival of this bacterium when the cheese was exposed to conditions simulating those found in the gastro-intestinal tract. Throughout the entire storage period of the cheese, the probiotic cell counts were higher than recommended levels for probiotic products. The probiotic bacterium exhibited satisfactory resistance to low pH values and to high concentrations of bile salts. The addition of probiotic cells and inulin generated no alterations in the physicochemical characteristics of cheese. By allowing the viable microorganism has characteristics desirable for incorporation of a probiotic strain. Probiotic cells could be added to the dressing, creamy liquid that surrounds the granules of cheese because after this step there is not exposition at high temperature.

Although cottage cheese is well adapted to the health requirements of modern populations, its consumption has been in decline over the past few years. By developing new production processes, cottage cheese, apart from carrying the nutritional qualities of milk, may also furnish consumers with a source of lactic acid bacteria, probiotic microorganisms and prebiotics. The lactic acid bacteria perform more critical functions in cottage cheese than just producing lactic acid. They also aid the manufacture process and increase the final rheological and sensorial qualities of the cheese. Controlling of the fermentation process with lactic acid bacteria allows for the enhancement of the sensorial quality of the cheese and could hence play a crucial role in increasing consumption of cottage cheese.

Souza, et al. (2008) and Souza and Saad (2009) studied the manufacture of Minas fresh cheese supplemented solely with the probiotic strain of *L. acidophilus* La-5. Cheeses manufactured solely with La-5 presented populations above 1×10^6 CFU/g, reaching 1×10^7 CFU/g on the 14th day of storage.

The Argentinean fresh cheese is a soft rindless cheese with a ripening period of 12 days at 5 ºC before its commercial distribution. This cheese presents the following physicochemical characteristics: pH 5.29, moisture 58% (w/w), fat 12% (w/w), proteins 23% (w/w), salt 0.9% (w/w), ashes 3.4% (w/w), dry matter 40.8% (w/w) and calcium 0.6% (w/w). This product has proven to be an adequate vehicle for probiotic bacteria during storage and until consumption. It offers offer a certain degree of protection of the viability of bacteria during the *in vitro* simulation of gastric transit (Vinderola et al., 2000).

Kasimoglu et al. (2004) have shown that *L. acidophilus* strain can be used for the manufacture of probiotic Turkish white cheese. The final numbers of *L. acidophilus* were greater than the minimum (10^7 cfu g^{-1}) required to make health benefits claims. Furthermore, *L. acidophilus* can be used to enhance flavor, texture, and a produce a high level of proteolysis. Moreover, probiotic cheese which was vacuum packed following salting was shown to be more acceptable than the corresponding cheese stored in brine following salting. Therefore, vacuum packaging is the preferred means for storing probiotic Turkish white cheeses.

6. Concluding remarks and future trends

In conclusion, probiotic microorganisms, including bacteria and yeasts, are attracting a growing interest due to their promising physiological effects as well as the value they add to probiotic-containing food products. There is a growing body of evidence that probiotics may play a beneficial role in human health (Ouwehand et al., 2002; Collado et al., 2009). Established effects in humans include alleviation of symptoms linked to lactose intolerance or to irritable bowel syndrome. They also include reduced diarrhea associated with antibiotic treatment, rotavirus or traveler's diseases. It should be emphasized that the beneficial properties of probiotic microorganisms are highly dependent on the strains, which means that each strain or product requires demonstration of the specific effects *in vivo*. The possibility of using certain probiotics to modulate the immune system, particularly at the mucosal level (O'Flaherty et al., 2010) is the most promising application. In this respect, promising healing effects were obtained using the probiotic mixture VSL#3 on ulcerative colitis patients (Miele et al., 2009; Huynh et al., 2009; Ng et al., 2010). These clinical studies, which still need to be confirmed by larger studies, strongly suggest that selected strains of probiotics may help in treating the bowel diseases which constitute a growing health concern in developing countries. Clearly, animal studies suggest other promising probiotic effects incuding inflammatory diseases, allergies and associated asthma, and colorectal cancer. These applications open exciting avenues that must be investigated at both molecular and clinical levels.

Understanding the impact of ingested bacteria on health, as well as the impact of gut microbiota perturbation (dysbiosis) on emerging diseases, including immune disorders and cancer remains a great challenge. In developed countries, gut microbiota have evolved with a reduced diversity of bacterial species (Yatsunenko et al., 2012). This is particularly true in Crohn's disease patients (Manichanh et al., 2006), who lack immunomodulatory anti-inflammatory bacteria, including *Faecalibacterium prausnitzii* (Sokol et al., 2008). A similar reduced diversity was also described in the case of colorectal cancer, (Chen et al., 2012) confirming the involvement of dysbiosis in digestive cancers (Azcarate-Peril et al., 2011). The composition of gut microbiota is linked to long term dietary patterns (Wu et al., 2011). This suggests that ingested bacteria can participate in the prevention and/or treatment of emerging diseases. This hypothesis has been reinforced by recent epidemiological studies which show that raw milk prevents the onset of allergy and asthma in children (Loss et al., 2011; Waser et al., 2007; Braun-Fahrlander et al., 2011). The authors suggested a protective immunomodulatory role of raw milk bacteria (Braun-Fahrlander et al., 2011).

Most interestingly, bacterial species used as dairy starters display promising properties in this field. For example, immunomodulatory anti-inflammatory properties were described in certain strains of *Propionibacterium freudenreichii* (Foligné et al., 2010; Deutsch et al., 2012), *Streptococcus thermophilus* (Ogita et al., 2011), *Lactobacillus delbrueckii* subsp. *bulgaricus* and subsp. *lactis* (Santos-Rocha et al., 2012), as well as *Lactobacillus helveticus* (Guglielmetti et al., 2010). Modulation of colon cancer cell growth was also reported in vitro and/or in animal models for *P. freudenreichii* (Cousin et al., 2010; Lan et al., 2008), when the cells were exposed to yogurt containing *S. thermophilus and L. bulgaricus* (Narushima et al., 2010; Perdigon et al., 2002) and *L. helveticus* (de Moreno et al., 2010). Future trends may thus include the development of specific fermented dairy products designed for specific population. These could use bacteria strains and employ both technological capabilities and probiotic potential to affect immune system modulation, gut physiology and cancer cells.

Author details

Emiliane Andrade Araújo
Universidade Federal de Viçosa, Campus Rio Paranaíba, Rio Paranaíba, MG, Brazil

Ana Clarissa dos Santos Pires and Antônio Fernandes de Carvalho*
Departamento de Tecnologia de Alimentos, Universidade Federal de Viçosa, Viçosa, MG, Brazil

Maximiliano Soares Pinto
Instituto de Ciências Agrárias, Universidade Federal de Minas Gerais, Montes Claros, MG, Brazil

Gwénaël Jan
INRA, UMR1253 Science et Technologie du Lait et de l'Œuf, Rennes, France

Acknowledgement

We would like to thank to Mary Margaret Chappell for reading and contributing. The authors are supported by grants from the FAPEMIG, CAPES and CNPq.

---

* Corresponding Author

7. References

Araujo, E. A., Carvalho, A. F., Leandro, E. S., Furtado, M.M., Moraes, C. A. (2010). Development of a symbiotic cottage cheese added with *Lactobacillus delbrueckii* UFV H2b20 and inulin. *Journal of Functional Foods*, 2, 85-89.

Azcarate-Peril, M. A., Sikes, M., Bruno-Barcena, J. M. (2011). The intestinal microbiota, gastrointestinal environment and colorectal cancer: a putative role for probiotics in prevention of colorectal cancer? *Am. J. Physiol Gastrointest. Liver Physiol,*, 301:G401-G424.

Benton, D., Williams, C., Brown, A. (2007). Impact of consuming a milk drink containing a probiotic on mood and cognition. *European Journal of Clinical Nutrition*, 61, 355–361.

Braun-Fahrlander, C., & Von, M. E. (2011). Can farm milk consumption prevent allergic diseases? *Clin. Exp. Allergy*, 41:29-35.

Charteris, W. P., Kelly, P. M., Morelli, L., Collins, J. K. (1998). Development and application of in vitro methodology to determine the transit tolerance of potentially probiotic *Lactobacillus* and *Bifidobacterium* species in the upper human gastrointestinal tract. *Journal of Applied Microbiology*, 84, 759–768.

Chen, W. J. L., Anderson, J. W., Jennings, D. (1984). Propionate may mediate the hypocholesterolemic effects of certain soluble plant fibers in cholesterol-fed rats. *Proc. Soc. Exp. Biol. Med*,175, 215-218.

Chen, W., Liu, F., Ling, Z., Tong, X., Xiang, C. (2012). Human intestinal lumen and mucosa-associated microbiota in patients with colorectal cancer. *PLoS. ONE.*, 7:e39743.

Clancy, R. (2003) Immunobiotics and the probiotic evolution. *FEMS Immunology and Medical Microbiology*, 38, 9-12.

Cliffe, A. J., Marks, J. D.; Mulholland, F. (1993). Isolation and characterization of non-volatile flavors from cheese: Peptide profile of flavor fractions from Cheddar cheese, determined by reverse-phase high performance liquid chromatography. *International Dairy Journal*, 3, 379–387.

Collado, M. C., Isolauri, E., Salminen, S., Sanz, Y. (2009). The impact of probiotic on gut health. *Curr. Drug Metab*, 10:68-78.

Costello, E. K., Lauber, C. L., Hamady, M., Fierer, N., Gordon, J. I., Knight, R. (2009) Bacterial community variation in human body habitats across space and time. *Science*, 326, 1694-1697.

Cousin, F. J., Jouan-Lanhouet, S., Dimanche-Boitrel, M. T., Corcos, L., Jan, G. (2012). Milk Fermented by *Propionibacterium freudenreichii* Induces Apoptosis of HGT-1 Human Gastric Cancer Cells. *PLoS. ONE.*, 7:e31892.

Crittenden, R. G. Prebiotics. In: Tannock, G. W. (Ed.). (1999). *Probiotics: a critical review*. Norfolk: Horizon Scientific Press, 141-156.

Cruz, A. G., Buriti, F. C. A., Souza, C. H. B., Faria, J. A. F., Saad, S. M. I. (2009a). Probiotic cheese: health benefits, technological and stability aspects. *Trends in Food Science & Technology*, 20, 344-354.

Cruz, A.G., Antunes, A.E.C., Sousa, A.L.O.P., Faria, J.A.F., Saad, S.M.I. (2009b). Ice-cream as a probiotic food Carrier. *Food Research International*, 42, 1233-1239.

Cruz, A.G., Faria, J.A.F., Van Dender, A.G.F. (2007). Packaging system and probiotic dairy foods. *Food Research International*, 40, 951–956.

Davidson, R.H., Duncan, S.E., Hackney, C.R., Eigel, W.N., Boling, J.W. (2000). Probiotic Culture Survival and Implications in Fermented Frozen Yogurt Characteristics. *Journal of Dairy Science*, 83, 666–673.

de Moreno, L. A., & Perdigon, G. (2010). The application of probiotic fermented milks in cancer and intestinal inflammation. *Proc. Nutr. Soc.*, 69:421-428.

Deutsch, S. M., Parayre, S., Bouchoux, A., Guyomarc'h, F., Dewulf, J., Dols-Lafargue, M., Baglinière, F., Cousin, F. J., Falentin, H., Jan, G., Foligné, B. (2012). Contribution of surface beta-glucan polysaccharide to physicochemical and immunomodulatory properties of *Propionibacterium freudenreichii*. *Appl. Environ. Microbiol.*, 78:1765-1775.

Espirito Santo, A.P., Perego, P., Converti, A., Oliveira, M.N. (2011). Influence of food matrices on probiotic viability: A review focusing on the fruity bases. *Trends in Food Science & Technology*, 22, 377-385.

Foligné, B., Deutsch, S. M., Breton, J., Cousin, F. J., Dewulf, J., Samson, M., Pot, B., Jan, G. (2010). Promising immunomodulatory effects of selected strains of dairy propionibacteria as evidenced *in vitro* and *in vivo*. *Appl. Environ. Microbiol.*, 76:8259-8264.

Fuller, R. (1989). Probiotics in man and animals. *Journal of Applied Bacteriology*, 66, 365–378.

Gadaga, T. H., Mutukumira, A. N., Narvhus, J. A., Feresu, S. B. (1999). A review of traditional fermented foods and beverages of Zimbabwe. *International Journal of Food Microbiology*, 53, 1–11.

Gardiner, G. E., Bouchier, P., O'sullivan, E., Kelly, J., Collins, K., Fitzgerald, G., Ross, R.P., Stanton, C. (2002). A spray-dried culture for porbiotic Cheddar chesse manufacture. *International Dairy Journal*, 12, 749-756.

Ghadimi, D., Folster-Holst, R., De Vrese, M., Winkler, P., Heller, K.J., Schrezenmeir, J. (2008). Effects of probiotic bacteria and their genomic DNA on TH1/TH2-cytokine production by peripheral blood mononuclear cells (PBMCs) of healthy and allergic subjects. *Immunobiology*, 213, 677–692.

Gibson, G. R., Fuller, R. (2000) Aspects of in vitro and in vivo research approaches directed toward identifying probiotics and prebiotics for human use. *Journal Nutrition*, 130, 391-395.

Godward, G., Sultana, K., Kailasapathy, K., Peiris, P., Arumugaswamy, R., & Reynolds, N. (2000). The importance of strain selection on the viability and survival of probiotic bacteria in dairy foods. *Milchwissenschaft*, 55, 441-445.

Guglielmetti, S., Taverniti, V., Minuzzo, M., Arioli, S., Zanoni, I., Stuknyte, M., Granucci, F., Karp, M., Mora, D. (2010). A dairy bacterium displays in vitro probiotic properties for the pharyngeal mucosa by antagonizing group A streptococci and modulating the immune response. *Infect. Immun.*, 78:4734-4743.

Holzapfel, W. H., Haberer, P., Snel, J., Schillinger, U., & Huis In't Velt, J. H. J. (1998). Overview of gut flora and probiotics. *International Journal of Food Microbiology*, 41, 85–101.

Huynh, H. Q., Debruyn, J., Guan, L., Diaz, H., Li, M., Girgis, S., Turner, J., Fedorak, R., Madsen, K. (2009). Probiotic preparation VSL#3 induces remission in children with mild to moderate acute ulcerative colitis: a pilot study. *Inflamm. Bowel. Dis.*, 15:760-768.

Hyun, C., Shin, H. (1998). Utilization of bovine plasma obtained from a slaughterhouse for economic production of probiotics. *Journal of Fermentation and Bioenginering*, 86, 34–37.

Jayamanne, V. S., & Adams, M. R. (2006). Determination of survival, identity, and stress resistance of probiotic bifidobacteria in bio-yoghurts. *Letters in Applied Microbiology*, 42(3),189-194.

Kailasapathy, K., Harmstorf, I., & Phillips, M. (2008). Survival of *Lactobacillus acidophilus* and *Bifidobacterium animalis* ssp *lactis* in stirred fruit yogurts. *LWT-Food Science and Technology*, 41, 1317-1322.

Karimi, R., Amiri-Rigi, A., 2010. *Probiotics in Dairy Products*. Marz Danesh Publication,Tehran.

Karimi, R., Mortazavian, A.M., Amiri-Rigi, A. (2012). Selective enumeration of probiotic microorganisms in cheese. *Food Microbiology*, 29,1-9.

Karimi, R., Mortazavian, A.M., Da Cruz, A.G. (2011). Viability of probiotic microorganisms in cheese during production and storage: a review. *Dairy Science and Technology*, 91, 283-308.

Kasimoglu, A., Goncuoglu, M., Akgun, S. (2004). Probiotic White cheese with *Lactobacillus acidophilus*. *International Dairy Journal*, 14, 1067-1073.

Lan, A., Bruneau, A., Bensaada, M., Philippe, C., Bellaud, P., Rabot, S., Jan, G. (2008). Increased induction of apoptosis by *Propionibacterium freudenreichii* TL133 in colonic mucosal crypts of human microbiota-associated rats treated with 1,2-dimethylhydrazine. *Br. J Nutr.*, 100:1251-1259.

Lopez, M., Li, N., Kataria, J., Russell, M., Neu, J. (2008). Live and ultraviolet-inactivated *Lactobacillus rhamnosus* GG decrease flagellin-induced interleukin-8 production in Caco-2 cells. *Journal of Nutrition*, 138, 2264–2268.

Loss, G., Apprich, S., Waser, M., Kneifel, W., Genuneit, J., Buchele, G., Weber, J., Sozanska, B., Danielewicz, H., Horak, E., Van Neerven, R. J., Heederik, D., Lorenzen, P. C., Von, M. E., Braun-Fahrlander, C. (2011). The protective effect of farm milk consumption on childhood asthma and atopy: the Gabriela study. *J. Allergy Clin. Immunol.*, 128:766-773.

Lourens-Hattingh,A., Viljoen, B.C. (2001a). Growth and survival of a probiotic yeast in dairy products. *Food Research International*, 34, 791-796.

Lourens-Hattingh,A., Viljoen, B.C. (2001b). Yogurt as probiotic carrier food. *International Dairy Journal*, 11, 1-17.

Lynch, C. M., Muir, D. D., Banks, J. M., Mcsweeney, P. L. H.; Fox, P. F. (1999). Influence of adjunct cultures *of Lactobacillus paracasei* ssp. *paracasei* or *Lactobacillus plantarum* on Cheddar cheese ripening. Journal of Dairy Science, 82, 1618–1628.

Macfarlane, G. T. Gibson, G. R. Cummings, J. H. (1992) Comparison of fermentation reactions in different regions of the human colon. *Journal Applied Bacteriology*, 72(3), 57-64.

Manichanh, C., Rigottier-Gois, L., Bonnaud, E., Gloux, K., Pelletier, E., Frangeul, L., Nalin, R., Jarrin, C., Chardon, P., Marteau, P., Roca, J., Dore, J. (2006). Reduced diversity of faecal microbiota in Crohn's disease revealed by a metagenomic approach. *Gut*, 55:205-211.

Margoles, A., Garcia, L. (2003). Characterisation of a bifidobacterium strain wish acquired resistance to cholate: A preliminary study. *International Journal of Food Microbiology*, 80, 191–198.

Medici, M., Vinderola, C. G., Perdigon, G. (2004). Gut mucosal immunomodulation by probiotic fresh chesse. *International Dairy Journal*, 14, 611-618.

Miele, E., Pascarella, F., Giannetti , E., Quaglietta , L Robert N. Baldassano , R. N., Annamaria Staiano , A. (2009). Effect of a Probiotic Preparation (VSL#3) on Induction and Maintenance of Remission in Children With Ulcerative Colitis. *American Journal of Gastroenterology*, 104, 437-443.

Miele, E., Pascarella, F., Giannetti, E., Quaglietta, L., Baldassano, R. N., Staiano, A. (2009). Effect of a probiotic preparation (VSL#3) on induction and maintenance of remission in children with ulcerative colitis. *Am. J. Gastroenterol.*, 104:437-443.

Moura, M.R. L., (2005). Alimentos Funcionais: seus benefícios e a legislação: Avaiable in: http://acd.ufrj.br/consumo/leituras/ld.htm#leituras.

Narushima, S., Sakata, T., Hioki, K., Itoh, T., Nomura, T., Itoh, K. (2010). Inhibitory effect of yogurt on aberrant crypt foci formation in the rat colon and colorectal tumorigenesis in RasH2 mice. *Exp. Anim.*, 59:487-494.

Ng, S. C., Plamondon, S., Kamm, M. A., Hart, A. L., Al-Hassi, H. O., Guenther, T., Stagg, A. J., Knight, S. C. (2010). Immunosuppressive effects via human intestinal dendritic cells of probiotic bacteria and steroids in the treatment of acute ulcerative colitis. *Inflamm. Bowel. Dis.*, 16:1286-1298.

O'flaherty, S., Saulnier, D. M., Pot, B., Versalovic, J. (2010). How can probiotics and prebiotics impact mucosal immunity? *Gut Microbes*, 1:293-300.

Ogita, T., Nakashima, M., Morita, H., Saito, Y., Suzuki, T., Tanabe, S. (2011). *Streptococcus thermophilus* ST28 ameliorates colitis in mice partially by suppression of inflammatory Th17 cells. *J. Biomed. Biotechnol.*, 2011:378417.

Ong, L., Henriksson, A., Shah, N.P. (2006) Development of probiotic Cheddar cheese containing *Lactobacillus acidophilus, Lb. casei, Lb. paracasei* and *Bifidobacterium* spp. and the influence of these bacteria on proteolytic patterns and production of organic acid. *International Dairy Journal* 16, 446–456.

Ong, L., Henrikssonb, A., Shaha, N. P. Chemical analysis and sensory evaluation of Cheddar cheese produced with *Lactobacillus acidophilus, Lb. casei, Lb. paracasei* or *Bifidobacterium* sp. *International Dairy Journal* 17 (2007) 937–945.

Ouwehand, A. C., Salminen, S., Isolauri, E. (2002). Probiotics: an overview of beneficial effects. *Anton. Leeuw. Int. J. G.*, 82:279-289.

Perdigon, G., De Moreno, D. L., Valdez, J., Rachid, M. (2002). Role of yoghurt in the prevention of colon cancer. *Eur. J. Clin. Nutr.*, 56 Suppl 3:S65-S68.

Prado, F.C., Parada, J.L., Pandey, A., Soccol, C.R. (2008). Trends in non-dairy probiotic beverages. *Food Research International*, 41, 111–123.

Rastall, R. A., Fuller, R., Gaskins H. R., Gibson G. R. (2000) Colonic functional foods. In *Functional Foods*, 71–89 [GR Gibson and CM Williams, editors]. Cambridge: Woodhead Publishing Limited.

Reddy, B. S., Rivenson, A. (1983) Inhibitory effect of Bifidobacterium longum on colon, mammary, and liver carcinogenesis induced by 2-amino-3-methyllimidazo [4,5-f]quinoline, a food mutagen. *Cancer Research*, 53, 3914-3918.

Reid G., Jessica A., Younes, J. A., Van Der Mei, H. C., Gloor, G. B., Knight, R., Busscher, H. J. (2011) Gut flora restoration: natural and supplemented recovery of human microbial communities. *Nature Reviews*. 9, 27-38.

Rodgers, S. (2008). Novel applications of live bacteria in food services: probiotics and protective cultures. *Trends Food Sci. Tech.* 19, 188-197.

Ross, R. P., Fitzgerald, G., Collins, K., Stanton, C. (2002). Cheese delivering biocultures: probiotic cheese. *Australian Journal of Dairy Technology*, 57(2), 71-78.

Saarela, M., Mogensen, G., Fonden, R., Matto, J., Mattila-Sandholm, T. (2000). Probiotic bacteria: safety, functional and technological properties. *Journal of Biotechnology*, 84, 197–215.

Samona, A., Robinson, R.K. (1994). Effect of yogurt cultures on the survival of bifidobacteria in fermented milks. *Journal of the Society of Dairy Technology* 47, 58-60.

Santos-Rocha C., Lakhdari, O., Blottiere, H. M., Blugeon, S., Sokol, H., Bermu'dez-Humara'n, L. G., Azevedo, V., Miyoshi, A., Dore, J., Langella, P., Maguin, E., Van De, G. M. (2012). Anti-inflammatory properties of dairy lactobacilli. *Inflamm. Bowel. Dis.*, 18:657-666.

Sendra, E., Fayos, P., Lario, Y., Fernandez-Lopez, J., Sayas-Barbera, E., & Perez-Alvarez, J. (2008). Incorporation of citrus fibers in fermented milk containing probiotic bacteria. *Food Microbiology*, 25, 13-21.

Shah, N.P., Lankaputhra, W.E.V., Britz, M.L., Kyle, W.S.A. (1995). Survival of *Lactobacillus acidophilus* and *Bifidobacterium bifidum* in commercial yoghurt during refrigerated storage. *International Dairy Journal*, 5, 515-521.

Sokol, H., Pigneur, B., Watterlot, L., Lakhdari, O., Bermudez-Humaran, L. G., Gratadoux, J. J., Blugeon, S., Bridonneau, C., Furet, J. P., Corthier, G., Grangette, C., Vasquez, N., Pochart, P., Trugnan, G., Thomas, G., Blottiere, H. M., Dore, J., Marteau, P., Seksik, P., Langella, P. (2008). *Faecalibacterium prausnitzii* is an anti-inflammatory commensal bacterium identified by gut microbiota analysis of Crohn disease patients. *Proc. Natl. Acad. Sci. U. S. A*, 105:16731-16736.

Souza, C. H. B., & Saad, S. M. I. (2009). Viability of Lactobacillus acidophilus La-5 added solely or in co-culture with a yoghurt starter culture and implications on physico-chemical and related properties of Minas fresh cheese during storage. *LWT e Food Science and Technology*, 42(2), 633-640.

Souza, C. H. B., Buriti, F. C. A., Behrens, J. H., & Saad, S. M. I. (2008). Sensory evaluation of probiotic Minas fresh cheese with *Lactobacillus acidophilus* added solely or in co-culture with a thermophilic starter culture. *International Journal of Food Science and Technology*, 43(5), 871-877.

Stapleton, A. E., Au-Yeung, M., Hooton, T. M., Fredricks, D. N., Roberts, P. L., Czaja, C. A., Yarova-Yarovaya, Y., Fiedler, T., Cox, M., Stamm, W. E. (2011). Randomized, Placebo-controlled Phase 2 Trial of a Lactobacillus crispatus Probiotic Given Intravaginally for Prevention of Recurrent Urinary Tract Infection. *Clinical Infectious Diseases*, 52 (10), 1212-1217.

Talwalkar, A., Kailasapathy, K. (2004). Comparison of selective and differential media for the accurate enumeration of strains of *Lactobacillus acidophilus*, *Bifidobacterium* spp. and Lactobacillus casei complex from commercial yoghurts. *International Dairy Journal*, 14, 142-149.

Talwalkar, A., Miller, C. W., Kailasapathy, K., & Nguyen, M. H. (2004). Effect of packaging materials and dissolved oxygen on the survival of probiotic bacteria in yoghurt. *International Journal of Food Science and Technology*, 39(6), 605-611.

Thamer, K. G.; Penna, A. L. B. (2005). Efeito do teor de soro, acucar e de frutooligossacarideos sobre a populacao de bacterias lacticas probioticas em bebidas fermentadas. *Revista Brasileira de Ciências Farmacêuticas*, 41(3), 393-400.

Topping, D. L. Clifton, P. M. (2001) SHorty-chain fatty acids and human colonic function: roles of resistant starch and nonstarch polysaccharides. *Physiological Reviews*, 81(3), 1031-1064.

Vinderola, C. G., Prosello, W., Ghiberto, D., Reinheimer, J. (2000). Viability of probiotic (*Bifidobacterium*, *Lactobacillus acidophilus* and *Lactobacillus casei*) and nonprobiotic microflora in argentinian Fresh cheese. *Journal of Dairy Science*, 83, 1905–1911.

Waser, M., Michels, K. B., Bieli, C., Floistrup, H., Pershagen, G., Von, M. E., Ege, M., Riedler, J., Schram-Bijkerk, D., Brunekreef, B., Van, H. M., Lauener, R., Braun-Fahrlander, C. (2007). Inverse association of farm milk consumption with asthma and allergy in rural and suburban populations across Europe. *Clin. Exp. Allergy*, 37:661-670.

Wohlgemuth, S., Gunnar Loh, G., Blaut, M. (2010). Recent developments and perspectives in the investigation of probiotic effects. *International Journal of Medical Microbiology*, 300, 3–10

Wu, G. D., Chen, J., Hoffmann, C., Bittinger, K., Chen, Y. Y., Keilbaugh, S. A., Bewtra, M., Knights, D., Walters, W. A., Knight, R., Sinha, R., Gilroy, E., Gupta, K., Baldassano, R., Nessel, L., Li, H., Bushman, F. D., Lewis, J. D. (2011). Linking long-term dietary patterns with gut microbial enterotypes. *Science*, 334:105-108.

Yan, F., Cao, H., Cover, T, L., Washington, M. K., Shi, Y, Liu, L., Chaturvedi, R., Peek Jr, R. M., Wilson, K. T., Polk, D. B. (2011). Colon-specific delivery of a probiotic-derived soluble protein ameliorates intestinal inflammation in mice through an EGFR-dependent mechanism. *Journal of Clinical Investigation*, 121(6), 2242-2253.

Yang, H., & Adams, M. C. (2004). In vitro assessment of the upper gastrointestinal tolerance of potential probiotic dairy propionibacteria. *International Journal of Food Microbiology*, 91, 253–260.

Yatsunenko, T., Rey, F. E., Manary, M. J., Trehan, I., Dominguez-Bello, M. G., Contreras, M., Magris, M., Hidalgo, G., Baldassano, R. N., Anokhin, A. P., Heath, A. C., Warner, B., Reeder, J., Kuczynski, J., Caporaso, J. G., Lozupone, C. A., Lauber, C., Clemente, J. C., Knights, D., Knight, R., Gordon, J. I. (2012). Human gut microbiome viewed across age and geography. *Nature*, 486:222-227.

Chapter 6

Dairy Probiotic Foods and Coronary Heart Disease: A Review on Mechanism of Action

Fariborz Akbarzadeh and Aziz Homayouni

Additional information is available at the end of the chapter

1. Introduction

Coronary heart disease (CHD) is one of the major causes of death in adults in the developed and developing countries which is referred to the condition in which the main coronary arteries supplying the heart are no longer able to supply sufficient blood and oxygen to the heart muscle (myocardium). The main cause of the reduced flow is an accumulation of plaques, mainly in the intima of arteries, a disease known as atherosclerosis (Akbarzadeh and Toufan, 2008). A number of risk factors known to affect an individual to CHD have been categorized such as hyperlipidaemia (high levels of lipids in the blood), hypertension (high blood pressure), obesity, cigarette smoking and lack of exercise. Probiotics as a live microbial food supplement beneficially affects the host by improving its intestinal microbial balance and is generally consumed as fermented milk products containing lactic acid bacteria such as bifidobacteria and/or lactobacilli. The supposed health benefits of probiotics include improved resistance to gastrointestinal infections, reduction in total cholesterol and TAG levels and stimulation of the immune system. A number of mechanisms have been proposed to explain their putative lipid-lowering capacity and these include a 'milk factor', which has been thought to inhibit HMG-CoA reductase and the assimilation of cholesterol by certain bacteria. The mechanism of action of probiotics on cholesterol reduction include physiological actions of the end products of fermentation SCFAs, cholesterol assimilation, deconjugation of bile acids and cholesterol binding to bacterial cell walls. It has been well documented that microbial bile acid metabolism is a peculiar probiotic effect involved in the therapeutic role of some bacteria. The deconjugation reaction is catalyzed by conjugated bile acid hydrolase enzyme, which is produced exclusively by bacteria. The mechanism of cholesterol binding to bacterial cell walls has also been suggested as a possible explanation for hypocholesterolaemic effects of probiotics. Probiotics have received attention for their beneficial effects on the gut microflora and links to their systemic effects on the lowering of lipids known to be risk factors for CHD, notably cholesterol and TAG. The incorporation of probiotics into dairy products such as fermented milk products controlled nutrition studies need to be carried out to determine the beneficial effects of prebiotics, probiotics and synbiotics before substantial health claims can be made (Ranjbar et al., 2007a).

2. Probiotics

Probiotics are distinct as live microorganisms which, when administered in sufficient amounts present a health benefit on the host (FAO/WHO, 2002; Homayouni, 2008a; Homayouni, 2009). In recent years probiotic bacteria have increasingly been incorporated into dairy foods as dietary adjuncts. *Lactobacillus* and *Bifidobacterium* are the most common species of probiotic bacteria that were used in the production of fermented and non-fermented dairy products. Consumption of probiotic bacteria via dairy food products is an ideal way to re-establish the intestinal microflora balance (Homayouni, 2008a).

Probiotics have been shown to be effective against a number of disorders. Some mostly documented effects are relieving diarrhea, improving lactose intolerance and its immunomodulatory, anticarcinogenic, antidiabetic, hypocholesterolemic and hypotensive properties (Shah, 2007; Mai, and Draganov, 2009; Lye, et al., 2009). Probiotic bacteria, by competing with enteric pathogens for available nutrients and binding sites, reducing the pH of the gut, producing a variety of chemicals which inactivate viruses, enhancing specific and non-specific immune responses and increasing mucin production, can reduce incidence, severity and duration of diarrhea (Homayouni, et al., 2007; Allen, et al., 2010; Ejtahed, and Homayouni Rad, 2010). Alleviation of lactose intolerance symptoms by probiotic bacteria is attributed to their intracellular β-galactosidase content (Mustapha, et al., 1997). Studies have revealed that probiotic bacteria can induce many immunological changes and affect both Th1 and Th2 cytokine production and that these effects are strongly strain-specific (Lebeer, et al., 2010). Some major routes through which probiotic bacteria have been assumed to prevent cancer are: binding to mutagenic compounds thus decreasing their absorption, suppression of the growth of bacteria which convert procarcinogens to carcinogens, decreasing the activity of enzymes predictive of neoplasm including β-glucuronidase, nitroreductase and choloylglycine hydrolase as well as enhancing immune responses (Roos, and Katan, 2000). Inflammation plays a major role in both initiation and progression of diabetes (Duncan, et al., 2003; Pickup, and Frcpath, 2004). By reducing inflammatory responses, probiotics have been shown to correct insulin sensitivity and reduce development of diabetes mellitus. This anti-inflammatory effect has been proposed to be rooted in immunomodulatory properties of probiotic bacteria (Lye, et al., 2009). By reducing cholesterol absorption in the gut, incorporation of cholesterol into cell membranes, enzymatically deconjugation of bile salts and conversion of cholesterol to coprostanol, probiotics can reduce blood cholesterol (Lye, et al., 2009; Ooi, and Liong, 2010). Release of angiotensin converting enzyme (ACE) inhibitory peptides from the parent protein through proteolytic action explains how probiotics can exert antihypertensive effects (Lye, et al., 2009).

3. Dairy probiotic foods

Dairy probiotic foods are scientifically documented as having physiological benefits beyond those of basic nutritional values. Dairy products such as ice cream, cheese, yogurt, acidophilus-bifidus-milk, ayran, kefir, kumis, doogh containing probiotics and milk having omega-3, phytosterols, isoflavins, CLA, minerals, and vitamins have an outstanding position in the development of functional foods (Homayouni, et al., 2008b; Homayouni, et al., 2008c). Dairy beverages (both fermented and non-fermented) have long been considered as important vehicles for the delivery of probiotics. In fermentation process, lactic acid, acetic acid and citric acid are naturally produced which are commonly used organic acids to enhance organoleptic qualities as well as safety of many food products. Lactic acid bacteria are found to be more tolerant to acidity and organic acids than most of the pathogens and spoilage microorganisms (Homayouni, et al., 2008d).

4. Coronary heart disease (CHD)

Coronary heart disease (CHD) is one of the major causes of death in adults in the developed and developing countries which is referred to the condition in which the main coronary arteries supplying the heart are no longer able to supply sufficient blood and oxygen to the heart muscle (myocardium). The main cause of the reduced flow is an accumulation of plaques, mainly in the intima of arteries, a disease known as atherosclerosis (Akbarzadeh etal., 2003; Ranjbar et al., 2007b; Akbarzadeh etal., 2010; Ghaffari etal., 2010).

5. Main risk factors of coronary heart disease

CHD has assumed almost epidemic proportions in wealthy societies, whereas rheumatic heart disease is common in developing countries (Akbarzadeh etal., 2003; Akbarzadeh etal., 2008). Known risk factors of CHD can be classified into those that cannot be modified (being male increasing age, genetic traits including lipid metabolism abnormalities, body build, ethnic origin), those that can be changed (cigarette smoking, hyperlipidaemia, low levels of high density lipoprotein, obesity, hypertension, low physical activity, increased thrombosis, stress, alcohol consumption), those associated with disease states (diabetes and glucose intolerance) and those related to geographic distribution (climate and season, cold weather, soft drinking water) (Lovegrove and Jackson, 2003; Akbarzadeh etal., 2009a). It has been demonstrated that there is a strong and consistent relationship between total plasma cholesterol and CHD risk (Martin et al., 1986). Accumulation of LDL in the plasma leads to a deposition of cholesterol in the arterial wall, a process that involves oxidative modification of the LDL particles. The oxidized LDL is taken up by macrophages, which finally become foam cells and forms the basis of the early atherosclerotic plaque. It has been estimated that every 1% increase in LDL cholesterol level leads to a 2-3% increase in CHD risk (Gensini et al., 1998; Akbarzadeh etal., 2009b). HDL cholesterol levels are higher in women than in men. Factors that may lead to reduced HDL cholesterol levels include smoking, low physical activity and diabetes mellitus; whereas those that increase levels include moderate alcohol consumption (Assmann et al., 1998; Akbarzadeh etal., 2009c).

6. Probiotics and CHD: Mechanism of action

Diet is considered to control the risk of CHD through its effects on certain risk factors including blood lipids, blood pressure and probably also through thrombogenic mechanisms. New evidences suggest a protective role for dietary antioxidants such as vitamins E and C and carotenes, possibly through a mechanism that prevents the oxidation of LDL cholesterol particles (Lovegrove and Jackson, 2003). The diet is one of the adjustable risk factors associated with CHD risk which is recommends to reduce total fat (especially saturated fat), increasing Non-starch polysaccharides (NSP) intake and consumption of fruit and vegetables is advice that is expected to be associated with overall benefits on health.

As a result of low consumer compliance of low-fat diets, attempts have been made to identify other dietary components that can reduce blood cholesterol levels. These have included investigations into the possible hypocholesterolaemic properties of milk products, especially in a fermented form. 18% fall in plasma cholesterol after feeding 4-5 liters of fermented milk per day for three weeks (Mann, and Spoerry, 1974).

The mechanisms of action of probiotics on cholesterol reduction are physiological actions of the end products of fermentation SCFAs, cholesterol assimilation, deconjugation of bile acids and cholesterol binding to bacterial cell walls. The SCFAs that are produced by the bacterial anaerobic breakdown of carbohydrate are acetic, propionic and butyric. It has been well documented that microbial bile acid metabolism is a irregular probiotic effect involved in the therapeutic role of some bacteria. The deconjugation reaction is catalyzed by conjugated bile acid hydrolase enzyme, which is produced exclusively by bacteria. Deconjugation ability is widely found in many intestinal bacteria including genera Enterococcus, Peptostreptococcus, Bifidobacterium, Fusobacterium, Clostridium, Bacteroides and Lactobacillus (Hylemond, 1985). This reaction releases the amino acid moiety and the deconjugated bile acid, thereby reducing cholesterol reabsorption, by increasing faecal excretion of the deconjugated bile acids. Many in vitro studies have investigated the ability of various bacteria to deconjugate a variety of different bile acids. Grill et al. (1995) reported Bifidobacterium longum as the most efficient bacterium when tested against six different bile salts. Another study reported that Lactobacillus species had varying abilities to deconjugate glycocholate and taurocholate (Gilliland et al., 1985). Studies performed on in vitro responses are useful but in vivo studies in animals and humans are required to determine the full contribution of bile acid deconjugation to cholesterol reduction. Intervention studies on animals and ileostomy patients have shown that oral administration of certain bacterial species led to an increased excretion of free and secondary bile salts (De Smet, et al., 1998; Marteau, et al., 1995).

There is also some in vitro evidence to support the hypothesis that certain bacteria can assimilate (take up) cholesterol. It was reported that L. acidophilus and B. bifidum had the ability to assimilate cholesterol in in vitro studies, but only in the presence of bile and under anaerobic conditions (Gilliland, et al., 1985; Rasic, et al., 1992). However, despite these reports there is uncertainty whether the bacteria are assimilating cholesterol or whether the cholesterol is co-precipitating with the bile salts. Studies have been performed to address this question. Klaver and Meer (1993) concluded that the removal of cholesterol from the growth medium in which L. acidophilus and a Bifidobacterium sp. were growing was not due to assimilation, but due to bacterial bile salt deconjugase activity. The same question was addressed by Tahri et al., (1995) with conflicting results, and they concluded that part of the removed cholesterol was found in the cell extracts and that cholesterol assimilation and bile acid deconjugase activity could occur simultaneously.

The mechanism of cholesterol binding to bacterial cell walls has also been suggested as a possible explanation for hypocholesterolaemic effects of probiotics. Hosona and Tono-oka (1995) reported Lactococcus lactis subsp. biovar had the highest binding capacity for cholesterol of bacteria tested in the study. It was speculated that the binding differences were due to chemical and structural properties of the cell walls, and that even killed cells may have the ability to bind cholesterol in the intestine. The mechanism of action of probiotics on cholesterol reduction could be one or all of the above mechanisms with the ability of different bacterial species to have varying effects on cholesterol lowering. However, more research is required to elucidate fully the effect and mechanism of probiotics and their possible hypocholesterolaemic action.

It has been demonstrated that microbial bile acid metabolism is a main effect in the therapeutic role of probiotic bacteria. The deconjugation reaction is catalysed by conjugated bile acid hydrolase enzyme, which is produced by Bifidobacterium and Lactobacillus. This reaction releases the amino acid and deconjugated bile acid, which is reducing cholesterol reabsorption, by increasing faecal elimination of the deconjugated bile acids.

7. Conclusions and future trends

Risk factors known to affect an individual to CHD have been categorized such as hyperlipidaemia, hypertension, obesity, cigarette smoking and lack of exercise. Probiotics may prevent coronary heart disease by cholesterol reduction and microbial bile acid metabolism. The mechanism of action of probiotics on cholesterol reduction include physiological actions of the end products of fermentation SCFAs, cholesterol assimilation, deconjugation of bile acids and cholesterol binding to bacterial cell walls. It has been demonstrated that microbial bile acid metabolism is a peculiar probiotic effect involved in the therapeutic role of some bacteria. Deconjugation reaction is catalyzed by conjugated bile acid hydrolase enzyme, which is produced exclusively by bacteria. The mechanism of cholesterol binding to bacterial cell walls has also been suggested as a possible explanation for hypocholesterolaemic effects of probiotics. Probiotics have beneficial effects on the gut microflora and links to their systemic effects on the lowering of lipids known to be risk factors for CHD, notably cholesterol and TAG. In recent years, several probiotic foods were produced industrially. These foods have received attention for their beneficial effects on the gut microflora and links to their systemic effects on the lowering of lipids known to be risk factors for CHD. For progress to be made, the consumers need to be educated about the various health benefits and how they will be able to use these products in their own diet without adverse consequences. Also to make these foods attractive to the consumer, the products need to be priced in such a way that they are accessible to the general public.

Author details

Fariborz Akbarzadeh*
Faculty of Medicine, Tabriz University of Medical Sciences, Tabriz, I.R. Iran
Cardiovascular Research Center, Tabriz University of Medical Sciences, Tabriz, Iran

Aziz Homayouni
Department of Food Science and Technology, Faculty of Health and Nutrition,
Tabriz University of Medical Sciences, Tabriz, I.R. Iran

8. References

Akbarzadeh, F. and Toufan, M. (2008). Atrioventricular Delays, Cardiac Output and Diastolic function in patient with implanted dual chamber pacing and sensing pacemakers, Pakistan Journal of Biological Sciences, 11 (20): 2407-2412.

Akbarzadeh, F., Hejazi, M. E., Koshavar, H. and Pezeshkian, M. (2003). Prevalence of cardiovascular diseases and cardiac risk factors in north western Tabriz, Medical Journal of Tabriz University of Medical Sciences, 11-15.

Akbarzadeh, F., Kazemi, B. and Pourafkari, L. (2009a). Supraventricular Arrhythmia Induction by an implantable cardioverter defibrillator in a patient with hypertrophic cardiomyopathy, Journal compilation, 1-5.

Akbarzadeh, F., Kazemi-arbat, B., Golmohammadi, A. and Pourafkari, L. (2009b). Biatrial Pacing vs. Intravenous amiodarone in prevention of atrial fibrillation after coronory artery bypass surgery, Pakistan Journal of Biological Sciences, 12 (19): 1325-1329.

Akbarzadeh, F., Pourafkari, L., Mohammad Hashemi Jazi, S., Hesami, L. and Habibi, H. (2010). Prevalence and severity of cad among hypertensive and normotensive patients undergoing elestive coronary angiographi in Tabrize madani heart center, ARYA Atherosclerosis Journal, 5: 1-5.

Akbarzadeh, F., Ranjbar kouchaksaraei, F., Bagheri, Z. and Ghezel, M. (2009c). Effect of Preoperative information and reassurance in decreasing anxiety of patients who are candidate for coronary artery bypass graft surgery, J. Cudirwsc. Thoruc. Rs. 25-28.

Akbarzadeh, F., Toufan, M. and Afsarpour, N. (2008). AV Interval and cardiac output in patient with implanted DDD pacemaker, Research Journal of Biological Sciences, 3 (12): 1381-1386.

Allen, S. J., Martinez, E. G., Gregorio, G. V. and Dans, L. F. (2010). Probiotics for treating acute infectious diarrhoea. Chocrane Collaboration.

Assmann, G., Cullen, P. and Schulte, H. (1998). The Münster Heart Study (PROCAM): Results of follow-up at 8 years, Eur. Heart J. 19: 2-11.

---

* Corresponding Author

De Smet, I., De Boever, P. and Verstraete, W. (1998). Cholesterol lowering in pigs through enhanced bacterial bile salt hydrolase activity, BJN, 79: 185-194.

Duncan, B. B, Schmidt, M. I., Pankow, J. S. and Ballantyne, C. M. (2003). Low-Grade Systemic Inflammation and the Development of Type 2 Diabetes. Diabetes; 52: 1799-1805.

Ejtahed, H. S. and Homayouni Rad, A. (2010). Effects of Probiotics on the Prevention and Treatment of Gastrointestinal Disorders. Microbial biotechnological journal of Islamic Azad University, 2(4): 53-60 [Persian].

Gensini, G. F., Comeglio, M. and Colella, A. (1998). Classical risk factors and emerging elements in the risk profile for coronary artery disease, Eur. Heart J. 19: 52-61.

Ghaffari, S., Akbarzadeh, F. and Pourafkari, L. (2010). Aneurysmal coronary arteriovenous fistula closing with covered stent deployment: A case report and review of literature, Cardiology Journal, 17: 1-4.

Gilliland, S. E., Nelson, C. R. and Maxwell, C. (1985). Assimilation of cholesterol by Lactobacillus acidophilus, Appl. Environ. Microbiol. 49(2): 377-381.

Grill, J. P., Manginot-durr, C., Schneider, F. and Ballongue, J. (1995). Bifidobacteria and probiotic effects: action of Bifidobacterium species on conjugated bile salts, Curr. Microbiol. 31: 23-27.

Homayouni, A. (2008a). Therapeutical effects of functional probiotic, prebiotic and symbiotic foods. (1st ed.). Tabriz University of Medical Sciences. Tabriz. Iran.

Homayouni, A. (2009). Letter to the editor. Food Chemistry, 114: 1073-1073.

Homayouni, A., Azizi, A., Ehsani, M. R., Razavi, S. H. and Yarmand, M. S. (2008b). Effect of microencapsulation and resistant starch on the probiotic survival and sensory properties of synbiotic ice cream. Food Chemistry, 111: 50-55.

Homayouni, A., Ehsani, M. R., Azizi, A, Yarmand, M. S. and Razavi, S. H. (2007). Effect of lecithin and calcium chloride solution on the microencapsulation process yield of calcium alginate beads. Iranian Polymer Journal, 16(9): 597-606.

Homayouni, A., Ehsani, M. R., Azizi, A., Razavi, S. H. and Yarmand, M. S. (2008c). Spectrophotometrically evaluation of probiotic growth in liquid media. Asian Journal of Chemistry, 20(3): 2414-2420.

Homayouni, A., Ehsani, M. R., Azizi, A., Razavi, S. H. and Yarmand, M. S. (2008d). Growth and survival of some probiotic strains in simulated ice cream conditions. Journal of Applied Sciences, 8(2): 379-382.

Hosono, A. and Tono-Oka T. (1995). Binding of cholesterol with lactic acid bacterial cells, Milchwissenschaft, 50(20): 556-560.

Hylemond, P. B. (1985). Metabolism of bile acids in intestinal microflora. In H. Danielson and J. Sjovall (eds), pp. 331-343, Sterols and Bile Acids, New York, Elsevier Science.

Klaver, F. A. M. and Van Der Meer, R. (1993). The assumed assimilation of cholesterol by lactobacilli and Bifidobacterium bifidum is due to their bile salt-deconjugating activity, Appl. Environ. Microbiol. 59(4): 1120-1124.

Lebeer, S., Vanderleyden, J. and Keersmaecker, S. C. J. (2010). Host interactions of probiotic bacterial surface molecules: comparison with commensals and pathogens. Nature Reviews Microbiology, 8: 171-184.

Lovegrove, J. and Jackson, K. (2003). Coronary heart disease in: Functional dairy products, (Eds: Tiina Mattila-Sandholm and Maria Saarela). Woodhead Publishing Ltd and CRC Press LLC. England, pp: 54-93.

Lye, H. S., Kuan, C. Y., Ewe, J. A., Fung, W. Y. and Liong, M. T. (2009). The improvement of hypertension by probiotics: effects on chelesterol, diabetes, renin and phytoesterogens. International Journal of Dairy Sciences, 10: 3755-3775.

Mai, V. and Draganov, P. V. (2009). Recent advances and remaining gaps in our knowledge of associations between gut microbiota and human health. World J Gastroenterol, 15(1): 81-85.

Mann, G. V. and Spoerry A. (1974). Studies of a surfactant and cholesteremia in the Maasai, Am J Clin Nutr 27: 464-469.

Marteau, P., Gerhardt, M. F., Myara, A., Bouvier, E., Trivin, F. and Rambaud, J. C. (1995). Metabolism of bile salts by alimentary bacteria during transit in human small intestine, Microbiol. Ecol. in Health and Disease, 8: 151-157.

Martin, M. J., Browener, W. S., Wentworth, J., Hulley, S. B. and Kuler, L. H. (1986). Serum cholesterol, blood pressure and mortality: implications from a cohort of 361662 men, Lancet, 2: 933-936.

Mustapha, A., Jiang, T. and Savaiano, D. A. (1997). Improvement of lactose digestion by humans following ingestion of unfermented acidophilus milk: influence of bile sensitivity, lactose transport and acid tolerance of lactobacilus acidophilus. Journal of Dairy Sciences, 80: 1537-1545.

Ooi, L. G. and Liong, M. T. (2010). Cholesterol-lowering effects of probiotics and prebiotics: a review of in vivo and in vitro findings. International Journal of molecular Sciences, 11: 2499-2522.

Pickup, J. C. and Frcpath, D. (2004). Inflammation and Activated Innate Immunity in the Pathogenesis of Type 2 Diabetes. Diabetes Care, 27: 813-823.

Ranjbar, F., Akbarzade, F. and Hashemi, M. (2007a). Quality of life of patients with impianted cardiac pacemakers in north west of Iran, ARYA Atherosclerosis Journal, 2 (4):197-203.

Ranjbar, F., Akbarzadeh, F., Kazemi, B. and Safaeiyan, A. (2007b). Relaxation therapy in the background of standard antihypertensive drug treatment is effective in management of moderate to severe essential hypertension, Relaxation therapy in management of hypertension, 32: 120-124.

Rasic, J. L., Vujicic, I. F., Skrinjar, M. and Vulic, M. (1992). Assimilation of cholesterol by some cultures of lactic acid bacteria and bifidobacteria, Biotech. Lett. 14 (1): 39-44.

Roos, N. M. and Katan, M. B. (2000). Effects of probiotic bacteria on diarrhea, lipid metabolism and carcinogenesis: a review of papers published between 1988 and 1998. American journal of clinical nutrition, 71: 405-411.

Shah, N. P. (2007). Functional cultures and health benefits. International dairy journal, 17: 1262-1277.

Tahri, K., Crocciani, J., Ballongue, J. and Schneider, F. (1995). Effects of three strains of bifidobacteria on cholesterol, Lett. Appl. Microbiol. 21: 149-151.

Chapter 7

Milk and Dairy Products:
Vectors to Create Probiotic Products

Gabriel-Danut Mocanu and Elisabeta Botez

Additional information is available at the end of the chapter

1. Introduction

The most important function of alimentation is represented by the assurance of human metabolic needs as well as wellbeing and satisfaction induced by sensorial characteristics of food. In the same time, by modulating some target functions of the body, the food components might have benefic psychological and physiological effects, beside the nutritional ones, already accepted.

In fact, food must contribute to health improving/protection and sustain systems of defence against different aggressions. We are situated at a new frontier of nutrition, in which the foods are evaluated by their biological potential and by their ability to reduce the risk of developing certain diseases. We can talk today about the fact that food for health represent an expanding field: *probiotic functional food*.

In essence, probiotic functional food are products that, by their biological active compounds and consumed in current diets, contribute to optimal human physical and psihycal health.

The appearance and development of functional probiotic food are the response of production field to the results of cellular and molecular biology field research, which demonstrates the implication of food components in proper functioning cellules and subcelular structures. The importance of these studies is essential in contemporaneous context in which the environment assaults by many ways the human body, fully stressing it's protection, adaption and equilibrium maintenance systems. By their specific action, the food components might contribute to the maintain the normal parameters of cellular edificium and of the human body equilibrium.

Nowadays we are assisting to an intensification of research in food – alimentation – health relationship field. The ideea that food might increase/defend health due to active biological components from it's composition conquers more and more acceptability in the scientific community and there are many publication in this field. Unlike the last years, the customers from many countries become more and more interested in health beneficial determined by alimentation, including probiotic functional food. In Romania, even before the adherence to UE, there were registered studies concerning manufacturing of probiotic functional foods, especially in dairy industry and explaining the induced benefits for health.

In this trend of food science are included some of the studies developed over the years by researchers from Galati Food Science and Engineering Faculty.

2. Probiotics: What are they?

2.1. Definitions

The name probiotic comes from the Greek „pro bios" which means „for life". The history of probiotics began with the history of man; cheese and fermented milk were well known to the Greeks and Romans, who recommended their consumption, especially for children and convalescents. Probiotics are defined as the living microorganisms administered in a sufficient number to survive in the intestinal ecosystem. They must have a positive effect on the host [1].

The term „probiotic" was first used by [2] in 1965 to describe the „substances secreted by one microorganism that stimulate the growth of another". A powerful evolution of this definition was coined by [3] in 1974, who proposed that probiotics are „organisms and substances which contribute to intestinal microbial balance" [4]. In more modern definitions, the concept of an action on the gut microflora, and even that of live microorganisms disappeared [5] in 1998 defined probiotics as the „food which contains live bacteria beneficial to health", whereas [6] in 2001 defined them as „microbial cell preparations or components of microbial cells that have a beneficial effect on the health and well-being".

Some modern definitions include more precisely a preventive or therapeutic action of probiotics. [7] in 1997 for example, defined probiotics as „microorganisms which, when ingested, may have a positive effect in the prevention and treatment of a specific pathologic condition". Finally, since probiotics have been found to be effective in the treatment of some gastrointestinal diseases [6], they can be considered to be therapeutic agents. It is clear that a number of definitions of the term „probiotic" have been used over the years but the one derived by the Food and Agriculture Organization of the United Nations/World Health Organization [8] and endorsed by the International Scientific Association for Probiotics and Prebiotics [9] best exemplifies the breadth and scope of probiotics as they are known today:"live microorganisms which, when administered in adequate amounts, confer a health benefit on the host".

This definition retains historical elements of the use of living organisms for health purposes but does not restrict the application of the term only to oral probiotics with intestinal outcomes [10]. Despite these numerous theoretical definitions, however, the practical question arises whether a given microorganism can be considered to be a probiotic or not.

Some strict criteria have been proposed. [11] in 1992, for example, proposed the following parameters to select a probiotic: total safety for the host, resistance to gastric acidity and pancreatic secretions, adhesion to epithelial cells, antimicrobial activity, inhibition of adhesion of pathogenic bacteria, evaluation of resistance to antibiotics, tolerance to food additives and stability in the food matrix.

The probiotics in use today have not been selected on the basis of all these criteria, but the most commonly used probiotics are the strains of lactic acid bacteria such as *Lactobacillus, Bifidobacterium* and *Streptococcus* (*S. thermophilus*); the first two are known to resist gastric acid, bile salts and pancreatic enzymes, to adhere to colonic mucosa and readily colonize the intestinal tract [4, 12].

2.2. Properties of lactic acid bacteria

The lactic acid bacteria are generally defined as a cluster of lactic acid-producing, low %G+C, non-spore-forming, Gram-positive rods and cocci that share many biochemical, physiological, and genetic properties. They are distinguished from other Gram positive bacteria that also produce lactic acid (e.g., *Bacillus, Listeria*, and *Bifidobacterium*) by virtue of numerous phenotypic and genotypic differences. According to current taxonomy, the lactic acid bacteria group consists of twelve genera (table 1). All are in the phylum *Firmicutes*, Order, *Lactobacillales*. Based on 16S rRNA sequencing and other molecular techniques, the lactic acid bacteria can be grouped into a broad phylogenetic cluster, positioned not far from other low G +C Gram positive bacteria.

Five sub-clusters are evident from this tree, including: (1) a *Streptococcus-Lactococcus* branch (Family *Streptococcaceae*), (2) a *Lactobacillus* branch (Family *Lactobacillaceae*), (3) a separate *Lactobacillus-Pediococcus* branch (Family *Lactobacillaceae*); (4) an *Oenococcus-Leuconostoc-Weisella* branch (Family *Leuconostocaceae*), and (5) a *Carnobacterium-Aerococcus-Enterococcus-Tetragenococcus-Vagococcus* branch (Families *Carnobacteriaceae, Aerococcaceae*, and *Enterococcaceae*).

Seven of the twelve genera of lactic acid bacteria, *Lactobacillus, Lactococcus, Leuconostoc, Oenococcus, Pediococcus, Streptococcus*, and *Tetragenococcus*, are used directly in food fermentations. Although *Enterococcus* sp. Are often found in fermented foods (e.g., cheese, sausage, fermented vegetables), except for a few occasions, they are not added directly. In fact, their presence is often undesirable, in part, because they are sometimes used as indicators of fecal contamination and also because some strains may harbor mobile antibioticresistance genes.

Importantly, some strains of *Enterococcus* are capable of causing infections in humans. Likewise, *Carnobacterium* are also undesirable, mainly because they are considered as spoilage organisms in fermented meat products. Finally, species of *Aerococcus, Vagococcus*, and *Weisella* are not widely found in foods, and their overall significance in food is unclear.

2.3. Probiotics as functional foods

In the last decades consumer demands in the field of food production has changed considerably. Consumers more and more believe that foods contribute directly to their health [13, 14]. Today foods are not intended to only satisfy hunger and to provide necessary nutrients for humans but also to prevent nutrition-related diseases and improve physical and mental well-being of the consumers [15, 16].

Genus	Cell morphology	Fermentation route	Growth at		Growth in NaCl at		Growth at pH		Lactic acid isomer
			10°C	45°C	6.5%	18%	4.4	9.6	
Lactobacillus	rods	homo/hetero[4]	±[5]	±	±	-	±	-	D, L, DL[6]
Lactococcus	cocci	homo	+	-	-	-	±	-	L
Leuconostoc	cocci	hetero	+	-	±	-	±	-	D
Oenococcus	cocci	hetero	+	+	±	-	±	-	D
Pediococcus	cocci (tetrads)	homo	±	±	±	-	+	-	D, L, DL
Streptococcus	cocci	homo	-	+	-	-	-	-	L
Tetragenococcus	cocci (tetrads)	homo	+	-	+	+	-	+	L
Aerococcus	cocci (tetrads)	homo	+	-	+	-	-	+	L
Carnobacterium	rods	hetero	+	-	-	-	-	-	L
Enterococcus	cocci	homo	+	+	+	-	+	+	L
Vagococcus	cocci	homo	+	-	-	-	±	-	L
Weisella	coccoid	hetero	+	-	±	-	±	-	D, L, DL

[1]Adapted from [17]
[2]Adapted from [18]
[3]Refers to the general properties of the genus; some exceptions may exist
[4]Species of Lactobacillus may be homofermentative, heterofermentative, or both
[5]This phenotype is variable, depending on the species
[6]Some species produce D-, L-, or a mixture of D- and L-lactic acid.

Table 1. Genera of lactic acid bacteria and their properties [1,2,3]

In this regard, functional foods play an outstanding role. The increasing demand on such foods can be explained by the increasing cost of healthcare, the steady increase in life expectancy, and the desire of older people for improved quality of their later years [19, 15, 20].

The term "functional food" itself was first used in Japan, in the 1980s, for food products fortified with special constituents that possess advantageous physiological effects [21, 22]. Functional foods may improve the general conditions of the body (e.g. pre- and probiotics), decrease the risk of some diseases (e.g. cholesterol-lowering products), and could even be used for curing some illnesses.

The European Commission's Concerted Action on Functional Food Science in Europe (FuFoSE), coordinated by International Life Science Institute (ILSI) Europe defined functional food as follows: "a food product can only be considered functional if together with the basic nutritional impact it has beneficial effects on one or more functions of the human organism thus either improving the general and physical conditions or/and decreasing the risk of the evolution of diseases. The amount of intake and form of the functional food should be as it is normally expected for dietary purposes. Therefore, it could not be in the form of pill or capsule just as normal food form" [23].

European legislation however, does not consider functional foods as specific food categories, but rather a concept [22, 24]. Therefore, the rules to be applied are numerous and depend on the nature of the foodstuff. Functional foods have been developed in virtually all food categories. From a product point of view, the functional property can be included in numerous different ways as it can be seen in table 2.

Type of functional food	Definition	Example
Fortified product	A food fortified with additional nutrients	Fruit juices fortified with vitamin C
Enriched products	A food with added new nutrients or components not normally found in a particular food	Margarine with plant sterol ester, probiotics, prebiotics
Altered products	A food from which a deleterious component has been removed, reduced or replaced with another substance with beneficial effects	Fibers as fat releasers in meat or ice cream products
Enhanced commodities	A food in which one of the components has been naturally enhanced through special growing conditions, new feed composition, genetic manipulation, or otherwise	Eggs with increased omega-3 content achieved by altered chicken feed

Table 2. Prominent types of functional food [20, 25, 26]

It should be emphasized however, that this is just one of the possible classifications. According to alternative classification, some functional products are (1) "add good to your life", e.g. improve the regular stomach and colon functions (pre- and probiotics) or "improve children's life" by supporting their learning capability and behaviour. It is difficult, however to find good biomarkers for cognitive, behavioural and psychological, functions. Other group (2) of functional food is designed for reducing an existing health risk problem such as high cholesterol or high blood pressure. A third group (3) consists of those products, which "makes your life easier" (e.g. lactose-free, gluten-free products) [27].

These products have been mainly launched in the dairy-, confectionery-, soft-drinks-, bakery- and baby-food market [16, 20, 26].

3. Health benefits of probiotics

Since Metchnikoff's era, a number of health benefits have been contributed to products containing probiotic organisms. While some of these benefits have been well documented and established, others have shown a promising potential in animal models, with human studies required to substantiate these claims. More importantly, health benefits imparted by probiotic bacteria are very strain specific; therefore, there is no universal strain that would provide all proposed benefits, not even strains of the same species. Moreover, not all the strains of the same species are effective against defined health conditions. Some of these strain specific health effects are presented in figure 1.

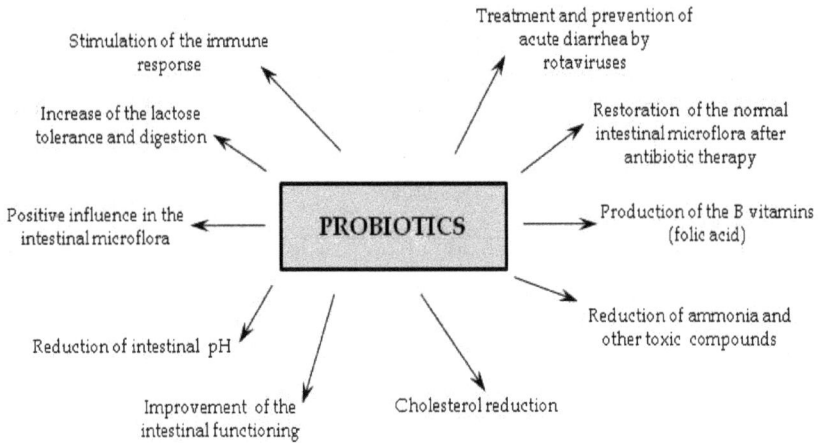

Figure 1. Probiotic beneficial effects on human health [28, 29]

4. Probiotic dairy products

Foods that affect specific functions or systems in the human body, providing health benefits beyond energy and nutrients—functional foods—have experienced rapid market growth in recent years. This growth is fueled by technological innovations, development of new products, and the increasing number of health-conscious consumers interested in products that improve life quality. Since the global market of functional foods is increasing annually, food product development is a key research priority and a challenge for both the industry and science sectors. Probiotics show considerable promise for the expansion of the dairy industry, especially in such specific sectors as yogurts, cheeses, beverages, ice creams, and other desserts. This book chapter presents an overview of functional foods and strategies for their development, with particular attention to probiotic dairy products.

4.1. Types of probiotic dairy product

The most common probiotic dairy products worldwide are various types of yogurt, other fermented dairy product, various lactic acid bacteria drinks and mixture of probiotic (fermented) milks and fruit juice. Probiotic cheese, both fresh and ripened, have also been launched recently. In table 3 are listed some dairy functional food products that have been developed recently in Faculty of Food Science and Engineering.

4.1.1. Fermented milks and beverages

Fermented milks and beverages make up an important contribution to the human diet in many countries because fermentation is an inexpensive technology, which preserves the food, improves its nutritional value and enhances its sensory properties.

Type of dairy functional food products	Description/Name
Fermented dairy products	Drink yogurts with La-5 and carrot juice/ BIOCOV
	Yogurt with La-5 and biomass of *Spirulina platensis*/YLaSP
	Yogurt with BB 12 and biomass of *Spirulina platensis*/YBbSP
	Yogurt with ABY 3/ABT 5 and medicinal plant extracts/ AFINOLACT
	Yogurt with ABY 3/ABT 5 and medicinal plant extracts/ CATINOLACT
	Yogurt with ABY 3/ABT 5 and medicinal plant extracts/ ROSALACT
Cheeses	Dessert based on fresh cheese and some fruit pulp
	Appetizer – type fresh cheese
	Probiotic Telemea cheese

Table 3. Some examples of dairy probiotic products developed

[30, 31] in 2011, proposed the realization of a probiotic dairy drink with added carrot juice. This probiotic product was obtained using goat milk (fat = 3.63%, proteins = 3.05%, lactose = 4.55%, dry matter = 12.05% and density = 1.030 $g \cdot mL^{-1}$) which has been pasteurized at a temperature of 72ºC, for 20 minutes, a probiotic culture type Nutrish containing *Lactobacillus acidophilus* La-5 and carrot juice (dry matter = 9.35%, pH = 6.23, titratable acidity = 0.14 malic acid/100g, ash = 0.7%). After pasteurization, milk was quickly cooled to inoculation temperature at 37°C. The incubation of obtained fermented dairy drink was made at 37°C for 5 hours.

The addition of carrot juice (at a percentage of 10%) had a positive effect on physical – chemical and microbiological parameters of fermented dairy drink. Combining goat milk with carrot juice can get some food with potential therapeutic role.

As a result of the lactose fermentation, the titratable acidity increased fast during the incubation period. At the end of the storage period (after 5 days), the highest value of titratable acidity was 61 ºT. The pH of the obtained new product decreased during incubation period, and will stabilize during storage period, pH = 5.1 after 5 days of storage. The evolution of the number of microorganisms was analyzed for each sample during incubation and storage period. It was observed that the fermented dairy drink with added carrot juice product had been preserving its functional properties during storage (over 10^8 $cfu \cdot mL^{-1}$ probiotic bacteria).

The products were analyzed in terms of fluid flow thus establishing their rheological behavior. The literature shows that the rheological properties of fermented dairy products depend on the development of lactic bacteria as a consequence of metabolic changes leading physicochemical substrate in milk.

In figure 2 is presented the variation of shearing stress (τ, Pa) according to the shearing rate ($\dot{\gamma}$, s^{-1}). There was determined that samples have a rheological behavior similar with the one of the non-Newtonian fluids, time independent, therefore a pseudoplastic behavior. Specific for a fluid with this type of behavior is the flow resistance decrease as a result of the fluid shearing rate increase.

For all samples, it was noted that for low values of shear rate, tangential shear stress variation depending on shear rate was increasing (regression coefficient R^2 values varies from 0.962 and 0.995).

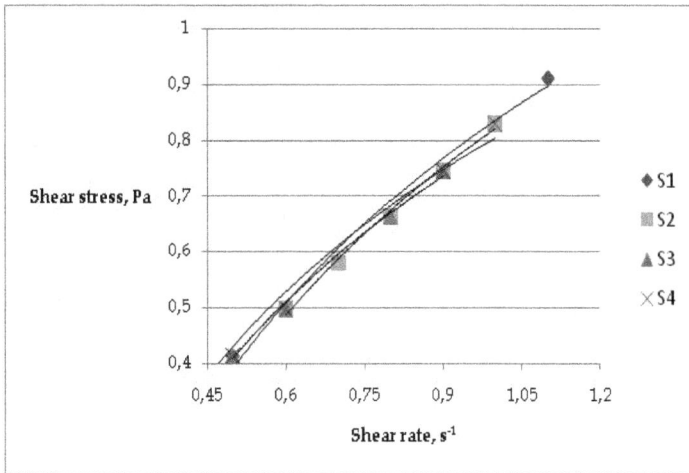

Figure 2. The shearing stress variation according to the shearing rate

To obtain yoghurt with *Spirulina platensis* biomass was used pasteurized cow milk (non fat dry matter = 9.08%, fat = 1.5%, proteins = 3.52%, lactose = 4.32%, mineral salts = 0.72%). Pasteurization of milk is achieved by maintaining standardized milk at 95 °C for 5 minutes. After pasteurization, milk was cooled to inoculation temperature at 42°C.

The inoculation of milk for obtaining these fermented dairy products is with a probiotic culture containing *Lactobacillus acidophilus* La-5 respectively *Bifidobacterium lactis* BB 12, at this time was added and biomass of *Spirulina platensis* (0.5 – 1% according to [32]).

After inoculation follows the distribution and packaging and incubation was made at 42°C for 6 hours in the thermostats set at the optimal temperature for the development of these bacteria. Meanwhile yoghurt gel gets a specific consistency. Cooling and storage of obtained yoghurts is performed at 6 °C for 15 days. In this storage period, coagulum is more compact, the flavor and taste become more pleasant. As a result of the lactose fermentation, the titratable acidity increased. This is slightly higher for the samples with La 5 from those with BB12.

All products with Spirulina platensis biomass have titratable acidity higher than control sample (1.1 times higher for samples with BB 12 and 1.2 times higher for samples with La 5).

The evolution of pH is correlated with lactose fermentation intensity and increased with titratable acidity, but in the same time it is influenced by the buffer substances that are found in *Spirulina platensis* biomass or formed during the manufacture of yoghurt. The pH of fermented dairy products fall between the values 4.11 and 4.53, values considered normal for such products.

The addition of *Spirulina platensis* biomass (figure 3) has positively influenced the number of viable probiotic microorganisms.

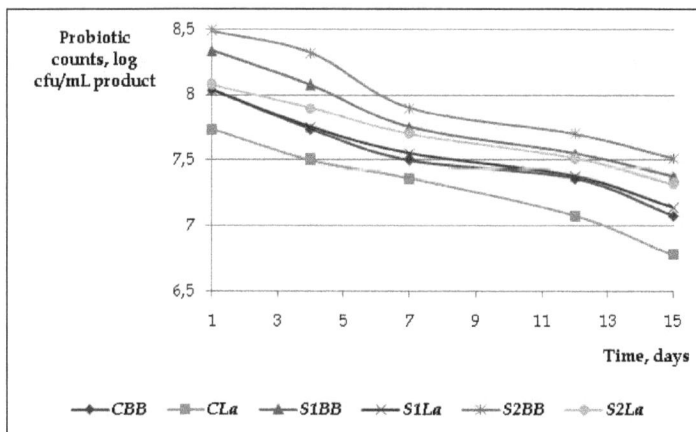

Figure 3. Viable counts variation during storage period

At the end of the storage period (after 15th days) the number of probiotic lactic bacteria for both, control samples and samples with *Spirulina platensis* biomass is still high, which shows that the product with *Spirulina platensis* biomass has been preserving its functional properties during storage period.

4.1.2. Cheeses

Perhaps no other fermented food starts with such a simple raw material and ends up with products having such an incredible diversity of color, flavor, texture, and appearance as does cheese. It is even more remarkable that milk, pale in color and bland in flavor, can be transformed into literally hundreds of different types of flavorful, colorful cheeses by manipulating just a few critical steps.

Just what happened to cause the milk to become transformed into a product with such a decidedly different appearance, texture, and flavor? To answer that question, it is first necessary to compare the composition of the starting material, milk, to that of the product, the finished cheese (figure 4).

In an attempt to diversify the range of probiotic dairy products, there has been made a series of research on the introduction of probiotic bacteria in cheese. According to [33], cheese is an

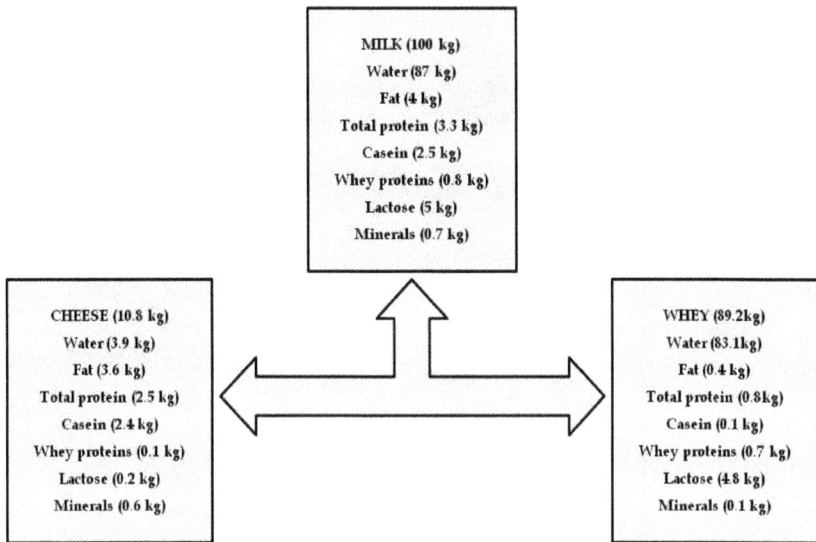

Figure 4. Partition of milk into cheese and whey (adapted from [18]).

interesting way of supplying probiotic bacteria due to the chemical composition of the raw milk that encourages their growth, metabolism and viability and also due to their relatively low acidity compared to other food products. The most of research has been focused on fresh cheese, but there are published some results on probiotic brined or ripened cheese, too.

Fresh cheese, mixt coagulated, is the most suitable cheese to carry probiotic bacteria, due to the high composition of nutrients, low acidity and low salt content. In 2009, [34] used probiotic fresh cheese and peach pulp in order to obtain a dessert, according to figure 5. Probiotic bacteria, *Lactobacillus acidophilus* La 5, was introduced in the fresh cheese as an agent of milk maturation, during coagulation stage. The product was rich in nutritive components (proteins: 10.9...11.3%; fat: 9.1...10.4% and minerals: 2...2.3%) and has a pseudoplastic rheological behaviour. This influenced the sensorial properties of the product, which achieved a creamy texture including in its structure the minced peach pulp and fat globules from the cream.

The research of the above mentioned authors continued, in the attempt to obtain a similar product using goat milk [35]. The amount of nutrients increased, comparing to the previous product (proteins: 12.4...12.5%; fat: 10.1...12.2% and minerals: 2.1...2.4%) but the rheological behaviour was not affected. Although there was expected a reserved attitude of the consumer because of the unpleasant flavour of goat milk, this was not observed.

In 2010 a new probiotic product based on fresh cheese was obtained, by mixing fresh cheese with caraway, cream and salt. The probiotic bacteria (*Bifidobacterium lactis* BB 12) were introduced in cheese at milk maturation stage. In figure 6 it can be observed that the caraway favourised the development of probiotic bacteria.

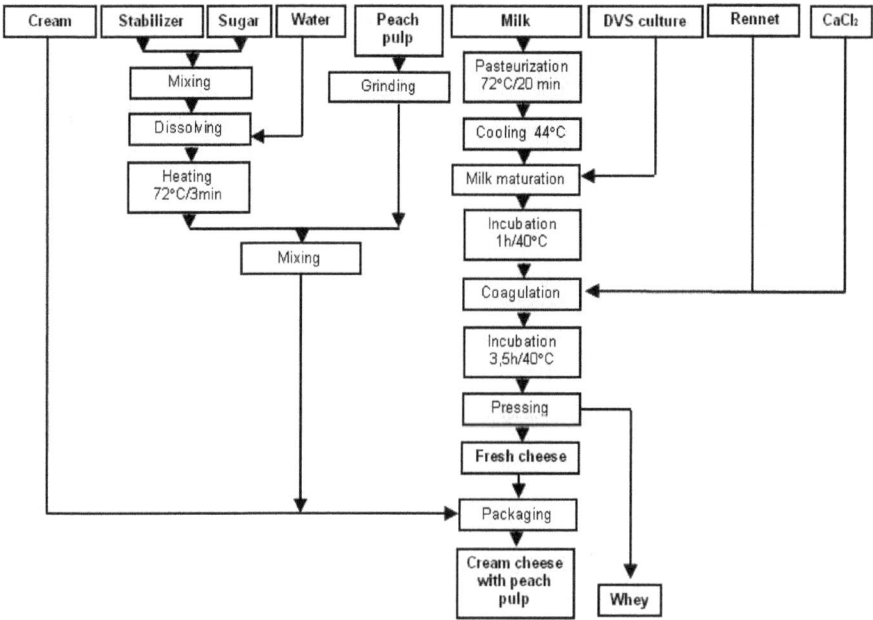

Figure 5. Technological flowchart for manufacturing the new product – Dessert based on fresh cheese and peach pulp

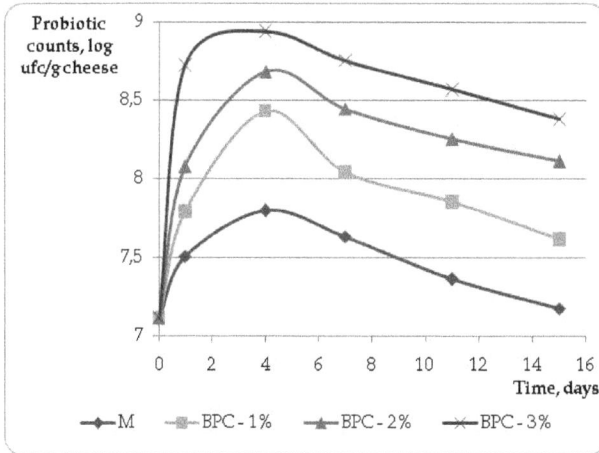

Figure 6. Evolution of bacteria during storage period

[36] and [37] studied the viability of probiotic bacteria *Bifidobacterium lactis*, *Lactobacillus acidophilus* and *Strepococcus thermophilus* in Telemea cheese during ripening and storage time. Telemea is a cheese variety originated in Romania, from where its manufacture spread

to other Balkan countries and Turkey [38]. The specific of this variety of cheese is ripening in brine. Evolution of probiotic bacteria during different stages of manufacturing process is presented in table 4. Conclusion of the study is that Telemea cheese can be considered a probiotic product, even if the high salt concentration disadvantages probiotic bacteria growth, as long as the number of viable cells remains above 10^7 cfu·g^{-1}.

Stage	Bifidobacterium lactis	Lactobacillus acidophilus	Lactobacillus bulgaricus	Streptococcus thermophilus
Inoculated milk	2.71	2.50	2.90	8
Milk, 10 minutes after renneting	2.68	3.21	4	12
Coagulum, before pressing	2.60	7.49	9.40	24.9
Pressed coagulum	2.40	7.29	9.50	24.3
Salted coagulum	2.20	7.20	9.60	22.1
Cheese ripened for 5 days	1.84	6.90	8.90	15
Cheese ripened for 10 days	1.75	6.36	8.40	14.2
Cheese ripened for 15 days	1.65	4.67	7.30	13.4
Cheese ripened for 20 days	1.57	4.21	6.70	12.6
Cheese ripened for 25 days	1.48	3.48	5.30	11.3
Cheese ripened for 30 days	1.41	2.90	4.20	9.1
Cheese ripened for 35 days	0.99	2.31	3.90	7.2
Cheese ripened for 40 days	0.60	2.21	3.50	6

Table 4. Evolution of probiotic bacteria during manufacturing of Telemea cheese (10^7 cfu·g^{-1})

There are registered many other studies about probiotic cheese and methods of manufacturing probiotic cheese. Most of them introduce probiotic bacteria in the milk maturation stage, but there are reports about introducing them after pressing [39] or immobilized on fruit pieces [40].

5. Improvement of benefical effect of probiotic dairy products through the use of bioactive compounds from plants

By sensorial analysis of several combinations milk-medicinal plants, as well as by physical and chemical analysis, there were selected the following medicinal plants: bilberry, sea-buckthorn, rosehip, liquorice, plants rich in active principles considered important for their pharmacological profile.

The research presented in this subchapter was realised on 14 variants of probiotic products (encoded according to table 5), manufactured from cow milk and medicinal plant extracts (bilberry, seabuckthorn, rosehip and liquorice), fermented by two types of probiotic cultures: ABY 3 (*Bifidobacterium lactis, Lactobacillus acidophilus, Lactobacillus delbrueckii* subsp. *bulgaricus* and *Streptococcus thermophilus*) and ABT 5 (*Bifidobacterium lactis, Lactobacillus acidophilus* and *Streptococcus thermophilus*).

Crt. No.	Product	Code	Culture	Description
1.	Control	M – 3		Milk + 0.02% DVS culture
2.	Afinolact	A – 3		Milk + 0.02% DVS culture + 6% bilberry extract
3.		LD+A – 3		Milk + 0.02% DVS culture + 6% bilberry extract + 6% liquorice extract
4.	Cătinolact	C – 3	ABY 3	Milk + 0.02% DVS culture + 6% seabuckthorn extract
5.		LD+C – 3		Milk + 0.02% DVS culture + 6% seabuckthorn extract + 6% liquorice extract
6.	Rosalact	Mă– 3		Milk + 0.02% DVS culture + 6% rosehip extract
7.		LD+Mă – 3		Milk + 0.02% DVS culture + 6% rosehip extract + 6% liquorice extract
8.	Control	M – 5		Milk + 0.02% DVS culture
9.	Afinolact	A – 5		Milk + 0.02% DVS culture + 6% bilberry extract
10.		LD+A – 5		Milk + 0.02% DVS culture + 6% bilberry extract + 6% liquorice extract
11.	Cătinolact	C – 5	ABT 5	Milk + 0.02% DVS culture + 6% seabuckthorn extract
12.		LD+C – 5		Milk + 0.02% DVS culture + 6% seabuckthorn extract + 6% liquorice extract
13.	Rosalact	Mă – 5		Milk + 0.02% DVS culture + 6% rosehip extract
14.		LD+Mă – 5		Milk + 0.02% DVS culture + 6% rosehip extract + 6% liquorice extract

Table 5. Experimental variants

The addition of aqueous medicinal plants extract positively influenced the number of viable probiotic microorganisms. At the end of storage period the number of probiotic lactic bacteria is high for both control samples and samples with medicinal plants, meaning that the products maintain their functional character [31, 41-46].

For the obtain products there was demonstrated the cytoprotective character, by studing the total antioxidant capacity, the total content of polyphenols, the superoxiddismutasic (SOD) activity, the minerals content, the ascorbic acid and anthocyaninis.

The results of the study reveal that probiotic dairy products with added medicinal plants contain a high level of total polyphenols and a high total antioxidant capacity. All these products are an excellent source of minerals with high biodisponibility in human diet. The addition of medicinal plants extract improved the SOD activity.

5.1. Identification of bioactive compounds from plants

Medicinal plants are extremely valuable biological currants. The valorification of this potential represents a never-ending source of raw materials for pharmaceutics and food industry. World Health Organisation has recently announced that 75-80% of world's population is treated with natural remedies.

The plants do not cure all the diseases but they might be extremely helpful in rational treating of some diseases and are not to dangerous. The plants have favourable effect to human body and unfavourable effect to some pathogen agents due to certain substances from their composition. In every plant species there must be known that substance or substances which assure them the therapeutic effect (the active principles).

In order to test the chemical composition of studied plants (bilberry, sea-buckthorn, rosehip and liquorice) there were determined by chemical analysis: ascorbic acid (for seabuckthorn and rosehip), glycyrrhizic acid (for liquorice) and anthocyaninis (for bilberry). The concentrations of the active principles in medicinal plants samples are reported in table 6.

Medicinal plants Active principles	Bilberry (*Vaccinium myrtillus L.*)	Sea-buckthorn (*Hippophaë rhamnoides L.*)	Liquorice (*Glycyrrhiza glabra L.*)	Rosehip (*Rosa canina L.*)
Anthocyanins expressed as cyanidin-3-glucoside chloride	0.38 ± 0.06* (0.32÷0.47)	-	-	-
Ascorbic acid	-	0.8 ± 0.09* (0.66÷0.89)	-	1.24 ± 0.06* (1.18÷1.32)
Glycyrrhizic acid	-	-	5.03 ± 0.32* (4.6÷5.32)	-

The values were expressed in mean ± standard errors of regression and values in parenthesis indicate minimum and maximum level recorded.

Table 6. Active principles in medicinal plants

Regarding the active principles content there was demonstrated that all the analysed medicinal plants respect the values presented in European Pharmacopee, V edition: minimum 0.3% cyanidin–3–glucozide chloride in bilberry, the analysed probes having a maximum content of 0.47%. The ascorbic acid in seabuckthorn must be minimum in 0.5% and in rosehip minimum 1%. The analysed samples registered values of 0.66÷0.98% for seabuckthorn and 1,18% for rosehip. The glycyrrhizic acid, the main active principle in liquorice, must be minimum 4% (according to European Pharmacopee) and the determined values varied between 4.6 and 5.38% [31, 41-46].

5.2. The action of bioactive compounds from plants on probiotic bacteria metabolism

To have a probiotic effect, the strains of probiotic bacteria must be present in the product enough number. It is generally considered that the daily dose of probiotic strains must be between $1 \cdot 10^8$ and $1 \cdot 10^9$ cells. A portion of 100 g, the probiotic product should contain between 10^6 and 10^7 cfu·mL^{-1} product. The addition of aqueous medicinal plant extracts has positively influenced the number of viable probiotic microorganisms due to the presence of fermentable sugars and some growth factors (mineral salts, non-protein nitrogen). At the end of incubation period (after 5 hours), for the samples with medicinal plant extracts the lowest number of microorganisms has established for the samples: Mă–3 ($7.8 \cdot 10^8$ cfu·mL^{-1} probiotic bacteria) or A–5 and C–5 ($1.8 \cdot 10^9$ cfu·mL^{-1} probiotic bacteria) instead the higher number of probiotic bacteria was registered for LD+Mă–3 ($4.5 \cdot 10^9$ cfu·mL^{-1} probiotic bacteria) and LD+Mă–5 ($5.4 \cdot 10^9$ cfu·mL^{-1} probiotic bacteria).

After 8th days of storage period (table 7) the higher number of viable microorganisms was found in the sample with ABT 5 culture (LD+A–5: $2.6 \cdot 10^8$ cfu·mL^{-1} probiotic bacteria), and lowest number of probiotic bacteria cells was recorded for sample with ABY 3 culture (C–3: $0.9 \cdot 10^8$ cfu·mL^{-1} probiotic bacteria). The storage in refrigerated conditions causes a reduction of the number of probiotic bacteria up to 4.37 times in the products obtained with ABY 3 culture and 3.62 times for those with ABT 5.

Microbiological characteristics			
Sample code	cfu·mL^{-1} product	Sample code	cfu·mL^{-1} product
M – 3	$3 \cdot 10^7$	M – 5	$8 \cdot 10^7$
A – 3	$1 \cdot 10^8$	A – 5	$1.4 \cdot 10^8$
LD+A – 3	$1.8 \cdot 10^8$	LD+A – 5	$2.6 \cdot 10^8$
C – 3	$9 \cdot 10^7$	C – 5	$1.1 \cdot 10^8$
LD+C – 3	$1.9 \cdot 10^8$	LD+C – 5	$1.8 \cdot 10^8$
Mă – 3	$1.2 \cdot 10^8$	Mă – 5	$1.3 \cdot 10^8$
LD+Mă – 3	$2.2 \cdot 10^8$	LD+Mă – 5	$2.1 \cdot 10^8$

Table 7. Microbiological characteristics of fermented dairy products wit ABY 3 or ABT 5 after 8th days of storage

At the end of storage period, the number of probiotic lactic acid bacteria for both control samples and for samples with medicinal plant extracts is still high ($1\cdot10^7\div1\cdot10^8$ cfu·mL^{-1} probiotic bacteria), which shows that the products has been preserving its functional properties during storage period. Both cultures can be used in the production of probiotic products [31, 41-46].

Besides the cytoprotective effect conferred by the presence of probiotic bacteria, research has shown that products with added medicinal plants have a increased cytoprotective nature and because the content of biologically active compounds. Experimental results showed that the probiotic fermented dairy product with added medicinal plant extracts have a high content of total polyphenols with beneficial effects on human health, which help to prevent various diseases, such as cardiovascular disease, diabetes [47, 48] and consequently a higher total antioxidant capacity.

The higher amount of total polyphenols (table 8) was determined for samples: LD+Mă–3 (280.78 µg·mL^{-1}) or LD+Mă–5 (285.56 µg·mL^{-1}).

Total polyphenols expressed as catechin, µg·mL^{-1}			
Sample code	ABY 3	Sample code	ABT 5
M – 3	62.086	M – 5	82.086
A – 3	99.91	A – 5	106
LD+A – 3	152.95	LD+A – 5	158.6
C – 3	72.086	C – 5	87.73
LD+C – 3	135.56	LD+C – 5	147.3
Mă – 3	262.95	Mă – 5	239.47
LD+Mă – 3	280.78	LD+Mă – 5	285.56

Table 8. The total polyphenols content for samples with ABY 3 or ABT 5 culture

Compared with control samples (not containing medicinal plant extracts) total antioxidant capacity (Table 9) increased by 3.25-9.94 times in products made with ABY 3 culture and 2.1-8.3 times the ABT 5 products.

TEAC, mM·L^{-1}			
Sample code	ABY 3	Sample code	ABT 5
M – 3	0.16	M – 5	0.2
A – 3	0.57	A – 5	0.43
LD+A – 3	0.70	LD+A – 5	0.73
C – 3	0.52	C – 5	0.48
LD+C – 3	0.81	LD+C – 5	0.62
Mă – 3	1.19	Mă – 5	1.27
LD+Mă – 3	1.59	LD+Mă – 5	1.66

Table 9. Total antioxidant capacity for sample with ABY 3 or ABT 5 culture

For products manufactured with ABY 3 culture and those with ABT 5 was observed that the total antioxidant capacity and total polyphenols content is higher for mixtures with liquorice extract, from the rest of the samples tested, except for samples Mă–3 şi Mă–5.

In addition to being an excellent source of protein, probiotic dairy products based on milk and medicinal plant extracts are a good source of minerals, calcium, potassium, phosphorus, magnesium, zinc. The minerals in these products are from raw milk, and medicinal plant extracts. Because the extracts of bilberry, sea-buckthorn, rosehip and liquorice have different mineral content, the products made have a different content in some microelements.

Distribution of broad in probiotic dairy products based on milk and medicinal plant extracts depends on the content of plant extracts and reactions/associations that occur during the technological process. The results of measurements are presented in Tables 10 and 11.

Crt. No.	Sample name	Microelements content, mg/100g product									
		Ca	Mg	Na	K	Mn	Fe	Zn	Cu	Pb	Cd
1.	M – 3	130	6	36	130	-	0.1	0.4	ND	ND	ND
2.	A – 3	135	7	39	115	0.1	0.15	0.45	ND	ND	ND
3.	C – 3	135	7.5	37.5	125	0.1	0.2	0.5	ND	ND	ND
4.	Mă – 3	137.5	9	41	135	0.1	0.27	0.5	ND	ND	ND
5.	LD+A – 3	140	7.8	47.5	135	0.1	0.21	0.5	ND	ND	ND
6.	LD+C – 3	141	7.8	40	140	0.1	0.25	0.5	ND	ND	ND
7.	LD+Mă - 3	139.5	9.3	46	150	0.1	0.3	0.5	ND	ND	ND

Table 10. Mineral concentration of fermented dairy products with ABY 3 culture

Crt. No.	Sample name	Microelements content, mg/100g product									
		Ca	Mg	Na	K	Mn	Fe	Zn	Cu	Pb	Cd
1.	M – 5	130	6	36	130	-	0.1	0.4	ND	ND	ND
2.	A – 5	135	7	34.5	110	0.1	0.14	0.45	ND	ND	ND
3.	C – 5	140	7.8	32.5	115	0.1	0.21	0.5	ND	ND	ND
4.	Mă – 5	140	8	35	120	0.1	0.25	0.5	ND	ND	ND
5.	LD+A – 5	150	7.5	39.5	140	0.1	0.17	0.5	ND	ND	ND
6.	LD+C – 5	145	8	38	135	0.1	0.23	0.5	ND	ND	ND
7.	LD+Mă–5	147	9	41	140	0.1	0.3	0.5	ND	ND	ND

Table 11. Mineral concentration of fermented dairy products with ABY 5 culture

Minerals in fermented dairy products based on milk and medicinal plant extract fulfill in human body the following functions:

- Are composed of hard tissue: Ca and Mg contribute in a major portion at the formation of the skeleton and teeth. Ca is also one of the most sensitive elements that regulate cellular functions. Is the regulator of enzymes involved in carbohydrate, lipid and protein metabolism, is also involved in important physiological processes such as muscle contraction, blood coagulation, apoptosis and necrosis;

- Are components of soft tissue: Fe and K in the form of organic compounds contribute to muscles, organs and blood. Fe are component of hemoglobin involved in oxygen transport, the of myoglobin, the body's oxygen tank. Fe is considered a major potential prooxidant metals from the human body;
- Are regulators of biological functions: as solubilized salts in body fluids contribute to sensitivity of nervous stimulus, maintain muscle elasticity, adjustment of pH digestive fluids and other secretions, maintaining of osmotic pressure.

Fermented dairy product based on milk and medicinal plant extracts had a higher superoxiddismutase activity. The relationship between the iron and SOD activity is presented in figures 7 and 8.

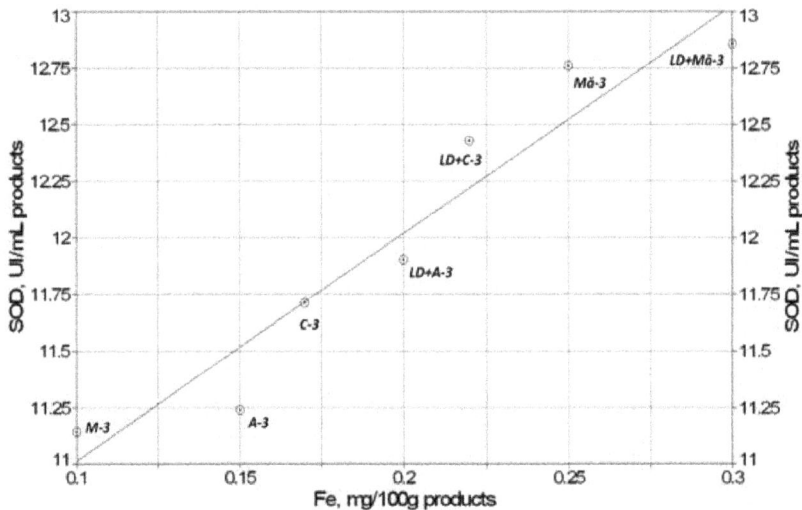

Figure 7. The relationship between SOD activity and iron content of products obtained with ABY 3 culture

For all samples of fermented dairy products with medicinal plant extracts is an increase in SOD activity compared with the control sample. Measured activity is total SOD-like activity (which contributes enzyme as such and superoxiddismutase-like activity of polyphenols and iron or zinc). SOD activity ranged from 11.142 to 12.857 IU·mL^{-1} product; it was maximum for the sample LD+Mă–3. Samples obtained with ABY 3 culture had a higher SOD activity than samples with ABT 5.

5.3. Probiotic dairy products with added plant extracts

To obtain the probiotic dairy products with medicinal plant extracts was used standardized cow milk to 1.5% fat. The technological process for production of fermented dairy products

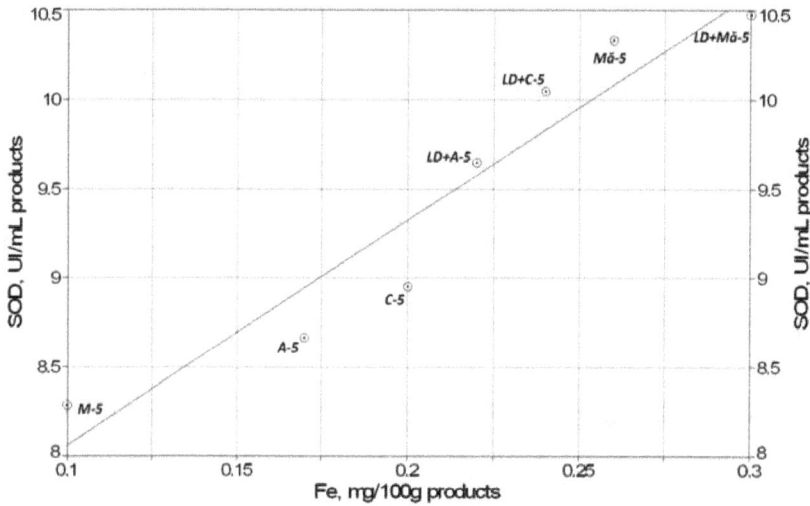

Figure 8. The relationship between SOD activity and iron content of products obtained with ABY 5 culture

Characteristics \ Sample	Bilberries extract	Sea-buckthorn extract	Rosehip extract	Liquorice extract
Dry matter, g/100g	4.84	4.84	5.29	4
Ash insoluble in hydrochloric acid, g/100g	0.74	0.83	0.67	0.81
Total carbohydrate, g/100g	4.69	0.2	7.19	7.29
Total proteins, g/100g	0.21	0.41	0.62	2.15
Calcium, mg/100g product	13.2	4.4	34.5	30
Magnesium, mg/100g product	15.4	4.4	13.8	60
Sodium, mg/100g product	6.6	4.4	8.05	9
Potassium, mg/100g product	132	110	300	230
Manganese, mg/100g product	2.2	2.2	1.38	0.4
Iron, mg/100g product	1.1	2.2	0.46	0.6
Zinc, mg/100g product	0.66	0.44	0.69	0.6
Copper, mg/100g product	0.22	0.22	0.23	0.6
Lead, mg/100g product	ND	ND	ND	ND
Cadmium, mg/100g product	ND	ND	ND	ND
Caffeic Acid, g/100g	1.47	1.69	1.63	0.54
Cyanidin-3-glucoside chloride, g/100g	0.55	-	-	-
Ascorbic acid, g/100g	-	0.26	0.18	-
Glycyrrhizic acid, g/100g	-	-	-	1.96

Table 12. Characteristics of concentrated medicinal plant extracts

with medicinal plant extracts is presented in figure 8. The pasteurization of milk is achieved by maintaining standardized milk at 95 °C for 5 minutes. After pasteurization, milk is cooled to a temperature of 42 °C. Milk inoculation for these probiotic dairy products was made with two Probio-Tec probiotic cultures type: ABY 3 respectively ABT 5, at this time were added and aqueous extracts of medicinal plants (bilberries, sea-buckthorn, rosehip and liquorice) that have a number of characteristics presented in table 12.

After inoculation follows the distribution and packaging and incubation was made at 42°C for 6 hours in the thermostats set at the optimal temperature for the development of these bacteria. Meanwhile yoghurt gel gets a specific consistency. Cooling and storage of obtained yoghurts is performed at 6 °C for 8 days. In this storage period, coagulum is more compact, the flavor and taste become more pleasant.

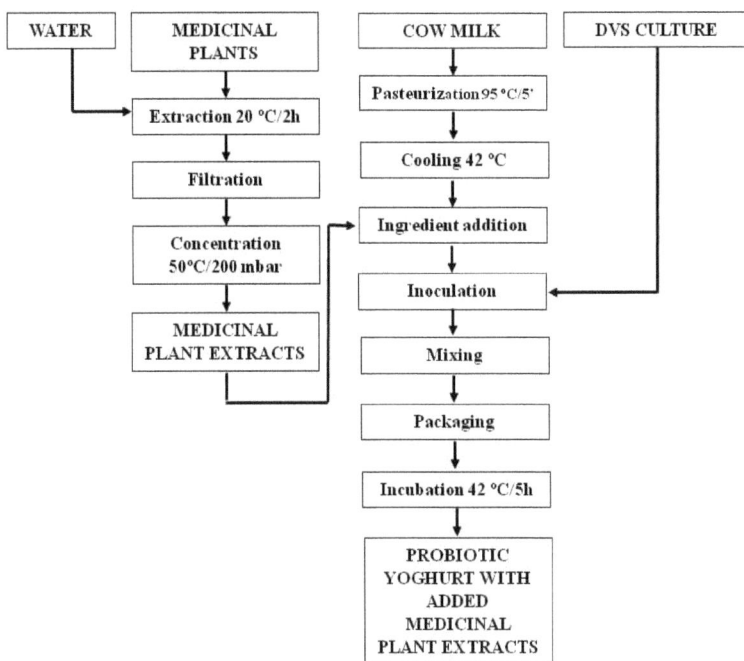

Figure 9. Technological flowchart for manufacturing the new product – Probiotic yoghurt with added medicinal plant extracts

The characteristics of fermented dairy products studied, in terms of chemical properties are:

- Total dry matter have values between 12.05% and 12.5% (lowest for products that contain liquorice extract), exceeding the minimum specified in Romanian standard for fermented dairy products (12%);
- The fat content of the samples vary between 0.6% and 1.3% lowest in products with liquorice compared with other, because smaller proportions of milk of these products;

- Lactic fermentation is faster for the samples with added plant extracts because of monosaccharides content (glucose, fructose, arabinose, xylose) and oligosaccharides (sucrose, raffinose, maltose, xiloglucan) from medicinal plants, which are fermented faster than lactose;
- Titratable acidity at the end of incubation period is between $67^{\circ}T$ and $78^{\circ}T$, with higher values for products liquorice extracts. After 8th days of storage period, the titratable acidity is between $84^{\circ}T$ and $97^{\circ}T$;
- The pH of products after incubation period varies between 5.035 and 5.287. After 8th days of storage it reaches values of 4.225-4.553, lowest value was obtained for the products with ABT 5 culture;
- ABT 5 probiotic culture which contains *Bifidobacterium lactis*, *Lactobacillus acidophilus* and *Strepococcus thermophilus* is more active than ABY 3 consists of *Bifidobacterium lactis*, *Lactobacillus acidophilus*, *Lactobacillus delbrueckii* subsp. *bulgaricus* and *Strepococcus thermophilus*;
- The established technological flowchart leads to obtaining some appropriate products in terms of physical-chemical characterization.

6. Conclusions

The researchers team of the Faculty of Food Science and Engineering, with many researchers in the scientific world, were concerned to investigate the possibility of obtaining probiotic products based on milk. Use milk as a vehicle for creating probiotic product was a constant concern of the staff of the Faculty of Food Science and Engineering in recent years. Probiotic character and functional role of probiotic products was obtained by adding fruit and vegetable juices, medicinal plant extracts, *Spirulina platensis* biomass, etc. We plan to continue research in this direction by investigating other products that may stimulate growth of probiotic bacteria.

Author details

Gabriel-Danut Mocanu and Elisabeta Botez
Department of Food Science, Food Engineering and Applied Biotechnology, Faculty of Food Science and Engineering, „Dunarea de Jos" University of Galati, Romania

Acknowledgement

Authors are grateful to the S.C. Hofigal Export – Import S.A. Bucharest for the material support of this work (medicinal plants, biomass of *Spirulina platensis*).

7. References

[1] Gismondo M.R. Drago L. Lombardi A. Review of probiotics available to modify gastrointestinal flora. International Journal of Antimicrobial Agents 1999; 12, 287–292.

[2]   Lilly D.M. Stillwell R.H. Probiotics: Growth-promoting factors produced by microorganisms. Science 1965; 147, 747–748.

[3]   Parker R.B. Probiotics, the other half of the antibiotic story. Animal Nutrition & Health 1974; 29, 4–8.

[4]   Fioramonti J. Theodorou V. Bueno L. Probiotics: What are they? What are their effects on gut physiology?. Best Practice & Research Clinical Gastroenterology 2003; 17, 711–724.

[5]   Salminen S. von Wright A. Morelli L. Marteau P. Brassart D. de Vos W.M. Fondén R. Saxelin M. Collins K. Mogensen G. Birkeland S.E. Mattila-Sandholm T. Demonstration of safety of probiotics – A review. International Journal of Food Microbiology 1998; 44, 93–106.

[6]   Marteau P.R. de Vrese M. Cellier C.J. Schrezenmeir J. Protection from gastrointestinal diseases with the use of probiotics. The American Journal of Clinical Nutrition (Suppl.) 2001; 73, 430–436.

[7]   Charteris W.P. Kelly P.M. Morelli L. Collins J.K. Selective detection, enumeration and identification of potentially probiotic *Lactobacillus* and *Bifidobacterium* species in mixed bacterial populations. International Journal of Food Microbiology 1997; 35,1–27.

[8]   Food and Agriculture Organization/World Health Organization (FAO/WHO), (2001). Health and nutritional properties of probiotics in food including powder milk with live lactic acid bacteria, Report of a Joint FAO/WHO Expert Consultation on Evaluation of Health and Nutritional Properties of Probiotics in Food including Powder Milk with Live Lactic Acid Bacteria, pp. 1-28, ISBN: 92-5-105513-0 Córdoba, Argentina, October 1-4, 2001

[9]   Reid G. Sanders M.E. Gaskins H.R. Gibson G.R. Mercenier A. Rastall R. New scientific paradigms for probiotics and prebiotics. Journal of Clinical Gastroenterology 2003; 37, 105–118

[10] Reid G. Safe and efficacious probiotics: What are they?. Trends in Microbiology 2006; 14, 348–352.

[11] Havenaar R. Ten Brink B. Huis in't Veld J.H.J. Selection of Strains for Probiotic Use. In: R. Fuller (ed.) Probiotics: The Scientific Basis. Chapman & Hall; 1992. p151-170.

[12] Soccol C.R. de Souza Vandenberghe L.P. Spier M.R. Pedroni Medeiros A.B. Yamaguishi C.T. De Dea Lindner J. Pandey A. Soccol V.T. The Potential of Probiotics. Food Technology and Biotechnology 2010;48(4) 413–434.

[13] Young Y. Functional foods and the European consumer. In: J. Buttriss & M. Saltmarsh (ed.) Functional foods. II. Claims and evidence. The Royal Society of Chemistry; 2000.

[14] Mollet B. Rowland I. Functional foods: At the frontier between food and pharma. Current Opinion in Biotechnology 2002;13, 483–485.

[15] Roberfroid M.B. An European consensus of scientific concepts of functional foods. The American Journal of Clinical Nutrition 2000b;16, 689–691.

[16] Menrad K. Market and marketing of functional food in Europe. Journal of Food Engineering 2003;56, 181–188.

[17] Axelsson L. Lactic acid bacteria: classification and physiology. In: Salminen, S., A. von Write, and A. Ouwehand, M. Dekker (ed.) Lactic Acid Bacteria Microbiological and Functional Aspects, Third Edition, Inc. New York; 2004. p1—66

[18] Hutkins R.W. Microorganisms and Metabolism. In: Microbiology and technology of fermented foods. Blackwell Publishing Professional; 2006. P.15-66.

[19] Roberfroid M.B. Concepts and strategy of functional food science: The European perspective. The American Journal of Clinical Nutrition 2000a;71, S1660–S1664.

[20] Kotilainen L. Rajalahti R. Ragasa C. Pehu E. Health enhancing foods: Opportunities for strengthening the sector in developing countries. Agriculture and Rural Development Discussion 2006;Paper 30.

[21] Kwak N.S. Jukes D.J. Functional foods. Part 1. The development of a regulatory concept. Food Control 2001a;12, 99–107.

[22] Stanton C. Ross R.P. Fitzgerald G.F. Van Sinderen D. Fermented functional foods based on probiotics and their biogenic metabolites. Current Opinion in Biotechnology 2005;16, 198–203.

[23] Diplock A.T. Aggett P.J. Ashwell M. Bornet F. Fern E.B. Roberfroid M.B. Scientific concepts of functional foods in Europe: Concensus document. British Journal of Nutrition 1999;81 (suppl. 1), S1–S27.

[24] Coppens P. Fernandes Da Silva M. Pettman S. European regulations on nutraceuticals, dietary supplements and functional foods: A framework based on safety. Toxicology 2006;221, 59–74.

[25] Spence J.T. Challenges related to the composition of functional foods. Journal of Food Composition and Analysis 2006;19, S4–S6.

[26] Siró I. Kápolna E. Kápolna B. Lugasi A. Functional food. Product development, marketing and consumer acceptance—A review. Appetite 2008;51, 456–467.

[27] Mäkinen-Aakula M. Trends in functional foods dairy market. In Proceedings of the third functional food net meeting 2006.

[28] Gibson G.R. Roberfroid M.B. Dietary modulation of the human colonic microbiota: Introducing the concept of prebiotics. Journal of Nutrition 1995;125, 1401–1412.

[29] Prado F.C. Parada J.L. Pandey A. Soccol C.R. Trends in non-dairy probiotic beverages – review. Food Research International 2008;41, 111-123.

[30] Mocanu G.D. Botez E. Andronoiu D.G. Gîtin L. Researches concerning the production of a fermented dairy drink with added carrot juice. Journal of Environmental Protection and Ecology 2011;12, 718-727.

[31] Mocanu G.D. Botez E. Nistor O.V. Andronoiu D.G. Characterization of probiotic yoghurt obtained with medicinal plant extracts and modelling of bacteria cell growth during its production. Journal of Agroalimentary Processes and Technologies 2011;17, 65-71.

[32] Guldas M. Irkin R. Influence of Spirulina platensis powder on the microflora of yoghurt and acidophilus milk. Mljekarstvo 2010;60, 237-243.

[33] Gomes M. Malcata F.X. Development of Probiotic Cheese Manufactured from Goat Milk: Response Surface Analysis via Technological Manipulation. Journal of Dairy Science, 1998;81, 1492–1507.

[34] Andronoiu D.G. Botez E. Nistor O.V. Mocanu G.D. Technological variants for obtaining of a dessert based on fresh probiotic chees. Journal of Agroalimentary Processes and Technologies 2009;XV, 102 – 106.

[35] Andronoiu D.G. Gîtin L. Botez E. Mocanu G.D. Researches Concerning the Production and Characterisation of a Dessert Based on Fresh Cheese and Peach Pulp. Journal of Environmental Protection and Ecology 2011;12, 502-508.

[36] Uliescu M. Rotaru G. Mocanu D. Stanciu V. Study of the probiotic telemea cheese maturation. The Annals of the University „Dunarea de Jos" Galaţi, Fascicle VI-Food Technology 2007;XXX, 92–99.

[37] Rotaru G. Mocanu D. Uliescu M. Andronoiu D. Research studies on cheese brine ripening. Innovative Romanian Food Biotechnology 2008;2, 30-39.

[38] Abd El-Salam M.H. Alichanidis E. Cheese Varieties Ripened in Brine. In: Fox, P.F.; P.L.H. McSweeney, T. M. Cogan, and T. P. Guinee (ed.) Cheese: chemistry, physics and microbiology, Third edition, volume 2, Elsevier Academic Press, 2004.

[39] Songisepp E. Kullisaar T. Hutt P. Elias P. Brilene T. Zilmer M. Mikelsaar M. A New Probiotic Cheese with Antioxidative and Antimicrobial Activity. Journal of Dairy Science 2004;87, 2017–2023.

[40] Kourkoutas Y. Bosnea L. Taboukos S. Baras C. Lambrou D. Kanellaki M. Probiotic Cheese Production Using Lactobacillus casei Cells Immobilized on Fruit Pieces. Journal of Dairy Science 2006;89, 1439–1451/

[41] Mocanu D.G. Rotaru G. Vasile A. Botez E. Andronoiu D.G. Nistor O. Vlăsceanu G. Dune A. Researches on maintaining functionality in the storage of probiotic dairy product – Afinolact. Journal of Agroalimentary Processes and Technologies 2009;15, 229 – 233.

[42] Mocanu D.G. Rotaru G. Vasile A. Botez E. Andronoiu D.G. Nistor O. Vlăsceanu G. Dune A. Studies on the production of probiotic dairy products based on milk and medicinal plant extracts. Journal of Agroalimentary Processes and Technologies 2009;15, 234 – 238.

[43] Mocanu G.D. Rotaru G. Botez E. Vasile A. Andronoiu D. Nistor O. Gîtin L. Vlăsceanu G. Dune A. Research concerning the production of a probiotic dairy product with added medicinal plant extracts. The Annals of the University „Dunărea de Jos" of Galaţi. Fascicle VI – Food Technology 2009;XXXII, 37 – 44.

[44] Mocanu G.D. Rotaru G. Botez E. Vasile A. Andronoiu D. Nistor O. Gîtin L. Vlăsceanu G. Dune A. Sensorial characteristics and rheological properties of probiotic product Cătinolact. The Annals of the University „Dunărea de Jos" of Galaţi. Fascicle VI – Food Technology 2009;XXXII, 64 – 69.

[45] Mocanu G.D. Rotaru G. Botez E. Gîtin L. Andronoiu D. Nistor O. Vlăsceanu G. Dune A. Sensory evaluation and rheological behavior of probiotic dairy products with Rosa canina L. and Glycyrriza glabra L. extracts. Innovative Romanian Food Biotechnology 2009;4, 32 – 39.

[46] Mocanu D. Rotaru G. Botez E. Andronoiu D. Nistor O. Probiotic yogurt with medicinal plants extract: Physical–chemical, microbiological and rheological characteristics. Journal of Agroalimentary Processes and Technologies 2010;16, 469-476.

[47] Manach C. Mazur A. Scalbert A. Polyphenols and prevention of cardiovascular diseases. Current Opinion in Lipidology. Nutrition and metabolism 2005;16, 1–7.

[48] Hărmănescu M. Moisuc A. Radu F. Drăgan S. Gergen I. Total polyphenols content determination in complex matrix of medical plants from Romania by NIR spectroscopy. Bulletin UASVM, Agriculture 2008;65, 123–128.

Chapter 8

Functional Dairy Probiotic Food Development: Trends, Concepts, and Products

Aziz Homayouni, Maedeh Alizadeh, Hossein Alikhah and Vahid Zijah

Additional information is available at the end of the chapter

1. Introduction

In recent years, scientific investigators have moved from primary role of food as the source of energy and nutrients to action of biologically active food components on human health. On the other hand, consumer interest about the active role of food in well-being and life prolongation has been increased. In this way, a novel term -functional food- was introduced which refers to preventional and/or curing effects of food beyond its nutritional value. There is a wide rage of functional foods that were developed recently and many of them are being produced in all over the world including probiotic, prebiotic and symbiotic foods as well as foods enriched with antioxidants, isoflavones, phytosterols, anthocyanins and fat-reduced, sugar-reduced or salt-reduced foods. Among these foods, probiotic functional food has exerted positive effects on the overall health. We can divide it in both probiotic dairy foods and probiotic non-dairy foods. The market of probiotic dairy foods is increasing annually. An increased demand for dairy probiotic products comes from health promotion effects of probiotic bacteria which are originally initiated from milk products, bioactive compounds of fermented dairy products and prevention of lactose intolerance. Therefore, development of these products is a key research priority for food design and a challenge for both industry and science sectors.

Literatures about probiotic application in pediatrics have some characteristics including numerous, randomized, controlled clinical trials or meta-analyses but the substantial heterogeneity of these works greatly complicates the interpretation of the results and thus makes it difficult to draw univocal and general conclusions. Despite these complications, it is possible to draw some conclusions about the clinical effectiveness of probiotics by examining the most significant literature on each pathology. In particular, there is strong evidence indicating that probiotics have preventive and therapeutic effect on pathologies such as acute diarrhea, antibiotic-associated diarrhea, NEC, and allergic pathology. It was reported that administration of L.GG to 50 infants, for a period of 6 weeks, did not improve abdominal pain but did reduce the incidence of abdominal tension compared to the placebo (Bausserman and Michail, 2005) But in other works it was clearly demonstrated that L. acidophilus did improve the symptoms in about half of the patients with IBS, that the blend of VLS#3 probiotics decreased abdominal swelling, while the combined use of L. plantarum and B. breve reduced pain intensity (Halpern, et al., 1996; Kim, et al., 2003; Saggioro, 2004). L. acidophilus and B. infantis for 4 weeks were administered alone or in combination with antibiotics ciprofloxacin for the first week to three different groups with IBS: diarrhea, constipation, and alternating diarrhea and constipation. Both therapeutic approaches have improved the quality of life and reduced symptoms in all three groups (Faber, 2000). In conclusion, although the use of some types of probiotics on IBS appears promising, additional studies are needed. Food supplementation with pre- and probiotics may reduce the prevalence for the infant in high-risk families developing an atopic eczema during the first 2 years of life. Those pregnant women should be advised to take probiotics (L. GG) in late pregnancy and the first 6 months postnatally during nursing. If breast-feeding is not possible, pro- or prebiotics can be supplemented to the infant. There are no known adverse reactions and it might prevent atopic eczema, especially in neonates after cesarean delivery. Therapeutic use of probiotics to improve atopic eczema is only supportive in infants 18 months and with IgE sensitization.

Recent experimental studies have shown that certain gut bacteria, in particular species of Lactobacillus and Bifidobacterium, may exert beneficial effects in the oral cavity by inhibiting Streptococci and Candida sp. Probiotic lactic acid bacteria can produce different antimicrobial components such as organic acids, hydrogen peroxide, carbon peroxide, diacetyl, low molecular weight antimicrobial substances, bacteriocins, and adhesion inhibitors, which also affect oral microflora. However, data is still sparse on the probiotic action in the oral cavity. More information is needed on the colonization of probiotics in the mouth and their possible effect on and within oral biofilms. There is every reason to believe that the putative probiotic mechanisms of action are the same in the mouth as they are in other parts of the gastrointestinal tract. Because of the increasing global problem with antimicrobial drug resistance, the concept of probiotic therapy is interesting and pertinent, and merits further research in the fields of oral medicine and dentistry (Meurman, 2005).

The number of microbial cells in the human gut is 10 times more than the number of cells in the adult body (Mountzouris and Gibson, 2003). So, the change of microbial balance in human intestine can impress the host health. The ratio between the beneficial microbes (probiotics) and harmful microbes would have an important effect on host health. One way to keeping up the probiotic cells in the gut, is to entering probiotics into the intestine through the regular consumption of food containing these bacteria. Among the functional foods, the dairy probiotic products, especially ice cream and cheese are good vehicle to transfer probiotics to the human intestinal tract (Homayouni, 2008a; Homayouni et al., 2012). Dairy products have an important role in human health and form the main part of the food pyramid. The therapeutical and health care characteristic of fermented dairy products has been used over long years. Another way to keeping up the probiotic cells in the gut is to entering prebiotics into the intestine through the regular consumption of foods containing these components. It is clear that versus probiotics the amounts of prebiotics do not changes during the passage from upper intestinal tract (Homayouni, 2008a).

The main role of food is providing enough nutrients to meet metabolic requirements in human body, while giving the consumer a satisfaction feeling and well-being (Homayouni, 2008a). Beyond meeting nutrition needs, food may have different physiological functions and may play detrimental or beneficial roles in some diseases (Koletzko et al., 1998). Functional foods were developed in order to promote a well-being state, improving health, and reducing the diseases risk. "Functional food" means; special foods which have preventional and/or curing effects beyond its nutritional (Homayouni, 2008a). There is a wide rage of functional foods that were developed recently and many of them are being produced in all over the world including probiotic, prebiotic and symbiotic foods as well as foods enriched with antioxidants, isoflavons, phytosterols, anthosyanins and fat-reduced, sugar-reduced or salt-reduced foods. Among these foods, probiotic functional foods are the first choice to exert positive effects on the human health. Probiotic functional foods were divided into dairy probiotic foods and non-dairy probiotic foods. Some of dairy probiotic foods including probiotic ice cream, frozen fermented dairy deserts, probiotic cheese, bio-yoghurt, drinking yoghurt, kefir, Freeze-dried yoghurt and spray dried milk powder have been employed as possible delivery vehicles for probiotic bacteria (Haynes and Playne, 2002; Homayouni et al., 2008b; Homayouni et al., 2012; Ejtahed et al., 2011; Ejtahed et al., 2012; Mirzaei et al., 2012 Kailasapathy and Rybka, 1997; Ravula and Shah, 1998; Stanton et al., 2001). Probiotics are distinct as live micro-organisms which, when administered in sufficient amounts present a health benefit on the host (Food and Agriculture Organization of United Nations; World Health Organization - FAO/WHO, 2002; Homayouni, 2009). In recent years probiotic bacteria have increasingly been incorporated into dairy foods as dietary adjuncts. *Lactobacillus* and *Bifidobacterium* are the most common probiotic bacterial cells that were used in the production of fermented and non-fermented dairy products.

Consumption of probiotic bacteria via dairy food products is an ideal way to re-establish the intestinal micro-floral balance. It must conform to certain requirements for a dairy food product to be considered as a valuable alternative for delivery of probiotic bacteria in one hand and for variety of probiotic cultures to use as a dietary adjunct and to exert a positive influence in the other hand. The culture must be native of the human gastrointestinal tract, having the ability to ferment prebiotics, survives passage through the stomach and small bowel in adequate numbers, be capable of colonizing in site of action, and have beneficial effects on human health. In order to survive, the strain must be resistant to acidic conditions (gastric pH 1-4), alkaline conditions (bile salts present in the small bowel), enzymes present in the intestine (lysozyme) and toxic metabolites produced during digestion (Homayouni et al., 2008d). For example in traditional yoghurt production, *Lactobacillus bulgaricus* and *Streptococcus thermophilus* were used as starter culture. These bacteria do not belong to the indigenous intestinal flora, are not bile-acid resistant and do not survive passage through the gut. So, the traditional yoghurt culture is not to be considering as probiotic. In the case of dairy food product to be considered as a valuable alternative for delivery of probiotics, it must to match definite necessities such as neutral pH, high enough total solids level, absence of oxygen and near to ambient temperatures (Homayouni et al., 2008b; Homayouni et al., 2008d; Homayouni et al., 2012). A number of dairy food bio-products have been employed and developed as delivery vehicles of probiotic bacteria. Around 80 bifido containing products are estimated to be on the world markets. Most of these products are from dairy origin including fresh milk, fermented milk, dairy beverages, ice cream, dairy desserts, cheese, cottage cheese and powdered milk (Tamime et al., 1995). Since the more interest in probiotics, different types of functional products were proposed as carrier foods for probiotic micro-organisms by which consumers can take in large amounts of probiotic bacteria for the therapeutic effects. Therefore, development of these products is a key research priority for food design and a challenge for both industry and science sectors. This chapter presents an overview of functional foods development with emphasizing probiotic dairy foods.

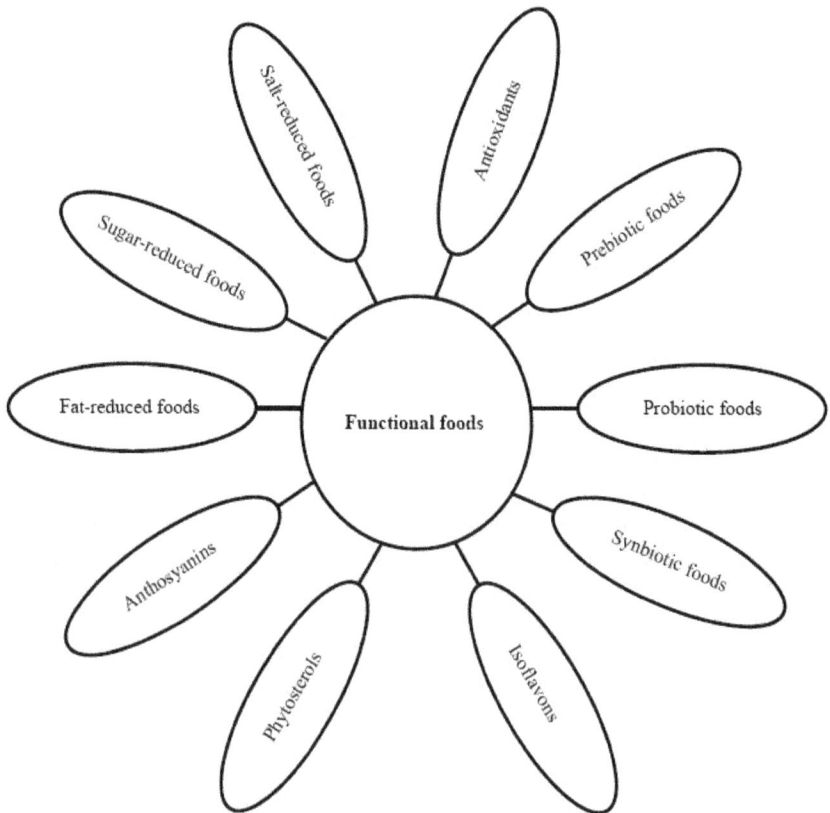

Figure 1. Classification of functional foods

2. Dairy probiotic foods

As mentioned before, dairy functional foods beyond its basic nutritional value has physiological benefits. Milk has an outstanding position in the development of functional foods because it has Omega-3, phytosterols, isoflavins, conjugated linoleic acid, minerals, and vitamins. Dairy products such as ice cream, cheese, yogurt, Acidophilus-Bifidus-milk, Ayran, Kefir, Kumis, Doogh containing probiotics and dairy beverages (both fermented and non-fermented) have long been considered as important vehicles for the delivery of probiotics. In fermentation process, acids such as lactic acid, acetic acid and citric acid are naturally produced. These acids are commonly used as organic acids to enhance organoleptic qualities as well as safety of food products. Lactic acid bacteria are found to be more tolerant to acidity and organic acids than most of the pathogens and spoilage micro-organisms.

2.1. Probiotic ice cream

Probiotic ice cream can be produced by incorporation of probiotic bacteria in both of fermented and unfermented mix (Homayouni et al., 2008b; Homayouni et al., 2012). Ice cream is ideal vehicle for delivery of these micro-organisms in the human diet (Akin et al., 2007; Kailasapathy and Sultana, 2003; Ravula and Shah, 1998; Homayouni et al., 2008d; Homayouni et al., 2012). *Lactobacillus* and *Bifidobacterium* are the most common species of lactic acid bacteria used as probiotics for fermented dairy products. Among the frozen dairy products with live probiotics, probiotic ice cream is also gaining popularity for its neutral pH. The pH of non-fermented ice cream is near to seven which is providing to survive probiotic bacteria (Akin et al., 2007; Christiansen et al., 1996; Homayouni et al., 2008b; Homayouni et al., 2008c; Homayouni et al., 2012). The high total solids level in ice cream including the fat and milk solids provides protection for the probiotic bacteria (Homayouni et al., 2012). Because the efficiency of added probiotic bacteria depends on dose level, type of dairy foods, presence of air and low temperature (Homayouni et al., 2008b), their viability must be maintained throughout the product's shelf-life and they must survive the gut environment (Kailasapathy and Chin, 2000). The therapeutic value of live probiotic bacteria is more than unviable cells; therefore, International Dairy Federation (IDF) recommends that a minimum of 10^7 probiotic bacterial cells should be alive at consumption time per gram/mililiter of product. Studies indicate, however, the bacteria may not survive in high enough numbers when incorporated into frozen dairy products unless a suitable method is used against freeze injury and oxygen toxicity (Dave and Shah, 1998; Kailasapathy and Sultana, 2003; Ravula and Shah, 1998; Homayouni et al., 2008d). The methods of increasing probiotic survival depend on type of food products. Selection of resistant probiotic strains to tolerate production, storage and gastrointestinal tract conditions, is one of the important methods (Homayouni et al., 2008d). Another way is to adjust the conditions of production and storage for more survival rates. The physical protection of probiotics by microencapsulation is a new method for increasing the survival of probiotics (Homayouni et al., 2007; Homayouni et al., 2008b). Encapsulation helps to isolate the bacterial cells from the adverse environment of the product and gastrointestinal tract, thus potentially reducing cell loss. Encapsulation thus may enhance the shelf-life of probiotic cultures in frozen dairy products (Kebary et al., 1998; Shah and Ravula, 2000; Homayouni et al., 2008b). Selecting of suitable probiotic strains depends to ability survive simulated conditions of ice cream (high sucrose concentrations, high oxygen, refrigeration and freezing temperatures), acidic (to simulate gastric) and alkaline conditions (to simulate intestinal). Microencapsulation of probiotics can further protect these bacteria from the mentioned conditions (Homayouni et al., 2008d).

Homayouni et al. (2008d) studied the survival of probiotics in simulated ice cream and gastrointestinal conditions in order to select appropriate probiotic strains for use in probiotic ice cream. The growth and survival rate of *Lactobacillus acidophilus, Lactobacillus casei, Bifidobacterium lactis* and *Bifidobacterium longum* in varying amount of sucrose concentrations (10, 15, 20 and 25%), oxygen scavengering components (0.05% L-cysteine and 0.05% L-ascorbate) and low temperatures (4°C and 20°C) during different periods of time (30, 60 and 90 days) in MRS-broth medium was studied. All of above stress factors have been able to influence the growth and survival of four probiotic strains. Results have demonstrated that it is possible to select the appropriate probiotic strains for use in probiotic ice cream. *Lactobacillus casei* (Lc01) and *Bifidobacterium lactis* (Bb12) had the highest resistance to simulated acidic, alkaline and ice cream conditions in comparison with other probiotic strains, making them suitable probiotic strains for use in probiotic ice cream (Homayouni et al., 2008b; Homayouni et al., 2008d).

2.2. Probiotic cheese

Survival in processing conditions, presence of oxygen, degree of acidity, ability to grow well in milk-based products and to rapidly acidify milk, thus reducing the fermentation time and, consequently, contamination risk during preparation of inoculums are important factors for probiotic bacteria such as *Lactobacillus spp.* and *Bifidobacterium spp* in order to apply these bacteria in probiotic dairy products. Probiotic bacterial cells have to fulfill the basic technological necessities when used in commercial probiotic dairy products. Since probiotic bacteria have to be presented in sufficient numbers in product at consumption time, their survival have to be maintained up to shelf-life date. In addition, no adverse effects on taste and aroma of the product should be exerted by the probiotic organisms. Various types of cheese have a good potential to maintain the probiotic survival. So, it is a good vehicle to transfer probiotics to the human intestinal tract. There are two ways for development of probiotic cheese: in the first step, the manufacture processes of cheese products may have to be modified and adapted to the requirements of probiotics and in second step, appropriate probiotic strains may be applied or new cheese products may have to be developed. Dairy products containing living bacteria have to be cooled during storage. Cooling is necessary to guarantee high survival rates of probiotics and to bring sufficient stability of the product (Roy et al., 1997). In addition, oxygen content and water activity of the probiotic cheese have to be considered in prepackaged cheese (Dave and Shah, 1997a). Interaction of the live probiotic microorganisms with the components of the cheese have to be inhibited by cooling of product. The degree of interaction depends on the kind and amount of carbohydrates available, degree of hydrolysis of milk proteins and thus availability of essential amino acids, and composition and degree of hydrolysis of milk lipids, determining the availability of short chain fatty acids (Fox et al., 1996). However, the proteolytic and lipolytic properties of the probiotic bacterial cells may have important effects on taste and flavor of the probiotic cheese (Kunji et al., 1996). The strength of interactions between probiotics and starter organisms in probiotic cheese depends on when the probiotics are added to the product. If they are added after fermentation, interactions may be kept to a minimum, since addition is possible immediately before or even after cooling below 8°C and metabolic activities of starters and probiotics are considerably reduced at refrigerated temperatures.

Antagonism between bacteria is often based on the production of metabolites that inhibit or inactivate more or less specifically other related starter organisms or even unrelated bacteria. While antagonism caused by bacteriocins, peptides, or proteins exhibiting antibiotic properties has been described as a limiting factor for combinations of starters and probiotics (Joseph et al., 1998), antagonism caused by hydrogen peroxide, benzoic acid, biogenic amines, and lactic acid may have considerable effects on probiotics in probiotic cheese. The physiological state of the probiotics may be of considerable importance for survival during ripening and/or storage if probiotics are added to the probiotic cheese after fermentation (Desmazeaud, 1996; Lankaputhra et al., 1996; Leuschner et al., 1998; Weber, 1996).

In probiotic cheese, probiotic cells must be able to grow and/or multiply in the human intestine and therefore should be able to survive during the passage through the gastrointestinal tract (GIT), which involves exposure to hydrochloric acid in stomach and bile in small intestine (Stanton et al., 2003). In fact, cheese provides a valuable vehicle for probiotic delivery, due to creation of a buffer against the high acidic environment in the gastrointestinal tract, and thus creates a more favorable environment for probiotic survival throughout the gastric transit, ought to higher pH. Moreover, the dense matrix and relatively high total solids as well as fat content of cheese may offer additional protection to probiotic bacteria in stomach (Bergamini et al., 2005; Ross et al., 2002). The presence of the prebiotics inulin and oligofructose can promote growth rates of *bifidobacteria* and *lactobacilli*, besides increased lactate and short chain fatty acids production in petit-suisse cheese (Cardarelli et al., 2007).

2.3. Probiotic yoghurt

Yoghurt has been historically recognized to be 'a healthy food' with therapeutically effects. There has been a considerable increase in the popularity of yoghurt especially probiotic yoghurt in recent years. The conventional yoghurt starter bacteria, *L. bulgaricus* and *Streptococcus thermophilus*, do not have ability to survive passage through intestinal tract and consequently so, they are not considered as probiotics. But the addition of *L. acidophilus* and *B. bifidum* into yoghurt can add extra nutritional and physiological values.

Similar processing to traditional yoghurt is applied for production of bio-yoghurt with incorporation of live probiotic starter cultures. Heat treated homogenized milk with an increased protein content (3.6–3.8%) is inoculated with the conventional starter culture at 45°C or 37°C and incubated for 3.5 and 9 h, respectively. The probiotic culture can be added prior to fermentation simultaneously with the conventional yoghurt cultures or after fermentation to cooled (4°C) product before packaging. Bio-yoghurt, containing *L. acidophilus* and *B. bifidum* is a potential vehicle for delivery of these probiotic cells to consumers. *L. acidophilus* and *B. bifidum* have to retain viability and activity in yoghurt as a probiotic at consumption time. Viability of probiotic bacteria in yoghurt products at refrigeration temperature is reported to be unsatisfactory over a long shelf life (Dave and Shah, 1997a). The survival of probiotic bacteria in fermented dairy products depends on the chemical composition of the fermentation medium (e.g. carbohydrate source), final acidity, milk solids content, availability of nutrients, growth promoters and inhibitors, strains used, interaction between species present, culture conditions, concentration of sugars (osmotic pressure), dissolved oxygen (especially for *Bifidobacterium* spp.), level of inoculation, incubation temperature, fermentation time and storage temperature. The lack of acid tolerance of some probiotic species and strains in fermented products based on milk is an important factor. During fermentation, pH levels decreases when the lactic acid content increases. 'Over-acidification' or 'post acidification' is due to decrease in pH after fermentation and during storage at refrigerated temperature. Excessive acidification is mainly due to the uncontrollable growth of strains of *L. bulgaricus* at low pH values and refrigerated temperatures. The 'overacidification' can be prevented to a limited extent by applying 'good manufacturing practice' and by using cultures with reduced 'over-acidification' behavior.

Viability of both *Lactobacillus* and *Bifidobacterium* species reduces at low pH levels during refrigerated storage. So, strain selection and survival monitoring are necessary to produce high quality bio-yoghurt. Probiotic yoghurt contains metabolic products secreted by starter microorganisms, which influence the viability of *L. acidophilus* and *B. bifidum*. The inhibition of *bifidobacteria* in probiotic yoghurt is due to antagonism effects among starter bacteria rather than hydrogen peroxide or organic acids (Dave and Shah, 1997a). The ideal procedure for probiotic yoghurt manufacturing is growing the *Bifidobacterium* spp. separately, followed by washing out of free metabolites and the transfer of the cells to the probiotic yoghurt. Oxygen toxicity is a critical problem for *Bifidobacterium* spp. because they are strictly anaerobic. Low initial oxygen content in milk may obtain the low redox potential required in the early phase of incubation to guarantee *Bifidobacteria* growth. Oxygen easily dissolves in milk during yoghurt production and also permeates through packages during storage. It has been suggested to inoculate *S. thermophilus* and *Bifidobacterium* simultaneously during fermentation to avoid the oxygen toxicity problem. *S. thermophilus* has a high oxygen utilization ability, which results in reduction of dissolved oxygen in probiotic yoghurt and an enhancement in viability of *bifidobacteria*. Higher survival rates of lactic acid bacteria were obtained at lower storage temperatures (Foschino et al., 1996). Low storage temperature restricts the growth of *L. bulgaricus* and consequently also over-acidification. *Bifidobacteria* are substantially less tolerant to low storage temperature when compared to *L. acidophilus*.

2.4. Probiotic milk

Lactobacillus acidophilus does not rapidly grow in milk because it is an acid-loving bacterium. Therefore, it is essential to maintain the inoculum active by daily transfers of mother culture in acidophilus milk production. The probiotic milk is to market in liquid form. During fermentation, milk pH often goes beyond the narrow range of optimal pH of *Lactobacillus acidophilus* (5.5-6.0). This eventually leads to decrease these bacterial counts. In traditional acidophilus milk production, the milk is heated at 95°C for 1 h or at 125°C for 15 min (Vedamuthu, 2006). Such a high heat treatment stimulates the growth of *Lactobacillus acidophilus* by providing denatured proteins and released peptides. High-heat-treated milk is cooled to 37°C and kept at this temperature for a period of 3-4 h to allow any spores present to germinate. Then, milk is re-sterilized to destroy almost all vegetative cells. Unless skim milk is used, the heat-treated milk is homogenized and cooled down to inoculation temperature (37°C). *Lactobacillus acidophilus* is added as active bulk culture. The level of inoculation is usually 2-5% and the inoculated milk is left to ferment until pH 5.5-6.0 or ~1.0% lactic acid is obtained, with no alcohol (Surono and Hosono, 2002). The fermentation takes about 18-24 h under inactive conditions. After the fermentation, the number of viable *Lactobacillus acidophilus* colonies is about 2-3×10^9 cfu mL^{-1}, but this number decreases up to consumption time. In extended incubation period reduction in counts of *Lactobacillus acidophilus* may occur. To overcome this problem, replacement of 25% of *Lactobacillus acidophilus* culture by a mixture of *Streptococcus thermophilus* and *Lactobacillus delbrueckii* subsp. *Bulgaricus* can be used. Following fermentation, the warm product is rapidly cooled to <7°C before agitation and pumped to a filler where it is filled into bottles or cartons (Kosikowski and Mistry, 1997; Vedamuthu, 2006). Protein quality and total amino acid content are similar in both fermented and non-fermented milk. Acidophilus milk has higher free amino acids than milk. As the milk lactose is hydrolyzed by β-galactosidase of *Lactobacillus acidophilus*, acidophilus milk is more suitable for individuals suffering from lactose intolerance. It is also possible to enrich acidophilus milk with calcium, iron and vitamins. Undesirable sour milk flavor caused acidophilus milk is gained limited popularity by consumers. So, sweet acidophilus milk has been developed. When *Lactobacillus acidophilus* is incorporated into pasteurized milk at about 5°C and bottled aseptically, these bacteria are able to keep their viability up to 14 days without reducing the pH of milk due to it does not grow at low temperatures (<10°C). Freeze-dried cultures may keep their viability up to 58% after 23 days at 4°C in sweet acidophilus milk. *Lactobacillus acidophilus* remained viable in sweet acidophilus milk over 28 days at 7°C. Addition of 200 g of frozen culture concentrate to 2000 L of pasteurized milk is satisfactory to reach the target level of *Lactobacillus acidophilus* in the probiotic milk (Vedamuthu, 2006).

Technology of bifidus milk and acidophilus-bifidus milk manufacturing is similar to acidophilus milk. Milk is standardized to desire protein and fat levels in both products. Then, for manufacture of bifidus milk, milk is heat-treated at 80-120°C for 5-30 min and rapidly cooled to 37°C. Heat-treated milk is inoculated with frozen culture of *Bifidobacterium bifidum* and *Bifidobacterium longum* at a level of 10% and left to ferment until pH 4.5. After fermentation, the product is cooled to <10°C and packaged. Final product has a slightly acidic flavor and the ratio of lactic acid to acetic acid is 2:3. Milk used for acidophilus-bifidus milk production is usually enriched with protein prior to fat standardization and homogenization. The standardized milk is heat-treated at 75°C for 15 s or 85°C for 30 min. After cooling the milk to 37°C, frozen cultures of *Lactobacillus acidophilus* and *Bifidobacterium bifidum* are inoculated and fermentation is allowed until pH 4.5–4.6 is reached (~16 h). Following fermentation, the fermented milk is cooled to <10°C. The shelf life of the product is about 20 days. Acidophilus-bifidus milk has a characteristic aroma and slightly acidic flavor. High viscosity of product cause to producing it in set form. It is also possible to produce probiotic milks by simply adding mix culture of *Lactobacillus acidophilus* and *Bifidobacterium bifidum* to cold pasteurized milk.

3. Development of functional dairy foods

Innovation is today's business demand and development of a new functional food is an expensive process and is very important for both food companies and consumers. Regulations should encourage food companies to follow functional food development. Development of dairy probiotic products requires detailed knowledge of both products and customers. It needs to manage customer knowledge effectively (Walzem, 2004; Jousse, 2008). Fundamental risks can affect the development of new functional food products and may leads to fail the development process. Development of new functional food products is very challenging and it has to complete the consumer's expectations for palatable and healthy products (Fogliano and Vitaglione, 2005; Granato et al., 2010; Shah, 2007). So, the development and commerce of functional food products is rather complex, expensive, and uncertain. Key points regarding for a successful functional food product development are consumer demands, technological conditions, and legislative regulatory background. However, consumer's knowledge of the health effects of specific ingredients can affect the acceptance of specific functional food. Therefore, functional ingredients that are in consumers mind for a long period of time, such as minerals, fiber, and vitamins, achieve considerably higher rates of consumer acceptance than new products, such as foods enriched with probiotics, prebiotics, flavonoids, carotenoids, and conjugated linilenic acid (CLA). Several ways to make a functional food product is to eliminating an allergenic protein, lactose, phenylanine and etc from the natural food product; by fortification with a micronutrient; by adding antioxidants, probiotics or prebiotics); by replacing a component, or by increasing bioavailability or stability of a component known to produce a functional effect or to reduce the disease-risk potential of the food (Roberfroid, 2000; Siro, et al., 2008; Granato, et al., 2010). Field of functional probiotic foods requires the cooperation of food technologists, nutritionists, medical doctors, and food chemists in order to obtain innovative products. In this way, these foods may be able to adjust physiological parameters related to health status or disease prevention in human. So, the design and development of functional probiotic foods is a scientific work (Hasler, 1998; Walzem, 2004; Fogliano and Vitaglione, 2005) which is an expensive and multistage process that takes into account many factors, such as sensory acceptance, physical and microbial stability, price, and chemical and other intrinsic functional properties to be successful in the marketplace. Moreover, consumer attitude toward the functional probiotic product also needs to be understood and taken into consideration.

4. Consumer attitude toward functional dairy foods

The development of functional probiotic foods is increasing, as their market increases day by day, although the consumer's information about these foods is increasing without relation to gender, age, and educational or economic levels of the consumers. The therapeutical effect of a functional probiotic food may depend on the consumer's characteristics and the type of carrier and enrichment considered. For instance, yoghurt is most preferred by its enrichment with calcium and fiber. Ingredients such as vitamins and minerals applied in fortification of functional foods are widely recognized and accepted by consumers, but new functional ingredients such as probiotics and prebiotics are not common to them. So, there is a need for increasing the consumer knowledge with respect to these new special ingredients (Hillian, 2000; Luckow and Delahunty, 2004; Ares and Gambaro, 2007; Vianna et al., 2008).

The sensory properties of prebiotic functional foods in comparison with conventional products can lead to different acceptance level. Oligofructose provides some suitable sensory properties such as rounder mouth feel, reduced aftertaste, and slight sweetness to the products. These properties are responsible for high score values for taste, creaminess, and overall acceptability of functional food products. The first important marker in choosing a functional food is flavor, and health consideration is in the second order. If the ingredients added give unpleasant flavors to the product, consumers are not interested in consume such functional probiotic food even if this results in health advantages. This means that flavor is correlated to intrinsic sensory properties of the product such as overall acceptability. In general, as functional products consumption increases, the acceptance of such products may increase, even if the sensory profiles are different from conventional products. When functional ingredients such as probiotics are added to dairy foods, consumers must be aware of probiotics health benefits in order to recognize the functional probiotic foods as being more beneficial than the conventional ones. Functional probiotic food industry should communicate with consumer in a clear way and this is one of the most important aspects for success (Tepper and Trail, 1998; Matilla-Sandholm et al., 1999; Roberfroid, 2000; Tuorila and Cardello, 2002; Nicolay, 2003; Vieira, 2003; Homayouni, 2008a).

5. Conclusion

The future success of functional probiotic dairy foods in marketplace depends on consumer acceptance of such products. The consumers must be convinced by its health claims through clear, honest, and definite messages to agree to pay the cost associated with functional probiotic dairy foods. Development of probiotic dairy products is a key research priority for food design and a challenge for both industry and science sectors. Among the functional foods, the dairy probiotic products, especially ice cream and cheese are good vehicle to transfer probiotics to the human intestinal tract. Additional way to keeping up the probiotic cells in the gut is to entering prebiotics into the intestine through the regular consumption of food containing these components. It is clear that versus probiotics the amounts of prebiotics do not changes during the passage from upper intestinal tract.

Author details

Aziz Homayouni
Department of Food Science and Technology, Faculty of Health and Nutrition,
Tabriz University of Medical Sciences, Tabriz, I.R. Iran

Maedeh Alizadeh
Pediatric Nursing, Faculty of Nursing and Midwifery of Maragheh,
Tabriz University of Medical Sciences, Tabriz, I.R. Iran

Hossein Alikhah
Faculty of Medicine, Tabriz University of Medical Sciences, Tabriz, I.R. Iran

Vahid Zijah*
Department of Dentistry, Behbood Hospital,
Tabriz University of Medical Sciences, Tabriz, I.R. Iran

6. References

Akin, M. B., Akin, M. S., and Kirmaci, Z. Effects of inulin and sugar levels on the viability of yogurt and probiotic bacteria and the physical and sensory characteristics in probiotic ice cream, *Food Chemistry* 104 (2007), pp. 93-99.

Ares, G., and G'ambaro, A. Influence of gender, age and motives underlying food choice on perceived healthiness and willingness to try functional foods, *Appetite* 49 (2007), pp. 148-158.

Bausserman, M. and Michail, S. (2005). The use of Lactobacillus GG in irritable bowel syndrome in children: a double-blind randomized control trial. The Journal of Pediatrics, 147(2): 197-200.

Bergamini, C. V., Hynes, E. R., Quiberoni, A., Sua'rez, V. B., and Zalazar, C. A. Probiotic bacteria as adjunct starters: influence of the addition methodology on their survival in a semi-hard Argentinean cheese, *Food Research International* 38(5) (2005), pp. 597-604.

Cardarelli, H. R., Saad, S. M. I., Gibson, G. R., and Vulevic, J. Functional petitsuisse cheese: Measure of the prebiotic effect, *Anaerobe* 13 (2007), pp. 200-207.

Christiansen, P. S., Edelsten, D., Kristiansen, J. R., and Nielsen, E. W. Some properties of ice cream containing Bifidobacterium bifidum and Lactobacillus acidophilus, *Milschwissenschaft* 51 (1996), pp. 502-504.

Cummings, J. H., Macfarlane, G. R., and Englyst, H. N. Prebiotic digestion and fermentation, *American Journal of Clinical Nutrition* 73 (2001), pp. 415-420.

* Corresponding Author

Dave, R., and Shah, N. P. Viability of probiotic bacteria in yoghurt made from commercial starter cultures, *International Dairy Journal* 7 (1997a), pp. 31-41.

Dave, R. I., and Shah, N. P. Effect of cysteine on the viability of yoghurt and probiotic bacteria in yoghurts made with commercial starter cultures, *International Dairy Journal* 7 (1997b), pp. 537-545.

Dave, R. I., and Shah, N. P. Ingredient supplementation effects on viability of probiotic bacteria in yogurt, *Journal of Dairy Science* 81 (1998), pp. 2804-2816.

Desmazeaud, M. (1996). *Growth inhibitors of lactic acid bacteria, in Dairy Starter Cultures, Cogan, T.M. and Accolas.* New York: VCH Publishers, (pp. 131–155).

Ejtahed, H. S., Mohtadi-Nia, J., Homayouni-Rad, A., Niafar, M., Asghari-Jafarabadi, M., Mofid, V. and Akbarian-Moghari, A. (2011). Effect of probiotic yogurt containing Lactobacillus acidophilus and Bifidobacterium lactis on lipid profile in individuals with type 2 diabetes mellitus. Journal of Dairy Science, 94: 3288-3294.

Ejtahed, H. S., Mohtadi-Nia, J., Homayouni-Rad, A., Niafar, M., Asghari-Jafarabadi, M. and Mofid, V. (2012). Probiotic yogurt improves antioxidant status in type 2 diabetic patients. Nutrition, 28: 539- 543.

Faber, S. M. (2000). Comparison of probiotics and antibiotics to probiotics alone in treatment of diarrhea predominant IBS (D-IBS), alternating (A-IBS) and constipation (C-IBS) patients. Gastroenterology, 118: 687-688.

Food and Agriculture Organization of United Nations; World Health Organization. FAO/WHO (2002). *Guidelines for the evaluation of probiotics in food, Food and Agriculture Organization of the United Nations and World Health Organization Expert Consultation Report.* Available from. http://www.who.int/foodsafety/publications/fs_management/probiotics2/en.

Fogliano, V., and Vitaglione, P. Functional foods: planning and development, *Molecular Nutrition and Food Research* 49 (2005), pp. 256-262.

Foschino, R., Fiori, E., and Galli, A. Survival and residual activity of Lactobacillus acidophilus frozen cultures under different conditions, *Journal of Dairy Research* 63 (1996), pp. 295-303.

Fox, P. F., Wallace, J. M., Morgan, S., Lynch, C. M., Niland, E. J., and Tobin, J. Acceleration of cheese ripening, *Antonie van Leeuwenhoek* 70 (1996), pp. 175-201.

Granato, D., Castro, I. A., Ellendersen, L. S. N., and Masson, M. L. Physical stability assessment and sensory optimization of a dairy-free emulsion using response surface methodology, *Journal of Food Science* 73 (2010), pp. 149-155.

Granato, D., Branco, G. F., Cruz, A. G., Faria, J. A. F., and Shah, N. P. Probiotic dairy products as functional foods, *Comperhensive reviews in Food Science and food safety* 9 (2010), pp. 455-470.

Halpern, G. M., Prindville, T. and Blankenburg, M. (1996). Treatment of irritable bowel syndrome with Lacteol forte: A randomized, double-blind, crossover trial. The American Journal of Gastroenterology, 91: 1579-1585.

Hansen, L. T., Wojtas, P. M. A., Jin, Y. L. and Paulson, A. T. Survival of Ca-alginate microencapsulated Bifidobacterium spp. In milk and simulated gastrointestinal conditions, *Food Microbiology* 19 (2002), pp. 35-45.

Hasler, C. M. Functional foods: their role in disease in developing new food products for a changing prevention and health promotion, *Food Technology* 52 (1998), pp. 57-62.

Haynes, I. N., and Playne, M. J. Survival of probiotic cultures in low-fat ice-cream, *Australian Journal of Dairy Technology* 57 (2002), pp. 10-14.

Hillian, M. Functional food: how big is the market? *World Food Ingredients* 12 (2000), pp. 50-53.

Homayouni, A., Ehsani, M. R., Azizi, A., Yarmand, M. S., and Razavi, S. H. Effect of lecithin and calcium chloride solution on the microencapsulation process yield of calcium alginate beads, *Iranian Polymer Journal* 16(9) (2007), pp. 597-606.

Homayouni, A. (2008a). *Therapeutical effects of functional probiotic, prebiotic and symbiotic foods.* (1st ed.). Tabriz: Tabriz University of Medical Sciences.

Homayouni, A., Azizi, A., Ehsani, M. R., Razavi, S. H. and Yarmand, M. S. Effect of microencapsulation and resistant starch on the probiotic survival and sensory properties of synbiotic ice cream, *Food Chemistry* 111 (2008b), pp. 50-55.

Homayouni, A., Ehsani, M. R., Azizi, A., Razavi, S. H., and Yarmand, M. S. Spectrophotometrically evaluation of probiotic growth in liquid media, *Asian Journal of Chemistry* 20(3) (2008c), pp. 2414-2420.

Homayouni, A., Ehsani, M. R., Azizi, A., Razavi, S. H., and Yarmand, M. S. Growth and survival of some probiotic strains in simulated ice cream conditions, *Journal of Applied Sciences* 8(2) (2008d), pp. 379-382.

Homayouni, A. Letter to the editor, *Food Chemistry* 114 (2009), pp. 1073.

Homayouni, A., Azizi, A., Javadi, M., Mahdipour, S. and Ejtahed, H. (2012). Factors influencing probiotic survival in ice cream: A Review. International Journal of Dairy Science, doi: 10.3923/ijds.2012.

Joseph, P. J., Dave, R. I., and Shah, N. P. Antagonism between yogurt bacteria and probiotic bacteria isolated from commercial starter cultures, commercial yogurts, and a probiotic capsule, *Food Australia* 50 (1998), pp. 20-23.

Jousse, F. Modeling to improve the efficiency of product and process development, *Comprihensive Review of Food Science and Food Safety* 7 (2008), pp. 175-181.

Kailasapathy, K., and Rybka, S. L. acidophilus and Bifidobacterium spp. Their therapeutic potential and survival in yoghurt, *Australian Journal of Dairy Technology* 52 (1997), pp. 28-35.

Kailasapathy, K., and Chin, J. Survival and therapeutic potential of probiotic organisms with reference to Lactobacillus acidophilus and Bifidobacterium spp., *Immunology and Cell Biology* 78 (2000), pp. 80-88.

Kailasapathy, K., and Sultana, K. Survival and β-D-galactosidase activity of encapsulated and free Lactobacillus acidophilus and Bifidobacterium lactis in ice cream, *Australian Journal of Dairy Technology* 58 (2003), pp. 223-227.

Kebary, K. M. K., Hussein, S. A., and Badawi, R. M. Improving viability of bifidobacterium and their effect on frozen ice milk, *Egyptian Journal of Dairy Science* 26 (1998), pp. 319-337.

Kim, H. J., Camilleri, M. and McKinzie, S. (2003). A randomized controlled trial of a probiotic, VSL 3, on gut transit and symptoms in diarrhoea-predominant irritable bowel syndrome. Alimentary Pharmacology and Therapeutics, 17: 895-904.

Koletzko, B., Aggett, P.J., and Bindels, J.G. Growth, development and differentiation: a functional food science approach, *Brazilian Journal of Nutrition* 80 (1998), pp. 35-45.

Kosikowski, F. V. and Mistry, V. V. (1997). *Cheese and fermented milk foods, in Origin and Principles: Fermented Milks*. Westport: F.V. Kosikowski, (pp. 57-74).

Kunji, E. R. S., Mierau, I., Hagting, A., Poolman, B., and Konings, W. N. The proteolytic systems of lactic acid bacteria, *Antonie van Leeuwenhoek* 70 (1996), pp. 187-221.

Lankaputhra, W. E. V., Shah, N. P., and Britz, M. L. Survival of bifidobacteria during refrigerated storage in the presence of acid and hydrogen peroxide, *Milchwissenschaft* 51 (1996), pp. 65-70.

Leuschner, R. G., Heidel, M., and Hammes, W. P. Histamine and tyramine degradation by food fermenting microorganisms, *International Journal of Food Microbiology* 39 (1998), pp. 1-10.

Luckow, T., and Delahunty, C. Consumer acceptance of orange juice containing functional ingredients, *Food Research International* 37 (2004), pp. 805-14.

Matilla-Sandholm, T., Blum, S., Collins, J.K., Crittenden, R., DeVos, W., Dunne, C., et al. Probiotics: towards demonstrating efficacy, *Trends in Food Science and Technology* 10 (1999), pp. 393-399.

Meurman, J. H. (2005). Probiotics: do they have a role in oral medicine and dentistry? Europian Journal of Oral Sciences, 113(3): 188-196.

Mirzaei, H., Pourjafar, H. and Homayouni, A. (2012). Effect of calcium alginate and resistant starch microencapsulation on the survival rate of Lactobacillus acidophilus La5 and sensory properties in Iranian white brined cheese. Food Chemistry, 132: 1966-1970.

Mountzouris, K. C. and Gibson, G. R. Colonization of the gastrointestinal tract, *Annales Nestle* 61 (2003), pp. 43-54.

Nicolay, C. Language is a key to marketing digestive health products, *Functional Foods and Nutraceuticals* 6 (2003), pp. 20-22.

Ravula, R. R. and Shah, N. P. Viability of probiotic bacteria in fermented frozen dairy desserts, *Food Australia* 50 (1998), pp. 136-139.

Roberfroid, M. (2000). *Inulin-type fructans*. Boca Raton: CRC Press.

Roberfroid, M.B. Concepts and strategy of functional food science: the European perspective, *American Journal of Clinical Nutrition* 71 (2000), pp. 1660-1664.

Ross, R. P., Fitzgerald, G., Collins, K., and Stanton, C. Cheese delivering biocultures: probiotic cheese, *Australian Journal of Dairy Technology* 57(2) (2002), pp. 71-78.

Roy, D., Mainville, I., and Mondou F. Bifidobacteria and their role in yogurt-related products, *Microecology Therapy* 26 (1997), pp. 167-180.

Saggioro, A. (2004). Probiotics in the treatment of irritable bowel syndrome. Journal of Clinical Gastroenterology, 38: 104-106.

Shah, N. P., and Ravula, R. R. Microencapsulation of probiotic bacteria and their survival in frozen fermented dairy desserts, *Australian Journal of Dairy Technology* 55 (2000), pp. 139-144.

Shah, N. P. Functional cultures and health benefits, *International Dairy Journal* 17 (2007), pp. 1262-1277.

Siro, I., Kapolna, E., Kapolna, B., and Lugasi, A. Functional food: product development, marketing and consumer acceptance-A review, *Appetite* 51 (2008), pp. 456-467.

Stanton, C., Gardiner, G., Meehan, H., Collins, K., Fitzgerald, G., Lynch, P. B., and et al. Market potential for probiotics, *American Journal of Clinical Nutrition* 73 (2001), pp. 4765-4835.

Stanton, C., Desmond, C., Coakley, M., Collins, J. K., Fitzgerald, G., and Ross, R. P. (2003). Challenges facing development of probioticcontaining functional foods. In E. R. Farnworth (Eds.). *Handbook of fermented functional foods* (pp. 27-58). Boca Ranton: CRC Press.

Surono, I.S. and Hosono, A. (2002). Fermented milks: Types and standards of identity. In H. Roginski, J. Fuquay, and P.F. Fox (Eds.). *Encyclopedia of Dairy Microbiology.* (pp. 1018-1023).

Tamime, A. Y., Marshall, V. M. E., and Robinson, R. K. Microbiological and technological aspects of milks fermented by bifidobacteria, *Journal of Dairy Research* 62 (1995), pp. 151-187.

Tepper, B., and Trail, A. Taste or health: a study on consumer acceptance of corn chips, *Food Quality and Preference* 9 (1998), pp. 267-272.

Tuorila, H., and Cardello, A. V. Consumer responses to an off-flavour in juice in the presence of specific health claims, *Food Quality and Preference* 13 (2002), pp. 561-569.

Vedamuthu, E.R. (2006). Other fermented and culture-containing milks. In R. Chandan, C.H. White, A. Kilara, and Y.H. Hui (Eds.), *Manufacturing Yogurt and Fermented Milks* (pp. 295-308). Blackwell Publishing.

Vernazza, C. L., Rabiu, B. A., and Gibson, G. R. (2006). Human colonic microbiology and the role of dietary intervention: Introduction to prebiotics. In G. R. Gibson and R. A. Rastall (Eds.), *Prebiotics: Development and application* (pp. 1-12). England: John Wiley and Sons Ltd.

Vianna, J. V., Cruz, A. G., Zoellner, S. S., Silva, R., and Batista, A. L. D. Probiotic foods: consumer perception and attitudes, *International Journal of Food Science and Technology* 43 (2008), pp. 1577-1580.

Vickers, Z., Mullan, L., and Holton, E. Impact of differences in taste ratings on the consumption of milk in both a laboratory and a foodservice setting, *Journal of Sensory Studies* 14 (1999), pp. 249-262.

Vieira, P. How to create brand awareness for new products, *Functional Foods and Nutraceuticals* 6 (2003), pp. 38-40.

Walzem, R. L. Functional foods, *Trends In Food Science and Technology* 15 (2004), pp. 518.

Weber, H. (1996). Starter cultures in dairy industry. In H. Weber (Eds.), *Mikrobiologie der Lebensmittel: Milch und Milchprodukte (in German)* (pp. 105-152). Hamburg: Behr's Verlag.

Chapter 9

Innovative Dairy Products Development Using Probiotics: Challenges and Limitations

Esteban Boza-Méndez, Rebeca López-Calvo and Marianela Cortés-Muñoz

Additional information is available at the end of the chapter

1. Introduction

Probiotic foods are food products that contain a living probiotic ingredient in an adequate matrix and in sufficient concentration, so that after their ingestion, the postulated effect is obtained, and is beyond that of usual nutrient suppliers (Saxelin et al., 2003).

Probiotic delivery has been consistently associated with foods (especially dairy). However, nowadays there is an increasing trend toward using probiotics in different food systems despite its original sources and even as nutraceuticals, such as in capsules. According to Ranadheera et al. (2010) this changing trend in delivering probiotics may lead to a reduction in functional efficacy due to the exclusion of the potential synergistic effect of the food. Selection of the adequate food system to deliver probiotics is a vital factor that should be considered when developing functional products.

Foods are carriers for the delivery of probiotic microorganisms to the human body. The growth and survival of probiotics during gastric transit is affected by the characteristics of the food carriers, like chemical composition and redox potential. Same probiotic strains could vary in functional and technological properties in the presence of different food ingredients or in different food environments (Ranadheera et al., 2010). Thus, variation between different strains' behavior in different conditions would be expected.

Dairy products have been considered as a good carrier for probiotics since fermented foods and dairy products have particularly a positive image. A major advantage is that consumers are already familiar with them and many believe that dairy products are healthy, natural products. Table 1 shows some of the beneficial physiological properties that have been associated with milk components.

Others advantages of dairy products as vehicles for probiotics are that fermentation acts to retain and optimize microbial viability and productivity, while simultaneously preserving the probiotic properties. Consumers are familiarized with the fact that a fermented dairy product contains living microorganisms, and they are also able to protect probiotics through the gastrointestinal transit. This protection comes as a result from the buffering capacity that increases survival chances. The refrigerated storage recommended for these products helps to stabilize probiotic bacteria (Ross et al., 2002; Stanton et al., 2003).

Ingredient	Source	Claim areas examples
Minerals	Calcium Casein peptides	Optimum body growth and development, dental health, osteoporosis
Fatty acids	Conjugated linoleic acid	Heart disease, cancer prevention, weight control
Prebiotics/carbohydrates	Galactooligosaccharides Lactulose Lactose	Digestion, pathogen prevention, gut flora balance, immunity, lactose intolerance
Probiotics	Lactic acid bacteria Bifidobacteria	Digestion, immunity, vitamin production, heart disease, antitumor activity, remission of inflammatory bowel disease, prevention of allergy, alleviation of diarrhea
Proteins/Peptides	Caseins, whey proteins, immunoglobulins, lactoferrin, glycoproteins, specific peptides	Immunomodulation, body growth, antibacterial activity, dental health, hypertension regulation (angiotensin inhibitors)

Table 1. Selection of ingredients and claims associated with functional dairy foods (adapted from Shortt et al., 2003).

Besides, according to Shortt et al. (2003) significant opportunities exist for dairy products whose functionalities have widespread appeal. This means that a product encapsulating the needs of every member of a family is extremely likely to be a success. The broad potential interest in functional dairy products is an important market advantage. Functional dairy products that affect conditions such as osteoporosis, heart disease and cancer are attractive specifically to adults, while products with claims on tooth health, bone health and immunity appeal to adults and children in a similar way. The possible range of sensory characteristics with dairy ingredients also allows the production of diverse textures and aromas, adding another benefit.

Current knowledge on probiotics support a number of potential health benefits. They help to maintain good balance and composition of intestinal flora increasing the ability to resist pathogens invasion and maintain the host's well being. Reduction of blood pressure, cholesterol and/or triglycerides levels, reduction of lactose intolerance problems, immune system enhancement, anti carcinogenic activity and improve nutrients utilization are well described in literature. The use of probiotics for preventing and treating illnesses related to gastrointestinal, respiratory and urogenital tracts have been studied. They have been widely used in therapeutic applications as constipation, diarrhea control, bowel syndrome, control of inflammatory processes, prevention of eczema, osteoporosis and food allergy (Aureli et al., 2011; Ranadheera et al., 2010; Rastall et al., 2000; Vasiljevic and Shah, 2008).

The most common probiotic strains used in dairy foods belong to *Lactobacillus* (*L. acidophillus, L. johnsonii, L. gasseri, L. crispatus, L. casei/paracasei, L. rhamnosus, L. reuteri, L.plantarum*) and *Bifidobacterium* (*Bifidobacterium lactis, B. bifidum, B. infantis, B. breve, B. animalis, B. adolescentis*) genera (Saxelin, 2008).

In Europe EFSA is responsible for the evaluation procedure that accepts or rejects applications for health and nutrition claims on food and beverages (EU Regulation 1924/2006). In recent years this European authority has rejected probiotic health claims adducing that there is no sufficient scientific evidence for the declared beneficial effects. This situation obliged food companies from probiotic industry to perform new clinical studies trying to generate solid scientific evidence for specific probiotic strains and health benefits for submission to the EFSA approval. Consumers still identify probiotic dairy products as healthy despite of this situation.

According to Shortt et al. (2003), the dairy industry is in an excellent position to develop and exploit the functional food market. These products are significant players in the functional food market; for example, they were estimated to account for approximately 60% of functional food sales in Europe by 2000. In 2008, consumers market for probiotic foods was over 1.4 billion Euros in Western Europe, and their annual sales growth was forecast at 7-8% for a 5 year period (Saxelin, 2008). Developing new technologies and new functional dairy products is nowadays relevant.

This chapter focuses on the development of innovative probiotic dairy products considering limiting factors for the survival of probiotics, techniques for the addition and protection of these microorganisms, the quality modifications of final products, the application of sensory analysis and finally how to determine probiotic populations in dairy products.

2. Limiting factors for the survival of probiotics

The food industry has an important market created by the incorporation of probiotic microorganisms into products. However, the addition of this kind of cultures in a food product could be difficult because of the bacteria conditions required in order to survive or to grow in food. Some authors have suggested that more research regarding the challenges that represent incorporating a probiotic culture is necessary because most of the information available is focused on health benefits of the probiotics (Champagne et al., 2005). Evaluation of technological traits such as growth and survival in milk-based media and during product manufacture and shelf life can be important considerations for the selection of strains for food applications (Stanton et al., 2003).

Successful marketing of probiotic products require a minimal amount of viable probiotic cells guaranteed throughout shelf life. To obtain the beneficial effects associated with this type of food, the bacteria must remain viable and in a proper concentration when the host consumes the product. This fact could determine the shelf life of the developed product, because the survival of the probiotics depends on many factors in the food (Talwaker and Kailasapathy, 2004).

Champagne et al. (2005) list seven factors that culture distributors and food manufacturers need to consider in order to add probiotics successfully into products. These factors include: type and form of the culture, the amount of bacteria required to obtain a beneficial effect, toxicity, production process effect on viability, the determination of probiotic cells used in the product, stability during storage and possible changes in sensory properties of the food.

To use a probiotic strain compatible with food production processes technologies is ideal. This means that the elaboration, distribution and commercialization of the product should not have any effect in the viability of bacteria. For example, in the specific case of dairy products, the probiotic should have the capacity to grow in milk (or dairy) but also have a low metabolic activity at low temperatures, in order to guarantee the proper amount of bacteria in the product with no significant changes in quality during shelf life. However, probiotic bacteria generally do not grow well in milk and are adversely affected by storage conditions in some dairy products (Champagne, 2008).

The compatibility and adaptability between the selected strain(s) and the food used as carrier is fundamental, and may represent a significant technological challenge since many probiotic microorganisms are sensitive to the concentration of oxygen, carbon dioxide and salt, high and freezing temperatures and acidic environments (Corrales et al., 2007; Cruz et al., 2009a; Fortin et al., 2011; Talwaker and Kailasapathy, 2004).

Since many dairy products are fermented, it is common to found levels of acidity that may affect the probiotics viability. Numerous studies have reported large losses in viability during storage of fermented milk, yogurt and alike (dairy products known as acid). It is believed that the pH is actually a critical stress factor in the probiotics viability through storage, although there are variations between species and strains for the survival in acidic environments (Roy, 2005). Donkor et al. (2006) evaluated the effect of the acidity of yogurt on the viability of some *Lactobacilli* and *Bifidobacteria* strains. They concluded that *Lactobacilli* strains showed a good cellular stability maintaining constant concentration throughout the storage period regardless of final pH. On the other hand, the cell counts of *Bifidobacteria* decreased by one log cycle at the end of the storage period, due to the high production of organic acids.

Boza et al. (2010) studied the effect of adding *Lactobacillus paracasei* subsp. *paracasei* to a semi hard cheese. Figure 1 presents the pH variation found in cheese during ripening at controlled conditions of 12°C and 85% RH. An important initial decrease is observed (day 0 to 13), pH values tend then to stabilize during cheese ageing process.

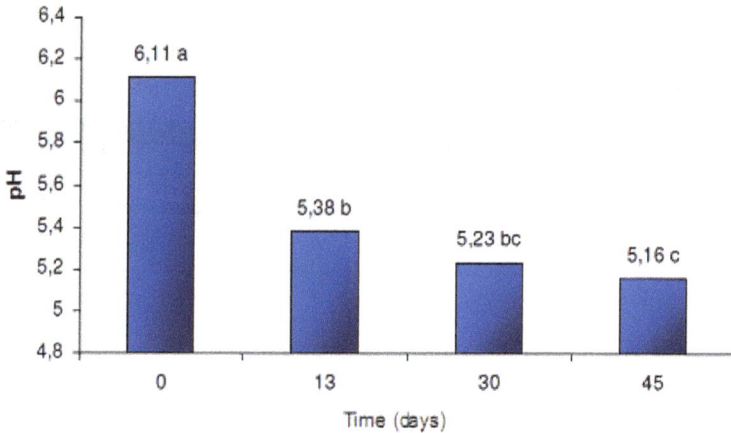

Figure 1. Values of pH for semi hard cheese with *Lactobacillus paracasei* subsp. *paracasei* aged for different periods at 12°C and 85% RH [18]. Different letters in the columns indicate significant differences ($P<0,05$).

Corriols (2004) studied the survival of *Bifidobacterium lactis* in a light sour cream (12% fat, w/w) during 40 days at 5°C. In this study, product behavior considering pH of a regular sour cream inoculated with a starter culture mix of *Lactococcus lactis* subsp. *cremoris*, *Lactococcus lactis* subsp. *lactis*, *Leuconostoc mesenteroides* subsp. *cremoris*, *Lactococcus lactis* subsp. *diacetylactis* and a probiotic sour cream (starter culture + *Bifidobacterium lactis*) was performed. Table 2 presents pH values for probiotic light sour cream during storage time at 4ºC. Evaluating pH at day 8, 15 and 22 showed that there was no significant difference ($P>0.05$) in these values.

Storage time (days)	pH
0	4.51 a
8	4.37 b
15	4.36 b
22	4.39 b

Table 2. Variation of pH for 12% fat (w/w) sour cream with *B. lactis* during refrigerated storage at 4ºC. Average of 5 measurements of three independent experiments. Values followed by the same letter within a column are not significant at $P<0.05$.

Since there was a slight product post-acidification (see table 2) *B. lactis* survival was possible as acidity could be a cause of probiotics viability loss in fermented products. No significant difference (*P*>0.05) was found in probiotic and regular sour cream pH values. Finally, this study showed that it was possible to preserve a probiotic population around 7 x 10^6 CFU/g after 40 days of storage indicating that this cheese could be considered a functional product along its shelf life. Author reported an increase of 12% on final cost of probiotic light sour cream when compared to regular product.

It is also important to note the relationship between probiotics and other fermenting microorganisms, as there may be synergistic or antagonistic effects between them (Heller, 1998). During the manufacture of cheese or yogurt, addition of the starters and probiotic cultures usually result in a slower growth of the probiotic strains. This is possibly because the starter cultures produce substances that inhibit not only pathogens and spoilage microorganisms but also probiotics, and because of the rapid growth of starter cultures, the nutrients availability for probiotics decreases (Roy, 2005). Champagne et al. (2005) mentioned that very few strategies have been proposed to reduce the starters' negative effects on the probiotic cultures, and that the most common is reducing starter dose (entirely or partially). However, precautions must be taken when lowering the dose of the starter microorganisms, because probiotics can also show a negative effect on these cultures and this would slow their activity.

Environments with a rich concentration of oxygen due to transportation systems and stirring or whipping procedures are also commonly found in dairy processing, especially in ice creams and some types of yogurts and fermented milks. The exposure of cultures to dissolved oxygen causes the accumulation of toxic metabolites such as superoxide, hydroxyl radicals and hydrogen peroxide, which eventually lead to cell death of the probiotic microorganisms that partially or completely lack of an electrons transport system. Regarding this oxygen toxic effect on probiotics, there are variations between species. For example, *Bifidobacterium* spp., strictly anaerobic in nature, is generally considered more vulnerable than strains of *Lactobacillus acidophilus* (Talwaker and Kailasapathy, 2004).

Another important issue concerning the addition of probiotic strains into food is temperature. Heating temperatures below 45°C are usually compatible with the cultures, although this depends on the time and the specific strain. Processes that include heating steps above 45°C result in destruction of at least a portion of the probiotic population (Roy, 2005).

On the other hand, low temperatures are generally used to delay the chemical reactions and growth of microorganisms found in foods, therefore a lower temperature implies greater bacterial inhibition growth. A temperature low enough will inhibit the growth of all microorganisms including probiotics. Because of their nature, dairy products, fermented or not, require low storage temperature for preservation, and this fact determines the survival and development of probiotics in these products. It is believed that freezing also leads to a considerable reduction in the number of viable microorganisms in food, although this reduction would depend on the freezing rate and the specific strain tolerance to low temperature.

Corrales et al. (2007) evaluated the effect of the dynamic freezing operation on the viability of two different probiotic strains, *Lactobacillus acidophilus* and *Bifidobacterium lactis,* during ice cream production. It was found that the reduction rate of both strains during this operation was not significant ($P>0.05$), but throughout the whole process of elaboration of the ice cream (dynamic freezing and then hardening at -30°C) there was a significant reduction on both populations.

Other unit operations like pressing and draining could also affect the bacterial counts in the products. The effect of pressing and draining in a cheese probiotic cells is obviously a loss of these cells in the whey, so the final concentration in the pressed cheese is difficult to control (Heller, 1998). Segura (2005) evaluated the effect of the pressing operation in a Turrialba cheese (typical Costarican fresh cheese, >60% water, w/w) added whith *Bifidobacterium lactis.* Probiotic population was determined before and after the pressing operation, and significant differences were found ($P<0.05$). A loss of approximately two logarithms on probiotic population was reported after the pressing operation.

Despite the above results, it is believed that cheese could be a very good vehicle for delivering probiotic strains into the organism, since cheese has a stable structure and usually a high fat content (case of aged cheeses), factors that can help bacteria to survive during product storage and transit on the gastro-intestinal tract.

When comparing with yogurt, the problem for cheese (especially semi-hard and hard cheese) acting as carrier for probiotics results from the high fat and salt content and the relatively low recommended daily intake. Also the concentration of probiotics in cheese should be about four to five times higher than in yogurt. However, this does not apply to fresh cheese, which can easily be adjusted to low fat and salt contents, and for which recommended daily intake is rather high (Cruz et al., 2009a).

Figure 2 shows the growth of a strain of *L. paracasei* subsp. *paracasei* in a semi hard cheese during a ripening period of 45 days at 12°C and 85% RH (Boza et al., 2010). Probiotic population increased during the ripening period reaching interesting levels according with the high levels population goal.

Figure 3 shows the stationary behavior of the same bacteria viability in the ripened cheese kept under refrigeration for 49 days. It should be noted that strains of *Lactobacillus paracasei* have been isolated from naturally ripened cheeses and recognized as non starter lactic acid bacteria (Lynch et al., 1999), indicating that the matrix of the cheese is a good substrate for the growth of this bacterium.

The trend in cheeses, as in yogurt and fermented milks, is that probiotic bacteria populations remain stable or loose viability during ripening and storage (Kılıc et al., 2009; Ong et al., 2006; Songisepp et al., 2004; Vinderola et al., 2000; Yilmaztekin et al., 2004). There are also studies that have shown the growth of some probiotics in cheese during ripening periods or storage under refrigerated conditions (Boza et al., 2010; Buriti et al., 2005; Gardiner et al., 2002; Gardiner et al., 1998; Segura, 2005). However, growth and survival of probiotic microorganisms in ripened cheeses are believed to depend on many factors (like ripening temperature and the probiotic strain interactions with other microorganisms found in cheese) hence hard to generalize.

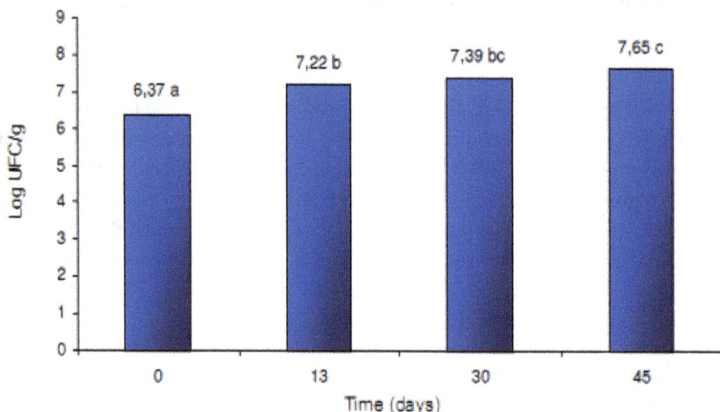

Figure 2. Logarithm of the number of colony forming units of *Lactobacillus paracasei* subsp. *paracasei* per gram of semi hard cheese for different time periods at 12°C and 85% RH. Different letters in the columns indicate significant differences (*P*<0,05).

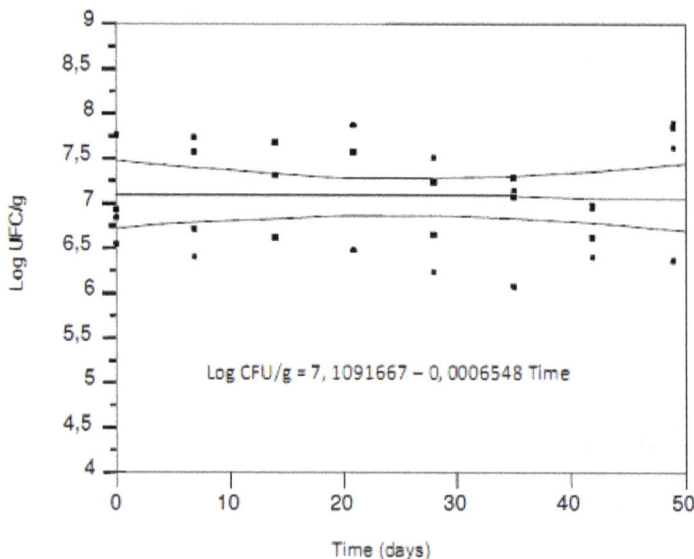

Figure 3. Logarithm of the number of colony forming units of *Lactobacillus paracasei* subsp. *paracasei* per gram of semi hard cheese vacuum packed and stored for 49 days at 5°C (Boza et al., 2010).

Indulgence products like ice-creams are potential probiotic vehicles as well, with the advantage of being appreciated by people belonging to all age groups and social levels (Cruz et al., 2009b). However, in these products, due to low storage temperatures and high concentration of dissolved oxygen, it is difficult for probiotic microorganisms to increase their number. The study conducted by Corrales et al. (2007) determined the behavior of two different probiotic strains, *L. acidophilus* and *B. lactis,* in ice cream throughout 85 days of storage at -30° C. Figure 4 (a and b) shows the behavior of probiotic strains.

The author found that freeze storage conditions affected significantly (P<0.05) the viability of the two microorganisms, and reported losses of 0.76 and 1.10 logarithmic units for *L. acidophilus* and *B. lactis* respectively. Functional shelf life (plate counts > 10^6 CFU/g) was found to be 90 days. An increase of 28% in variable costs was calculated for the product.

Salem et al. (2005) manufactured ice cream with different strains of *Lactobacilli* and *Bifidobacteria.* The probiotic ice cream was evaluated for cultures survival during 12 weeks of frozen storage at -26°C. Initial freezing of ice cream mix followed by hardening caused a reduction of less than one log cycle in viable counts of probiotics. The viable counts decreased during frozen storage by 2.23, 1.68, 1.54, 1.23 and 1.77 log for *Lactobacillus acidophilus, Bifidobacterium bifidum, Lactobacillus reuteri, Lactobacillus gasseri* and *Lactobacillus rhamnosus,* respectively. Although there was a decrease in the number of viable cells, the investigators considered the ice cream as a probiotic food during 12 weeks of storage, since the viable population remained above the recommended minimum limit of 1 x 10^6 CFU /g.

Feraz and colleagues (2012) investigated the survival of *L. acidophilus* in ice cream with different overrun levels during a 60 day storage period. All the ice creams presented a minimum count of 1 x 10^6 CFU/g at the end of 60 days of frozen storage.

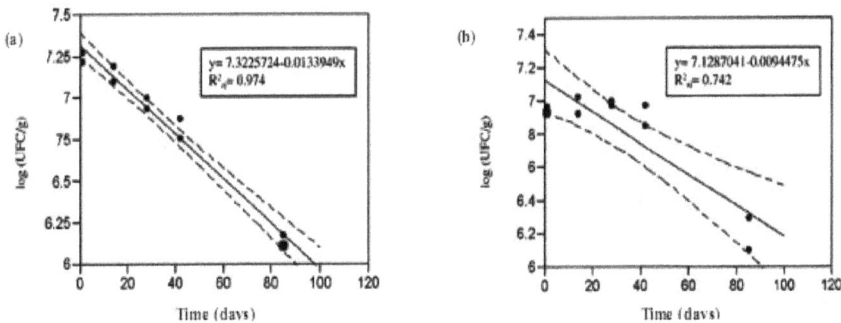

Figure 4. Behavior of *Lactobacillus acidophilus* (a) and *Bifidobacterium lactis* (b) during ice cream storage at -30°C (Corrales et al., 2007).

3. Techniques for the addition and protection of probiotics in dairy products

Controlled growth of probiotic bacteria in a dairy product during ripening or fermentation periods are desirable and interesting from a productive and economic point of view. This ideal situation may allow food producers to use a lower initial dose of inoculum, or may help to replace the microorganisms that could have been eliminated or destroyed during a specific step of the production process like thermal treatment, dynamic freezing or draining.

It has been already explained that probiotics generally do not grow well in milk, and in fact, as mentioned before, the populations of many probiotic bacteria are not even stable during storage of dairy products. However, it is possible to find variations among strains of the same species, and the current trend is the development of new dairy products by using new ingredients that favor the growth of these microorganisms, such as yeasts, tomato juice, rice and soy milk (Champagne et al., 2005; Liu and Tsao, 2009).

Champagne (2008) suggests some ways to address stability problems, and these include: strain selection, ingredients selection (flavours, enzymes, fruits or vegetables, prebiotics) and packaging. All these techniques can be used to innovate and develop new products. Other techniques may include the microencapsulation with lipid materials, alginate and prebiotics (Akhiar, 2010; Siuta-Cruce and Goulet, 2001), the addition of antioxidants such as ascorbate and L-Cysteine, and the elimination from the environment of strains producing hydrogen peroxide (Champagne et al. 2005).

It was mentioned (Cruz et al., 2009a) that one strategy for enhancing bacterial tolerance toward stresses such as temperature, pH or bile salts is prior exposure to sub-lethal levels of the given stress. Cruz et al. (2009a) proposed as alternative to avoid destruction by heat the addition of the probiotic after pasteurization, microencapsulation, pre-adaptation of cells to stress and changing technologies by a slight decrease in temperature.

In order to use probiotic bacteria with proven health benefits in the manufacture of dairy products, sometimes the process has to be modified and adapted for the strains, due to their high sensitivity. According to Cruz et al. (2009a) there are two options for the addition of probiotic bacteria during cheese processing which can directly affect the survival rate of these microorganisms: probiotic bacteria can be added before the fermentation (together with the starter culture), or after it.

Daigle et al. (1999) produced Cheddar cheese from microfiltered milk standardized with cream and fermented with *Bifidobacterium infantis*. In this case, bifidobacteria showed good survival (> 3 x 10^6 CFU/g) on cheese packaged under vacuum and kept at 4°C for 84 days. Cheddar cheese was also successfully produced with a spray dried adjunct of powder milk containing a strain of *Lactobacillus paracasei*. Data obtained demonstrated that probiotic spray-dried powder is a good option of probiotic addition to dairy products (Daigle et al, 1999).

Other research group (Songisepp et al., 2004) added *Lactobacillus fermentum* ME-3, which has been shown to possess antimicrobial and antioxidative properties, to a "Pikantne" cheese which is a semi-soft Estonian cheese with an open texture. They tested two different methods: adding the probiotic combination with the starter culture and adding the probiotic on the drained curd. The cheese produced using the first method showed better sensory characteristics and therefore was chosen to carry out stability tests of probiotic during ripening and storage. The results showed that the strain used was well suited to the process (levels of 5×10^7 CFU/g on ripened cheese) and maintained its probiotic effects.

Lactobacillus casei cells were immobilized on fruit pieces (apple and pear) and used them in the production of Feta cheese (Kourkoutas et al., 2005). Cheese was also produced with free cells of *L. casei*. At the end of the ripening period the authors concluded that the immobilized cells remained viable in the fruit, and in higher counts than in the cheese. Therefore, it is believed that these pieces of fruit were an effective support for the incorporation of probiotics in this type of product.

Ong and other researchers (2006) added combinations of *Lactobacillus acidophilus, L. casei* and *Bifidobacterium longum*; and *L. acidophilus, L. paracasei and B. Lactis* to Cheddar cheese. In this case cheese was produce following a standard procedure, in which milk, after being standardized was tempered to 31°C before inoculation with cheese starter culture and probiotic bacteria. All probiotic adjuncts survived manufacturing process and maintained their viability until the end of the ripening process.

Segura (2005) elaborated a probiotic fresh cheese (>60% water), adding *Bifidobacterium lactis* either to the milk before fermentation or to the curd (mixed with salt). It was found that a large number of bacteria were lost in subsequent operations such as pressing, but this phenomenon was lower when the probiotic culture was added to the curd (see Table 3).

Boza et al. (2010) modified the traditional process of semi hard cheese to avoid larger losses of probiotic in the whey. They added a strain of *Lactobacillus paracasei* mixed with salt after a preliminary pressing of the curd, wherein a major portion of whey was removed, obtaining a cheese with a viable probiotic cell number greater than 1×10^6 CFU/g.

Logarithm of the population of *B. lactis*			
Inoculation technique	Before pressing the curd	After pressing the curd	Variation in the logarithm of the probiotic population
Addition after pasteurization	8.51 [a1]	2.95 [b1]	5.56
Addition to the curd	9.81 [a2]	6.09 [b2]	3.72

[a, b]... Different letters between columns indicate significant differences (P<0,05).
[1, 2]... Different numbers between rows indicate significant differences (P<0,05).

Table 3. *Bifidobacterium lactis* population logarithmic variation before and after the pressing stage of a fresh cheese using two inoculation techniques.

Evaluation of the effect of inoculation time of the probiotics on viable counts of five bacteria in curds and whey during Cheddar cheese manufacture was performed (Fortin et al., 2011). These authors found that inoculation of probiotics in milk before renneting resulted in almost half the cell losses in whey compared with the addition just before the cheddarization step, and they also discovered that addition of probiotics in milk improved their subsequent stability by about 1 log over the 20 days storage period as compared with cells added at cheddarization. Specifically, significantly higher populations of *Bifidobacteria* in curds were detected when the probiotic culture was added to milk. They found that although the quantity of whey generated during cheddarization is much lower than that obtained after the first cutting, the population of probiotics in the whey was ten times higher than after the first cutting when probiotics were added to milk. The authors proposed that cells were not as well entrapped in the curd mass at cheddarization than at renneting.

Arguedas (2010) added *L. paracasei* subesp.*paracasei* in a Philadelphia type cheese (24% fat, w/w) and evaluated their survival behavior during 40 days at 5ºC. This author found that it was possible to reach a population around 7 x 10^6 CFU/g after 40 days of storage, and this cheese could be considered a functional product along the shelf life. Considering that during the Philadelphia type cheese production there is a pasteurization step followed by homogenization and fermentation, probiotic culture was added during the stirring step just before packaging. Figure 5 presents the modified production process. The author reported an increase of 11% on the final cost of the probiotic cream cheese when compared with the regular product.

When producing ice cream with probiotics, cultures may be added in two ways, considering that they are of the DVS (Direct Vat Set) type for direct addition to the product during its manufacture: either adding them directly to the pasteurized mix or using the milk as a substrate for fermentation, producing frozen yoghurt ice cream (Cruz et al., 2009b).

Corrales et al. (2007) developed a process of ice cream adding *Bifidobacterium lactis* and *Lactobacillus acidophilus*. Figure 6 presents the followed steps for the product preparation. The frozen bacteria was dispersed in 1 L of pasteurized milk (2% fat content), and then added the milk to the ice cream mix with constant stirring.

In a similar way, free and encapsulated cells of *L.casei* and *B.lactis* were added to ice cream to evaluate the effect of microencapsulation and resistant starch on the probiotic survival (Homayouni et al., 2008). In general, the results indicated that encapsulation can significantly increase the survival rate of probiotic bacteria on ice cream over an extended shelf-life.

Functional ice creams have been produced by mixing fortified milk fermented with probiotic strains with an ice cream mix, followed by freezing (Salem et al., 2005). Probiotic ice cream has been also produced by the addition of probiotic yogurt to the mix prior the dynamic freezing-step (Soukoulis et al., 2010).

More recently, the effect of different overrun levels on probiotics survival on ice cream has been studied by Ferraz et al. (2012), incorporating *Lactobacillus acidophilus* into a vanilla flavored product. *L. acidophilus* was added to the mix with constant stirring just before freezing. Ice creams were processed with overruns of 45%, 60%, and 90%. Although all presented a minimum count of 1 x 10^6 CFU/g at the end of 60 days of frozen storage, higher overrun levels negatively influenced cell viability, being reported a decrease of 2 log units for the 90% overrun treatment. The authors suggest that lower overrun levels should be adopted during the manufacture of ice cream with probiotics in order to maintain its functional status through the shelf life.

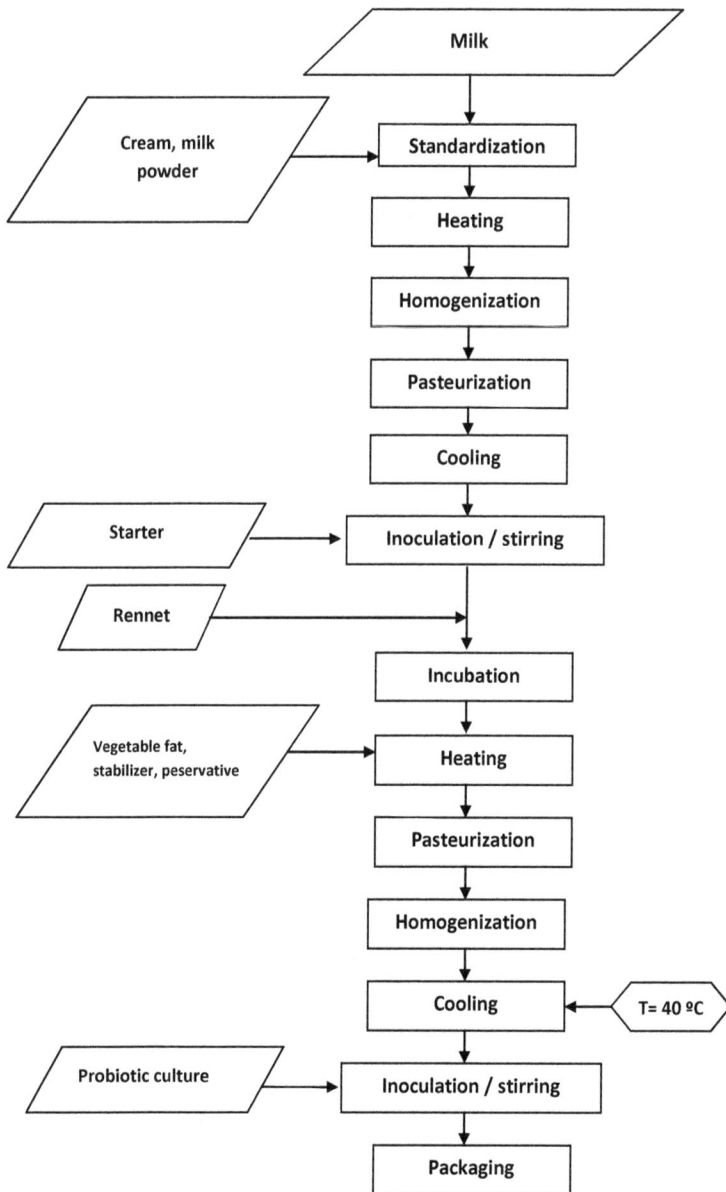

Figure 5. Production flow chart for Philadelphia type cheese with probiotics.

```
┌─────────────────────────────────┐
│ Standardization of the mixture for │
│           ice cream             │
└─────────────────────────────────┘
                │
        ┌───────────────────┐
        │   Pasteurization   │
        │     85° C/ 15 s    │
        └───────────────────┘
                │
      ┌─────────────────────────┐
      │     Homogenization       │
      │ 70-75 °C, 17 – 18.5 MPa  │
      └─────────────────────────┘
                │
        ┌───────────────────┐
        │     Ripening       │
        │   3-5 °C, 10-24 h  │
        └───────────────────┘
                │
   ┌──────────────────────────────────┐
   │ Preparation and probiotic addition │
   │     Stirring 10 min., 4-6 °C      │
   └──────────────────────────────────┘
                │
   ┌──────────────────────────────────┐
   │         Stirring-freezing         │
   │  -4.3 -3.8 °C / 80-90 % Overrun   │
   └──────────────────────────────────┘
                │
        ┌───────────────────┐
        │     Packaging      │
        └───────────────────┘
                │
      ┌─────────────────────────┐
      │        Freezing          │
      │  -25 to -30 °C/ 10-20h   │
      └─────────────────────────┘
```

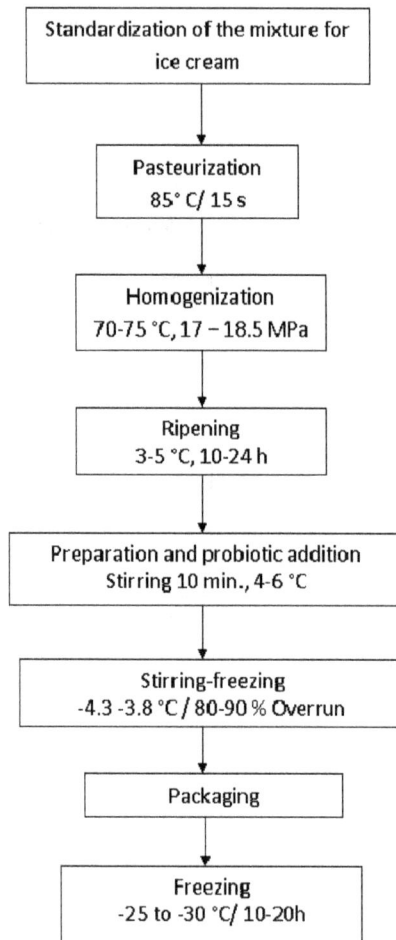

Figure 6. Production flow chart for ice cream with probiotics.

4. Quality modifications of products and sensory analysis

The products chosen for probiotic incorporation must be carefully studied, since the addition and/or multiplication of probiotic microorganisms could produce undesirable characteristics in the products (Dias and Mix, 2008; Komatsu et al., 2008). For many products the addition of probiotics may represent changes that significantly impact its physico-chemical properties, due to the metabolic activity of these living microorganisms and/or changes made on standard food processing procedures. Hence, careful selection of strains is necessary to minimize quality losses caused by alterations to flavor and texture of foods.

According to Champagne et al. (2005) many studies have shown that for some products the addition of probiotics do not lead to significant differences in the sensory properties, although changes in chemical composition and texture may occur these do not necessary have a relevant effect on flavor for some foods (depending on the extent of probiotic growth). This seems to be the case for fermented cheeses.

Natural cheeses are known for their complex microbial ecosystem which is in a constant state of flux as the cheese ages (Dias and mix, 2008). In general, a probiotic cheese should have the same acceptance as a conventional cheese: the incorporation of probiotic bacteria should not imply a loss of quality of the product. In this context, the level of proteolysis and lipolysis must be the same or even greater than cheese which does not have this functional status (Cruz et al., 2009a).

Buriti et al. (2005) evaluated the effect of *Lactobacillus acidophilus* on the instrumental texture profile and related properties of Minas fresh cheese (>65% water, w/w) during storage at 5°C up to 21 days. Parameters measured included hardness, elasticity, cohesiveness, chewiness and gumminess. Four cheese-making trials (T) were prepared, two supplemented with a mesophilic type O culture (T1, T2) and two with lactic acid (T3, T4). *L. acidophilus* was added in T2 and T3. Probiotic cheeses T3 were firmer by the end of storage, due to higher values of pH and hardness, and according to the authors also had better results in the sensory evaluation (preference-ranking test). Differences detected were attributed to the starter, rather than to *L. acidophilus*. In this study percentage of syneresis and the proteolytic index were also determined after the different storage times, finding no relevant differences.

For this same type of cheese, it was proved that the use of a probiotic culture (containing *L. acidophilus*, *B. animalis* and *S. thermophilus*) complementary to lactic acid, aiming to substitute tradicionally employed culture for Minas cheese production, is advantageous (Buriti et al., 2007). Cheeses with added probiotic culture showed to be less brittle and with more favorable sensory characteristics than those made with the traditional lactic acid culture. Researchers conducted an instrumental texture profile analysis of cheeses and a preference-ranking test.

In other study the influence of probiotic bacteria on proteolytic patterns and production of organic acid during ripening period of 6 months on Cheddar cheese at 4°C was evaluated (Ong et al., 2006). No significant differences (P>0.05) were observed in composition (fat, protein, moisture, salt content), but acetic acid concentration was higher in probiotic cheeses. The assessment of proteolysis during ripening showed no significant differences in the level of water-soluble nitrogen (primary proteolysis), but the concentration of free amino acids were significantly higher in probiotic cheeses (secondary proteolysis).

More recently, the survival and influence on sensory characteristics of probiotic strains of *Lactobacillus fermentum* and *Lactobacillus plantarum*, all derived from human faces, were investigated in Turkish Beyaz cheese production. Quantification of volatile aroma components by gas chromatography was performed as well as sensory evaluation. The results showed that tested probiotic culture mix was successfully used in cheese production without adversely affecting cheese quality during ripening. The chemical composition and sensory quality of probiotic cheeses were also comparable with traditional cheeses (Kılıç et al., 2009).

Arguedas (2010) analyzed the effect of adding *L. paracasei* subesp.*paracasei* in a Philadelphia type cheese (24% fat, w/w) on product texture during the shelf life. Table 4 shows the results obtained on hardness, cohesivity, adhesivity and gumminess (instrumental analysis) at day 2 and 44 for samples of regular and probiotic cheese at refrigerated storage (5ºC).

There was no significant difference (P> 0.05) in any parameter between regular and probiotic cream cheese although there was a variation as a function of time on hardness, cohesivity and gumminess for the samples analyzed. In general, these three parameters decreased along storage probably due to syneresis. Since there was no interaction between the time effect and the type of product effect, the decrease on these parameters is not related with the probiotic presence.

Treatment		Hardness (N)	Cohesivity	Adhesivity (erg)	Gumminess (N)
With probiotics	2 days	7,9970	0,3194	-141475,0	2,5964
	44 days	5,6058	0,2115	-120637,5	1,1735
Without probiotics	2 days	6,5627	0,2584	-139880,0	1,6967
	44 days	6,0673	0,2285	-115408,3	1,3882

Table 4. Philadelphia type cheese texture average values obtained during refrigerated storage at days 2 and 44 (Arguedas, 2010).

There was no significant difference (*P*> 0.05) in any parameter between regular and probiotic cream cheese although there was a variation as a function of time on hardness, cohesivity and gumminess for the samples analyzed. In general, these three parameters decreased along storage probably due to syneresis. Since there was no interaction between the time effect and the type of product effect, decreased on these parameters is not related with the probiotic presence.

Consumers rated taste liking degree for cheese during refrigerated storage (5ºC) at days 2, 16, 30 and 44. Figure 7 shows the average results for probiotic Philadelphia cheese type during this period of time. No significant differences (*P*>0.05) were found along shelf life considering taste liking degree for Philadelphia cheese type with *Lactobacillus paracasei* subsp. *paracase*. Average liking degree was 6.5.

Ice cream and ice milk appear to be good products for the delivery of probiotic bacteria. When the cream blend is prepared by adding a fermented milk, the resulting flavor of the product can be affected (Champagne et al., 2005; Cruz et al., 2009b). However, when small quantities of concentrated cultures are introduced, the sensory properties are not affected. Strain or species do seem to be important, since ice creams manufactured with *L. reuteri* cultures have shown to be "more sour" than those made from corresponding cultures of *L. acidophilus*, *L. rhamnosus*, or *B. bifidum* (Champagne et al., 2005). Also, products like non-fermented probiotic ice-cream will not normally present problems resulting from the microbial metabolism, since they are stored at very low temperatures, minimizing the probiotic microorganisms' biochemical reactions (Cruz et al., 2009b).

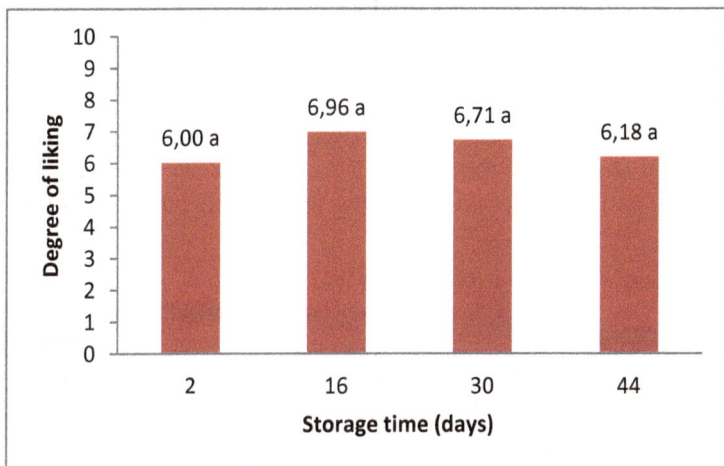

Figure 7. Consumers average taste liking degree of Philadelphia cheese type with *Lactobacillus paracasei* subsp. *paracasei* during storage (Arguedas, 2010). Different letters in the columns indicate significant differences ($P<0,05$).

Corrales et al. (2007) conducted a sensory evaluation of the ice cream flavor, using the duo-trio differentiation technique with 30 semi-trained panelists. It was found that 17 of the 30 semi-trained panelists were able to detect the sample that was equal to the pattern, indicating that no significant difference ($P > 0.05$) was found in the ice creams flavor with and without probiotics. This result supports the conclusion that the consumer did not detect changes in the flavor of ice cream, contributing to the product acceptance.

According to Soukoulis et al. (2010), probiotic ice cream is a functional frozen dairy dessert with particular sensory characteristics combining the flavor and taste of fermented milks with the texture of ice cream. In their study, the effects of compositional parameters (hydrocolloids type and amount, yogurt and milk fat content) on texture and flavor of a probiotic ice cream were evaluated. In such a product, the use of hydrocolloids like xanthan gum and low acidified formulations are recommended to improved creamy sensation, high textural quality and enhanced flavor. They found that based on hedonic and descriptive evaluation, consumers' acceptability of probiotic ice cream is mainly affected by ten sensory drivers including "sweet", "sour", "astringent", "vanilla flavor", "gummy", "coarse", "watery", "creamy", and "foamy".

The effect of several probiotic strains on the sensory acceptance of ice cream was evaluated by Salem et al. (2005). Probiotic ice cream was manufactured by mixing fortified milk fermented with probiotic strains with an ice cream mix. They found that all the ice cream samples received a high score in the sensory evaluation. Ice cream containing *Lactobacillus reuteri* was judged to be sourer and reached a higher score for "probiotic" flavor.

Two types of synbiotic ice cream containing 1% (w/w) resistant starch with free and encapsulated *Lactobacillus casei* and *Bifidobacterium lactis* were manufactured by Homayouni et al. (2008). The synbiotic ice cream samples were sensory assessed by 32 panelists. According to the authors, total evaluations in term of color, texture and taste of all samples were positive and did not have any marked off-flavor during the storage period. None of the ice creams were judged to be crumbly, weak, fluffy or sandy.

Finally, Ferraz et al. (2012) supplemented a vanilla ice cream with *Lactobacillus acidophilus* at different overrun levels (45%, 60%, and 90%). They did not report an influence for any overrun level ($P>0.05$) on acceptability regarding appearance, aroma, and taste of the ice creams.

Performing sensory evaluation is certainly an important step in probiotic dairy products development before the launch of the product into the market. As new products with probiotics may change some characteristics studying the behavior of trained panelists and consumers toward the developed product is a key factor and might represent a powerful tool to recover information that could support a product launch.

Another central issue in new probiotic products is to guarantee enough microorganism population in order to allow consumers to experience the beneficial effects described before. Probiotic quantification with an appropriate technique is a must in the product process development.

5. Probiotic quantification techniques

Proper selection of an analytical method for the probiotic microorganism's enumeration in food is critical since confirmation of whether the product has the minimum required amount of bacteria to provide the health benefits associated will depend on the result obtained.

The choice of culture medium and methodology for selective enumeration of commercial probiotic strains in combination with starters depends strongly on the product matrix, the target group and the taxonomic diversity of the bacterial background flora in the product (Van de Casteele et al., 2006). There is a wide variety of analysis methods that consider all these aspects and are extensively documented by various authors.

Several media have been suggested for the enumeration of probiotic bacteria alone or in combination in commercial cultures or products (Vinderola and Reinheimer, 2000). MRS agar is the media most commonly used and is normally supplemented with different sugars as maltose or glucose and with antibiotics solutions such as dicloxacillin, clindamycin, vancomycin, nalidixic acid, among many others. It is also common to add inhibitory agents as LiCl, NaCl, acids, bile salts and sorbitol. Supplements selection is made depending on the microorganism of interest and strains that wanted to be inhibited, for this purpose combination of both is very common. RCA agar with different antibiotics and salts is likewise used.

For *Bifidobacterium* sp. count, an incubation of plates under anaerobic conditions is required while Lactobacillus sp. strains can be recover both aerobically and anaerobically. Therefore one criterion for selecting the correct method is not only the strain of interest oxygen requirement but also accompanying flora characteristics. Similarly, temperature and incubation time varies between methods. Most of probiotic cultures are recovered at 37°C but increasing incubation temperature at 43°C is often use to inhibit mesophilic flora. Incubation times typically range from three to six days.

An important aspect to consider is that probiotic microorganisms viable cells amount should be kept at the minimum accepted level in order to be considered as a functional food during its entire shelf life. Therefore, in new product development probiotic bacteria count should be performed in fresh product and throughout shelf life. In many cases, shelf life of such products is determined as a function of time in which availability of minimum required concentration of probiotics can be guarantee.

In the scientific literature, populations of 10^6 - 10^7 CFU/g in the final product are established as therapeutic quantities of probiotic cultures in processed foods (Talwaker et al., 2004), reaching 10^8 - 10^9 CFU, provided by a daily consumption of 100 g or 100 ml of food, hence benefiting human health (Jayamanne and Adams, 2006). For example, in Brazil, the present legislation states that the minimum viable quantity of probiotic cultura should be between 10^8 and 10^9 CFU per daily portion of product and that the probiotic population should be stated on the product label (Brazilian Agency of Sanitary Surveillance, 2012).

6. Conclusion

The use of products like yogurt, fermented milks, different cheeses and ice cream as probiotic food carrier opened a valuable alternative for dairy industry. To meet consumers demand for probiotic foods in different countries, different types of products are needed. Research has demonstrated that is possible to incorporate successfully probiotics reaching the recommended amounts in order for consumers to experience the described health benefits. It is also possible to reach a reasonable shelf life according to the expected product characteristics.

From a technological point of view adding probiotics into dairy products could represent a difficult task depending on the type of product or microorganisms. Knowledge of all unit operations involved in processing and adaptations in traditional dairy process are helpful. Preliminary test to follow product and bacteria behavior provide useful information and sometimes it is necessary to change process parameters or inoculation step.

Proper techniques for population determination must be used to follow probiotic behavior during production and storage time and correctly predict shelf life. Performing physico-chemical analysis is decisive since characterization of product gives important information of probiotic effects and finally appropriate sensory techniques help to determine if attributes may have an influence on consumer acceptance. Since final product quality modifications could occur it is important to perform sensorial test with trained, semi-trained judges or directly with consumers at this stage. Results obtained in a product developing process are indeed specific for the product, microorganism or mixture of microorganisms and technology involved. It is not possible to generalize them to other products, strains or elaboration techniques.

Developing successful functional dairy food requires to be supported by scientific research. Product development in this field should consider knowing the consumer expectations, the technological process, the appropriate analyzing techniques and marketing. Nutrition advantages of dairy products need to be emphasized and information should be focused on consumers but also need to consider health care professionals.

Industry needs relevant regulation of physiological claims and health claims and nowadays some companies are performing clinical studies with particular strains to prove specific benefits but it is clear that production of functional dairy foods following the rules of medicine production is hardly of interest.

Considering the healthy population there may be potential to develop targeted products for different age groups. In the reduction of risk and treatments of various diseases, probiotics have resulting in promising benefits. However, it is important to understand the mechanisms behind the effects on our well-being. Information regarding the interaction between bacteria and dairy is focused on growth and survival of probiotics during production, storage and gastric transit therefore more research is needed to determine the effect of food substrate on metabolic activities of probiotics associated with their beneficial properties.

Author details

Esteban Boza-Méndez, Rebeca López-Calvo and Marianela Cortés-Muñoz*
*National Research Center of Food Science and Technology (CITA),
University of Costa Rica, San José, Costa Rica*

7. References

Akhiar, N.S. (2010). Enhancement of probiotics survival by microencapsulation with alginate and prebiotics. *Basic Biotechnology*, Vol.6, pp.13-18.

Arguedas, N. (2010). Determinación de la sobrevivencia del cultivo probiótico *Lactobacillus paracasei* subesp.*paracasei* (LC-01®) en un queso crema durante su almacenamiento y su influencia sobre la aceptación por consumidores, el pH, la textura y los costos variables. Thesis Lic. in Food Technology. Universidad de Costa Rica.

Aureli, P.; Capurso, L.; Castellazzi, A.M.; Clerici, M.; Giovannini, M.; Morelli, L.; Poli A.; Pregliasco, F.; Salvini, F.; Zuccotti, G.V. (2011). Probiotic and health: an evidence-based review. *Pharmacological Research*, Vol.63, No.5, pp. 366-376.

---

* Corresponding Author

Boza, E.; Morales, I.; Henderson, M. (2010). Development of mature cheese with the addition of the probiotic culture *Lactobacillus paracasei* subsp. *paracasei* Lc-01. *Revista Chilena de Nutrición*, Vol.37, No.2, pp.215-223.

Brazilian Agency of Sanitary Surveillance. (May 2012). Food with health claims, new foods/ingredients, bioactive compounds and probiotics. In: *Alimentos*, 05. 5. 2012, Available from http://www.anvisa.gov.br/alimentos/comissoes/tecno_lista_alega.htm

Buriti, F.; Da Rocha, J.; Saad, S. (2005). Incorporation of Lactobacillus acidophilus in Minas fresh cheese and its implications for textural and sensorial properties during storage. *International Dairy Journal*; Vol.15, pp.1279-1288.

Buriti, F.; Okazaki, T.; Alegro, J.; Saad, S. (2007). Effect of a probiotic mixed culture on texture profile and sensory performance of Minas fresh cheese in comparison with the traditional products. *Archivos Latinoamericanos de Nutrición*, Vol.57, No.2, pp. 179-185.

Champagne, C. (2008) Development of yoghurt and specialty milks containing probiotics. *Journal of Animal Science*, Vol.86, E-Suppl.2, pp.367-368.

Champagne, C.; Gardner, N.; Roy, D. (2005). Challenges in the addition of probiotic cultures to foods. *Critical Reviews in Food Science and Nutrition*, Vol.45, No.1, pp. 61-84.

Corrales, A.; Henderson, M.; Morales, I. (2007). Survival of probiotic microorganisms *Lactobacillus acidophilus* and *Bifidobacterium lactis* in whipped ice cream. Revista Chilena de Nutrición, Vol.34, No.2, pp.157-163.

Corriols, M. (2004). Determinación de la sobrevivencia del *Bifidobacterium lactis* en una natilla liviana durante el período de almacenamiento. Thesis Lic. in Food Technology. Universidad de Costa Rica.

Cruz, A.; Buriti, F.; Souza, C.; Faria, J.; Saad, S. (2009a). Probiotic cheese: health benefits, technological and stability aspects. *Trends in Food Science & Technology*, Vol.20, pp.344-354.

Cruz, A.; Antunes, A.; Sousa, A.; Faria, J.; Saad, S. (2009b). Ice-cream as a probiotic food carrier. *Food Research International*, Vol.42, pp.1233–1239.

Daigle, A.; Roy, D.; Belanger, D.; Vuillemard, J. (1999) Production of Probiotic Cheese (Cheddar Like Cheese) using enriched cream fermented by *Bifidobacterium infantis*. *Journal of Dairy Science*, Vol.82, pp.1081-1091.

Dias, B.; Mix, N. (2008) Probiotics in natural cheese. *Journal of Animal Science*, Vol.86, E-Suppl.2, pp.367-368.

Donkor, O.; Henriksson, A.; Vasiljevic, J.; Shah, N. (2006). Effect of acidification on the activity of probiotics in yoghurt during cold storage. *International Dairy Journal*, Vol.16, pp.1181-1189.

Ferraz, J.; Cruz, A.; Cadena, R.; Freitas, M.; Pinto, U.; Carvalho, C.; Faria, J.; Bolini, H. (2012). Sensory acceptance and survival of probiotic bacteria in ice cream produced with different overrun levels. *Journal of Food Science*, Vol. 71, No. 1, pp. 524-528.

Fortin, M.; Champagne, C.; St-Gelais, D.; Britten, M.; Fustier, P.; Lacroix, M. (2011). Effect of time of inoculation, starter addition, oxygen level and salting on the viability of probiotic cultures during Cheddar cheese production. *International Dairy Journal*, Vol.21, pp.75-82.

Gardiner, G.; Roos, R.P.; Collins, J.; Fitzgerald, G.; Stanton, C. (1998). Development of a probiotic Cheddar cheese containing human-derived *Lactobacillus paracasei* strains. *Applied and Environmental Microbiology*, Vol.64, No.6, pp.2192-2199.

Gardiner, G.; Bouchier, P.; O'Sullivan, E.; Kelly, J.; Collins, K.; Fitzgerald, G.; Ross, R.P.; Stanton, C. (2002). A spray-dried culture for probiotic Cheddar cheese manufacture. *International Dairy Journal*, Vol.12, pp.749-756.

Heller, J. (1998). Starterorganismen und Produktcharakteristika. *Deutsche Molkereizeitung*, Vol.12, pp.598-604.

Homayouni, A.; Azizi, A.; Ehsani, M.; Yarmand, M.; Razavi, S. (2008). Effect of microencapsulation and resistant starch on the probiotic survival and sensory properties of synbiotic ice cream. *Food Chemistry*, Vol.111, pp.50–55.

Jayamanne, V. S.; Adams, M. R. (2006). Determination of survival, identity, and stress resistance of probiotic bifidobacteria in bio-yoghurts. *Letters in Applied Microbiology*, Vol.42, No.3, pp. 189 -194.

Kılıc G.B, Kuleaşan H, Eralp I, Karahan A.G. (2009). Manufacture of Turkish Beyaz cheese added with probiotic strains. *LWT - Food Science and Technology*, Vol.42, pp.1003-1008.

Komatsu, T.; Buriti, F.; Saad, S. (2008). Inovação, persistência e criatividade superando barreiras no desenvolvimento de alimentos probióticos. *Brazilian Journal of Pharmaceutical Sciences*, Vol.44, No.3, pp. 329-347.

Kourkoutas, Y.; Xolias, V.; Kallis, M.; Bezirtzoglou, E.; Kanellaki, M. (2005) *Lactobacillus casei* cell immobilization on fruit pieces for probiotic additive, fermented milk and lactic acid production. *Process Biochemistry*, Vol.40, pp.411-416.

Liu, S-Q.; Tsao, M. (2009). Enhancement of survival of probiotic and non-probiotic lactic acid bacteria by yeasts in fermented milk under non-refrigerated conditions. *International Journal of Food Microbiology*, Vol.135, pp.34–38.

Lynch, C.; Muir, D.; Banks, J.; McSweeney, P.; Fox, P. (1999). Influence of adjunct cultures of *Lactobacillus paracasei* ssp. *paracasei* or *Lactobacillus plantarum* on Cheddar cheese ripening. *Journal of Dairy Science*, Vol.82, pp.1618-1628.

Ong, L.; Henriksson, A.; Shah, N. (2006). Development of probiotic Cheddar cheese containing *L. acidophilus*, *L. casei*, *L. paracasei* and *Bifidobacterium* sp. and the influence of these bacteria in proteolytic patterns and organic acid production. *International Dairy Journal*, Vol.16, pp.446-456.

Ranadheera R.D.C.S.; Baines, S.K.; Adams, M.C. (2010). Importance of food in probiotic efficacy. *Food Research International*, Vol.43, pp.1-7.

Rastall, R. A.; Fuller, R., Gaskins, H. R. (2000). Colonic functional foods. In: *Dairy Processing*, Gibson G.R., Williams C.M. (eds.), pp. 71-89, CRC Press, Boca Raton.

Ross, R.P.; Fitzgerald, G.F.; Collins, J.K.; Stanton, C. (2002). Cheese delivering biocultures-probiotic cheese. *Australian Journal of Dairy Technology*, Vol.57, No.2, pp.71-78.

Roy, D. (2005). Technological aspects related to the use of bifidobacteria in dairy products. *Lait*, Vol.85, pp.39-56.

Salem, M.; Fathi, F.; Awad, R. Production of probiotic ice cream. (2005). Polish Journal of Food and Nutrition Sciences, Vol.14, No.3, pp.267-271.

Saxelin, M.; Korpela, R.; Mäyrä-Mäkinen, A. Functional dairy products. In: *Dairy Processing. Improving Quality*, Smit, G. (ed.), pp.229-245, CRC Press, Boca Raton.

Saxelin, M. (2008). Probiotic Formulations and Applications, the Current Probiotics Market, and Changes in the Marketplace: A European Perspective. *Clinical Infectious Diseases*, Vol.46, pp.76-79.

Segura, N. (2005). Elaboración de queso fresco tipo Turrialba con probióticos. Thesis Lic. in Food Technology. Universidad de Costa Rica.

Shortt, C.; Shaw, D.; Mazza, G. (2003). Overview of opportunities for health-enhancing functional dairy products. In: *Handbook of Functional Dairy Products*, Shortt, C.; O'Brien, J. (eds), pp. 1-13, CR Press.

Siuta-Cruce, P.; Goulet, J. (2001). Improving probiotic survival rates. *Food Technology*, Vol.55, No.10, pp.36-42.

Songisepp, E.; Kullisaar, T.; Elias, P.; Hütt, P.; Zilmer, M.; Mikelsaar, M. (2004). A new probiotic cheese with antioxidative and antimicrobial activity. Journal of Dairy Science, Vol.87, pp.2017-2023.

Soukoulis, C.; Lyroni, E., Tzia, C. (2010). Sensory profiling and hedonic judgement of probiotic ice cream as a function of hydrocolloids, yogurt and milk fat content. *LWT-Food Science and Technology*, Vol.43, pp.1351-1358.

Stanton, C., Colette, D.; Coakley, M., Collins, K., Fitzgerald, G., Ross, P. (2003). Challenges facing development of probiotic-containing functional foods. In: *Handbook of Fermented Functional Foods*, Farnworth, E. (ed), pp.27-58, CR Press.

Talwaker, A.; Kailasapathy, K. (2004). A review of oxygen toxicity in probiotic yogurts: Influence on the survival of probiotic bacteria and protective techniques. *Comprehensive Reviews in Food Science and Food Safety*, Vol.3, pp.117-123.

Talwalkar, A.; Miller, C. W.; Kailasapathy, K.; Nguyen, M. H. (2004). Effect of packaging materials and dissolved oxygen on the survival of probiotic bacteria in yoghurt. *International Journal of Food Science and Technology*, Vol.39, No.6, pp.605 - 611.

Van de Casteele, S.; Vanheuverzwijn, T.; Ruyssen, T.; Van Assche, P.; Swings, J.; Huy, G. (2006). Evaluation of cultura media for selective enumeration of probiotic strains of lactobacilli and bifidobacteria in combination with yogurt or cheese starters. *International Dairy Journal*, Vol.16, pp. 1470-1476.

Vasiljevic, T., Shah N P. (2008). Probiotics –From Metchnikoff to bioactives. *International Dairy Journal*, Vol.18, pp.714-728.

Vinderola, C.; Prosello, W.; Ghiberto, D.; Reinheimer J. (2000). Viability of probiotic (Bifidobacterium, Lactobacillus acidophilus and Lactobacillus casei) and nonprobiotic microflora in Argentinian Fresco cheese. *Journal of Dairy Science*, Vol.83, pp.1905-1911.

Vinderola, C. G.; Reinheimer, J. A. (2000). Enumeration of Lactobacillus casei in the presence of *L. acidophilus*, bifidobacteria and lactic starter bacteria in fermented dairy products. *International Dairy Journal*, Vol.10, pp. 271-275.

Yilmaztekin, M.; Ozer, B.; Atasoy, F. (2004). Survival of *Lactobacillus acidophilus* LA-5 and *Bifidobacterium bifidum* BB-02 in white-brined cheese. *International Journal of Food Sciences and Nutrition*, Vol.55, No.1, pp.53-60.

Chapter 10

Cereal-Based Functional Foods

R. Nyanzi and P.J. Jooste

Additional information is available at the end of the chapter

1. Introduction

Functional foods are defined as foods that, in addition to their basic nutrients, contain biologically active components, in adequate amounts, that can have a positive impact on the health of the consumer [1, 2, 3, 4]. Such foods should improve the general and physical conditions of the human organism and/or decrease the risk of occurrence of disease [5]. Functional foods have also been referred to as medicinal foods, nutritional foods, nutraceuticals, prescriptive foods, therapeutic foods, super-foods, designer foods, foodceuticals and medifoods [4]. These foods generally contain health-promoting components beyond traditional nutrients [1]. Various criteria for defining functional foods have been mooted by [6] and a number of published reports have indicated the benefits of functional foods to the consumer [7, 8].

One way of creating a functional food is by inclusion of ingredients such as probiotics and prebiotics to levels that enable the consumer to derive optimal health benefits [2]. Probiotics are defined as live microorganisms which upon ingestion in adequate numbers impart health benefits to the host animal beyond inherent basic nutrition [4, 9,10]. Most of the probiotic species belong to the genera *Lactobacillus* and *Bifidobacterium* [11, 12,13]. Benefits of probiotic intake include prevention and treatment of infantile diarrhoea, travelers' diarrhoea, antibiotic induced diarrhoea, colon cancer, constipation, hypercholesterolaemia, lactose intolerance, vaginitis and intestinal infections [14, 15, 16]. Prebiotics, on the other hand, are non-digestible food ingredients that affect the host by selectively targeting the growth and/or activity of one or a limited number of beneficial bacteria in the colon, and thus have the potential to improve health [2, 7, 17, 18, 19]. Potential benefits of prebiotic intake include reduction of cholesterol absorption, control of constipation, bioavailability of minerals and reduction in blood glucose levels when used to replace sucrose in diabetic diets [8, 15, 20, 21]. The main aim of this chapter is therefore to discuss the possibility of converting cereal-based fermented foods into functional foods similar to the existing commercial dairy products. The fermentation of cereal based foods and the beneficial attributes of such foods will be discussed. The latter attributes include the use of such foods as delivery vehicles for probiotic bacteria to the consumer.

2. Fermentation of cereal based foods

Generally, fermentation is a food preservation method intended to extend shelf-life, improve palatability, digestibility and the nutritive value of food [22, 23, 24]. Lactic acid fermentation comprises of the chemical changes in foods accelerated by enzymes of lactic acid bacteria resulting in a variety of fermented foods [11, 25]. Lactic acid fermentation processes are the oldest and most important economical forms of production and preservation of food for human consumption ([11, 23, 26, 27]. It is, therefore, not surprising that fermented foods and beverages make a big contribution to people's diets in Africa [28]. It is reported that fermented foods globally contribute 20 to 40% of the food supply and usually, a third of the food consumed by man is fermented [29]. This renders fermented foods and beverages a significant component of people's diets globally. It is estimated that the largest spectrum of lactic acid fermented foods occurs in Africa [23, 30]. However, in Africa, fermented foods and beverages are often prepared by employing spontaneous fermentation processes at household level or by small-scale industries using maize, sorghum and millet as the main cereals [11, 31, 32]. In sections 3 and 4 of this chapter, a description will be given of acid-fermented cereal-based foods and beverages and the major bacteria involved in the fermentation of such foods. In section 5 of this chapter, probiotic cereal beverages will be dealt with.

2.1. Some beneficial attributes of African fermented cereal-based foods

Lactobacillus species are the predominant organisms involved in the fermentation of cereal-based foods and beverages in Africa (see section 4.1). These organisms are reported to have bacteriostatic, bactericidal, viricidal, anti-leukaemic and antitumor effects in the consumer [25, 28, 33]. Beneficial starter cultures are not usually used in the fermentation of traditional cereal-based foods and beverages. However, it is reported that fermented foods have a probiotic potential [34] due to the probiotic *Lactobacillus* species that may be contained in them, some of which are of human intestinal origin [11].

The quality of some traditional African fermented products (see section 3.2) can be enhanced using beneficial cultures. '*Dogik*' for example is '*ogi*' enhanced with a lactic acid starter culture reputed to have antimicrobial activities against diarrhoeagenic bacteria [11]. *Lactobacillus paracasei* ssp. *paracasei*, a probiotic *Lactobacillus* species [11] was present together with other LAB in *uji* [35]. Strains of *Lb. acidophilus*, which are probiotic, were also isolated from an African sorghum-based product in which accelerated natural lactic fermentation was observed [36].

Improved production of milk by nursing mothers has been attributed to consumption of fermented *uji*, one of the traditional fermented beverages in Africa. *Kanun-Zaki*, a fermented non-alcoholic cereal-based beverage widely consumed in Northern Nigeria is also popularly believed to enhance lactation in nursing mothers [37]. Restoration of the normal blood level and resultant compensation for blood lost during traditional tribal circumcision operations in parts of Africa is attributed to drinking large quantities of fermented *uji* [38].

It is reported that several B vitamins including niacin (B3), panthothenic acid (B5), folic acid (B9), and also vitamins B1, B2, B6 and B12 are released by LAB in fermented foods. These vitamins are co-factors in some metabolic reactions, for instance, folates prevent neural tube defects in babies and provide protection against cardiovascular disease and some cancers [39].

2.1.1. Shelf-life extension and improved nutritional and sensory properties

Generally, shelf-life, texture, taste, aroma and nutritional value of food products can be improved by fermentation [11, 23, 25, 40, 41]. The metabolic activities of microbial fermenters are responsible for the improvement in taste, aroma, appearance and texture [23, 30]. During fermentation, there is production of lactic, acetic and other acids and this enhances the flavour and lowers the pH of the final product. The acids also prolong food shelf-life by lowering the pH to below 4 and this restricts the growth and survival of spoilage organisms and some pathogenic organisms such as *Shigella, Salmonella* and *E. coli* [11, 25, 28, 33, 42]. Fermented foods, unlike non-fermented foods, have a longer shelf-life, making fermentation a key factor in the preservation of such foods [23, 43]. Because fermentation improves keeping quality and nutritional value, it is a predominant food processing and preservation process [44, 45]. During fermentation, enzymes such as lipases, proteases, amylases and phytases are produced and these in turn hydrolyse lipids, proteins, polysaccharides and phytates respectively [46]. The released nutrients contribute to the enhancement of sensory quality and nutritional value of the product [46, 47].

2.1.2. Inhibition of pathogenic microorganisms in fermented foods.

Spontaneous fermentation may involve species of *Lactobacillus, Lactococcus, Pediococcus* as well as certain yeasts and moulds [48]. Lactic acid bacteria involved in fermentation are able to produce hydrogen peroxide, but lack the true catalase to break down the hydrogen peroxide. The hydrogen peroxide can, therefore, accumulate and be inhibitory to some harmful bacteria and to the LAB themselves [11].

The organic acids released (e.g. lactic, acetic, propionic and butyric acids), as by-products during lactic acid fermentation, lower the pH to levels of 3 to 4 with a titratable acidity of about 0.6% (as lactic acid) [23, 40, 48]. The undissociated forms of the acetic and lactic acids at low pH exhibit inhibitory activities against a wide range of pathogens [23 48]. This improves food safety by restricting the growth and survival, in fermented cereal beverages, of spoilage organisms and some pathogenic organisms such as *Shigella, Salmonella* and *E. coli* [11, 25, 28, 33, 43, 47]. Fermented maize gruel and high-tannin sorghum gruel at pH 3.8 inhibited *E. coli, Campylobacter jejuni, Shigella flexneri, Salmonella typhimurium* and *Staphylococcus aureus* [30]. When starter cultures were used to ferment sour maize bread, it was found out that *Lb. plantarum* lowered the pH to 3.05 [40]. The fermented maize dough also showed growth inhibitory activity against *Salmonella typhi, S. aureus, E. coli*, and the aflatoxigenic *Aspergillus flavus* [40].

Although *Koko* sour water (KSW) fed to Ghanaian children did not seem to halt diarrhoea, improved well-being was claimed after 14 days of consumption of this product [44]. Conflicting results about the efficacy of fermented beverages against pathogens and diarrhoea is attributed to the unpredictable nature of spontaneous fermentation. Spontaneous fermentation results in a variety of species and strains with varying degrees of antibacterial activity and ability to adhere to intestinal membranes [44]. Other studies have however, reported positive outcomes of consuming fermented cereal beverages. It was reported that a fermented cereal gruel in Tanzania reduced diarrhoea by 40% in consuming children compared to those children that did not consume it over a period of 9 months [44, 48]. This was attributed to better beverage microbial safety as well as protection against intestinal enteropathogenic colonization [48]. In a review by [25] information gathered revealed that fermented cereal-based products which contained *Lactobacillus* spp. and lactic acid had viricidal, anti-leukemic, antitumor and antibacterial activities. .

Lactobacillus isolates including *Lb. fermentum*, and *Lb. plantarum*, from maize-based ogi (West Africa) and *Lb. fermentum, Lb. paracasei* and *Lb. rhamnosus* from maize-based *boza* (Eastern Europe) were active against potential pathogens such as *Escherichia coli, Klebsiella pneumoniae, Pseudomonas aeruginosa, Enterococcus faecalis and Bacillus cereus* due to the low pH in these products and the production of bacteriocins by the *Lactobacillus* spp [49].

2.1.3. Production of bacteriocins by lactic acid bacteria

Bacteriocinogenic lactic acid bacteria (LAB) isolated from fermented foods produce proteinaceous, antimicrobial substances (Table 1) called bacteriocins [23, 31, 50, 51]. It was reported that bacteriocinogenic LAB prevent the growth of pathogens such as *Listeria monocytogenes, Bacillus cereus, Staphylococcus aureus* and *Clostridium dificile* [23].

Bacteriocins have the ability to form pores in the membrane of target bacteria, in this way exerting bactericidal and bacteriostatic effects against the growth of pathogens in the intestinal tract [52]. Bacteriocins also reduce or prevent post-production microbial contamination of feed and food fermentation products in the food chain [51]. It was observed that bacteriocins from *Lb. plantarum* and *Lb. casei* isolated from fermented maize products, *kenkey* and *ogi* respectively inhibited and acted against a number of food borne pathogens [51]. However, bacteriocins have a narrow antimicrobial spectrum and of all bacteriocins, nisin produced by *Lactococcus lactis* is the only one generally used as a preservative by food manufacturers [46, 50]. A range of characterized bacteriocins that have potential benefits, have been reported to be produced by the *Lactobacillus* spp. and these are referred to in Table 1. While some LAB may show bacteriocin-linked inhibition of food spoilage and pathogenic bacteria *in vitro* in laboratory media, inhibitory activity in the food matrices may not be equally effective. This may be due to poorer diffusion of the bacteriocin into the cells of pathogenic bacteria in the food matrix or be the result of bacteriocin inactivation by nutrient components in the food [53].

Bacteriocin	Bacterial Species	Active against
Bulgarican	*Lb. delbrueckii* subsp. *bulgaricus*	Broad, including G (-).
N.N	*Lb. fermentum*	Broad G (+) incl *Listeria* spp
Acodophillin	*Lb. acidophilus* DDS 1	Disease-causing M/Os
Lactocidin	*Lb. acidophilus*	Disease-causing M/Os
Acidolin	*Lb. acidophilus*	Disease-causing M/Os
Lactobacillin	*Lb. acidophilus*	Disease-causing M/Os
Lactacin B	*Lb. acidophilus*	LAB
Nisin	*Lactococcus lactis*	Broad G(+) incl *Listeria* spp
Lactabacillin	*Lb. brevis*	LAB
Brevicin	*Lb. brevis*	LAB
Caseicin 80	*Lb. casei*	*Lb. brevis*
Plantaricin A	*Lb. plantarum*	LAB
Reuterin	*Lb. reuteri*	Broad G (+), G (-) and fungi

Source: [22, 27, 52, 119], G+, Gram positive bacteria; G-, Gram negative bacteria; MOs, microorganisms

Table 1. Some of the bacteriocins produced by lactic acid bacteria (LAB)

2.1.4. The effect of fermentation on toxic, antinutritional and indigestible compounds in cereal foods

During fermentation, microbial activity may lead to the elimination of toxic compounds from food products [28, 31]. For example it was reported that fermentation with *Lb. plantarum* starter cultures significantly reduced the cyanogenic glucoside content of cassava [23]. High cyanide content in a diet can cause acute poisoning, tropical ataxic neuropathy and konzo (a paralytic disease). It may also exacerbate iodine deficiency resulting in goitre and cretinism [54]. During 'gari' and 'lafun' production from cassava, the cyanogenic glucoside, linamarin, is hydrolysed by the linamarinase enzyme to glucose and cyanohydrin. The latter product is then broken down to acetone and hydrocyanic acid by hydroxynitrile lyase at pH 5-6 and the free cyanide is released faster by gentle heating [25, 55]. If the cyanogenic glucoside linamarin were to be hydrolysed in the gastro-intestinal tract (GIT), the released cyanide anion would be absorbed and halt the functioning of cytochrome oxidase enzymes in the body [23, 29].

Legumes and cereals contain indigestible oligosaccharides such as stachyose, verbascose, and raffinose which cause flatulence, diarrhoea and digestion problems [23]. The α-D-galactosidic bonds in the above-mentioned sugars are relatively heat-resistant, but they can be degraded by the galactosidase enzymes of some LAB including strains of *Lb. fermentum, Lb. plantarum, Lb. salivarius, Lb. brevis, Lb. buchneri* and *Lb. cellobiosus* [23]. During fermentation, the microorganisms disintegrate these flatulence-causing and indigestible oligosaccharides into utilisable di- and mono-saccharides [25, 29, 53].

Phytic acid, tannins and phenolic acids are polyphenols that are considered to be antinutritional factors (ANFs) and are found in cereals and legumes and the foods prepared therefrom [56]. The ANFs contribute to malnutrition and reduced growth rate due to the promotion of poor protein digestibility and by limiting mineral bioavailability [23, 46, 56, 57]. Phytic acid in cereals and legumes, for example, (Table 2) affects the nutritional quality due to chelation of phosphorus and other minerals such as Ca, Mg, Fe, Zn, and Mo [41, 56, 58, 59]. The resultant low mineral bioavailability can result in mineral deficiency [47, 59]. Deficiency in a mineral such as iron can result in anaemia, a decrease in immunity against disease and impaired mental development. Poor calcium bioavailability on the other hand prevents optimal bone development and can cause osteoporosis in adults. Insufficient zinc brings about recurring diarrhoea and retarded growth [59].

Product	Range (%)
Sorghum	0.57-0.96
Maize	0.44-1.2
Millet	0.85-1.1
Cowpeas	0.89-1.5

Adapted from reference [30]

Table 2. Approximate phytate content of sorghum, maize, millet and cowpeas

Other negative effects of the presence of phytate in the diet, include the reduction of the activity of digestive enzymes such as trypsin, alpha-amylase and beta-galactosidase in the GIT. This is due to the formation of complexes of phytate with the enzymes and other nutrients that negatively affect digestive processes [57, 58]. Similarly tannins and polyphenols are enzyme inhibitors of plant origin that form complexes with proteins, resulting in deactivation of digestive enzymes, reduction in protein solubility and digestibility and reduction of absorbable ions [57, 60, 61]. The enzymes inhibited by tannins and/or polyphenols include pepsin, trypsin, chymotrypsin, lipases, glucosidase and amylase [57, 62]. Inhibition of the amylase enzymes results in low starch breakdown and hence, less sugar release in the GIT [117]. In fermented products this amylase inhibition by tannins impairs microbial proliferation [83]. This in turn decelerates pH decrease and acidity production in the medium [83].

Fermentation, by certain LAB and yeasts, removes or reduces the levels of antinutritional factors such as phytic acid, tannins and polyphenols present in some cereals meant for weaning purposes [23, 31, 41, 47, 53, 56, 59, 63]. During fermentation, optimal pH conditions prevail for enzymatic degradation of the antinutritional factors. This results in better bioavailability of minerals such as iron, zinc and calcium [11, 23]. Strains of *Lb. plantarum* degraded phytic acid in the cereals after incubation at 37 °C for 120 hours [23]. This degradation can be ascribed to the hydrolysis of the phosphate group by phytases from the raw cereal substrate and produced by the fermenting microorganisms [46, 47, 57]. Fermentation alone reduced the phytate content by 39%. The combined effect of fermentation plus the addition of exogenous phytase, resulted in a reduction of 88% of the phytates in tannin sorghum gruel [47].

Fermentation reduced phenolic compounds and tannins in finger millet by 20% and 52% respectively [60]. Fermentation coupled with methods such as decortication, soaking and germination reduced the tannins in sorghum, other cereals and in beverages made from these cereals [57, 60, 61, 62, 83]. Fermentation of porridges from whole and decorticated tannin sorghum led to significant reduction of total phenols [61].

The use of *Rhizopus oligosporus* to ferment cooked soybean in *tempe* production reduced residual trypsin inhibitor activity (TIA) by 91% in addition to the 86.4% reduction attributed to steaming [57]. The reduction of the TIA was ascribed to hydrolysis of the trypsin inhibitor by the fungi fermenting the *tempe* [57]. In another study [63], *Lb. brevis*, *Lb. fermentum*, *Streptococcus thermophilus* and *Pediococcus pentosaceus* were observed to have improved the nutritional quality of fermented sorghum products. Table 3 shows that some strains of LAB significantly degraded trypsin inhibitors. This illustrates the possibility that using carefully selected probiotic bacteria to ferment cereal foods may reduce the antinutritional factors in such products.

Fermentation can also decrease the activity of the proteinase and amylase inhibitors in cereals resulting in an increase in the availability of starch and essential amino acids such as lysine, leucine, isoleucine and methionine [23, 46, 53]. The protein quality and nutritive value of fermented products such as *kenkey*; *iru*; and *ugba* [25] and *ogi* [64] was improved during fermentation due to either microbial protein synthesis or loss of non-protein material. In support of the above, [39] reported that fermenting with *Lb. plantarum* OG 261-5 significantly improved the levels of tryptophan, lysine and tyrosine even though other amino acids such as isoleucine, leucine, valine and phenylalanine decreased.

LAB isolate	Reduction of TI (mg)	Percent reduction
Lb. plantarum 91	2.41	48.0
Lb. fermentum 103	1.22	24.4
Pediococcus sp. 90	0.89	17.8
Pediococcus sp. 19	1.08	21.6
Leuconostoc sp. 106	2.68	53.6
Lactobacillus sp. 41	0.65	13.0
Lactobacillus sp. 17	1.86	37.2
Lactobacillus sp. 62	1.34	26.8

Adapted from references [23, 30]; *Aflata* is a gelatinized maize paste intermediate in kenkey production.

Table 3. Degradation of trypsin inhibitor (TI) by lactic acid bacteria isolated from *aflata* in Ghana

Fermentation in many instances results in an increased vitamin content of the final product [23]. Lactobacilli involved in fermentation may require vitamins for growth, but several of them are capable of bio-synthesizing B-vitamins in excess. It is reported that several B vitamins including niacin (B3), panthothenic acid (B5), folic acid (B9), and also vitamins B1, B2, B6 and B12 are released by LAB in fermented foods [39]. Cereal-based products such as *ogi*; *mageu*; and *kenkey* have thus been reported to have an improved B-vitamin content [25, 29]. Fermentation therefore improves the nutritive value of cereal foods.

2.1.5. Reduction, binding or detoxification of mycotoxins in fermented foods

Maize (*Zea mays*), sorghum (*Sorghum vulgare*), pearl millet (*Pennisetum glaucum*) and finger millet (*Eleusine coracana*) constitute the most important cereals for the preparation of fermented foods in the developing world [41, 65, 66, 67]. These cereal grains are however, exposed to pre- and post-harvest mycotoxin contamination which end up in the fermented foods [23, 54. 67]. Among the cereals, maize is the most prone to mycotoxin contamination [66].

Mycotoxins are secondary metabolites released into cereal grains and legume seeds by species of the genera *Aspergillus, Fusarium* and *Penicillium* [54, 66]. Aflatoxins and fumonisins are the mycotoxins, in cereals, of major health and economic concern in the developing world [23, 24, 48, 54, 66, 68, 69]. Table 4 shows the deaths linked to mycotoxins in foods. Aflatoxin B1 (AFB1) is toxic, carcinogenic, mutagenic and teratogenic [45, 69]. Fumonisins have been linked to oesophageal cancer in South Africa and liver cancer in China [66, 68]. Kwashiorkor in children is aggravated by long term exposure to aflatoxin [66]. The development and propagation of cereal-based probiotic and/or synbiotic (prebiotics and probiotics combined) beverages may consequently, to some extent, be hampered by mycotoxin-contamination of the cereals used in making such beverages.

Bacterial and fungal (biological) decontamination is one of the mycotoxin-reducing strategies that have been and are being investigated [24]. *Flavobacterium aurantiacum* (*Nocardia corynebacterioides*), *Corynebacterium rubrum, Saccharomyces cerevisiae, Candida lipolitica, Candida krusei, Aspergillus niger, Mucor* spp., *Rhizopus* spp., *Nurospora* spp., *Amillariella tabescens,* and *Trichoderma viride* are bacterial and fungal species reported to have the capability to degrade mycotoxins enzymatically ([23, 24, 45, 69]. Extracellular extracts of *Rhodococcus erythropolis* reduced Aflatoxin B1 (AFB1) by 66.8% after 72 hours of incubation [69]. Fermentation by *R. oryzae* and *R. oligosporus* was reported to reduce aflatoxins to aflatoxicol A which, under conditions created by organic acids, gets permanently converted to aflatoxicol B [54]. It was claimed that aflatoxin B1 is 18 times more toxic than aflatoxicol B and it is also possible that the former, during lactic acid fermentation to pH < 4.0, gets transformed into a less toxic isomer, aflatoxin B2 [54].

A heat-treated *Saccharomyces* yeast species was said to absorb more than 90 % (w/w) of ochratoxin A in grape juice while live cells could only bind 35 % (w/w) [24, 45]. Other workers have indicated that binding of Aflatoxin B1 was better at low pH and when cells were subjected to acid or heat treatment [24]. The implication is that food beverage preparation, which involves cooking after fermentation, together with the highly acidic conditions of the fermented food beverage, may physically alter the microbial cell structure thereby increasing the binding sites for AFB1 [45]. This provides a way of reducing aflatoxins in African fermented foods and beverages. However, some of the microorganisms indicated in the above paragraphs may not necessarily be GRAS (generally recognised as safe) in the human GIT.

Country	Year	Food source	Mycotoxin content	Percentage of samples contaminated	Mycotoxin	Deaths	Case patients
India	1974	maize	NA	NA	Aflatoxin B1	106	397
Kenya	1981	maize	NA	NA	Aflatoxin B1	NA	20
Kenya	2004	maize	~4400ppb	NA	Aflatoxin B1	215	317
Nigeria	2005	maize	NA	NA	Aflatoxin B1	100	NA
Kenya	2005	maize	NA	NA	Aflatoxin B1	30	8
Kenya	2006	maize	NA	NA	Aflatoxin B1	9	NA
Kenya	NA	3 maize brands	0.4-2.0 µg/Kg	NA	Aflatoxins	NA	NA
South Africa	NA	Peanut butter	< 300 ppb	NA	Aflatoxin B1	NA	NA
Togo, Benin	NA	Household maize	NA	30%	Aflatoxin B1	NA	NA
Nigeria	NA	Maize samples	NA	33%	Aflatoxin B1	NA	NA
Benin	NA	Agro-zone sample	> 5 µg/Kg	9.9 - 32.2%	Aflatoxins	NA	NA
Ghana	NA	Maize silos	20-335 µg/Kg	NA	Aflatoxins	NA	NA
Togo, Benin	NA	Maize samples	> 100 ppb	50%	Aflatoxins	NA	NA

Source: reference [66]

Table 4. Deaths and ill health linked to mycotoxin contamination of samples in African countries

Aflatoxin B1 could not be detected in fermented maize porridge (*amahewu*) that had been made from maize meal samples containing 0.55 and 0.84 µg/g aflatoxin B1. In the same study, the levels of fumonisin B1, in contaminated maize meal samples containing 12.1, 24.6, 4.1, 20.6, 47.2 µg/g of this mycotoxin, were drastically reduced in fermented maize porridge to levels of 1.4, 1.4, 0, 6.9, 6.3 µg/g respectively [46]. This exemplifies the detoxification potential for cereal beverages by lactic acid fermentation. The mechanism of mycotoxin removal from fermented food matrices is not clear.

Without forgetting the above paragraph relating to the effect of probiotic fermentation on mycotoxin levels, some reports on fermentation-linked reduction of aflatoxins in cereal food matrices are controversial. There are reports indicating no significant aflatoxin reduction during fermentation [54]. It was observed that fermentation only enabled a reduction of 18% and 13% of aflatoxin and fumonisin respectively in *ogi* [68]. It was reported that under acidic conditions, aflatoxins persist due to aflatoxin precursors and on the other hand, aflatoxin only undergoes reformation but not reduction under acidic conditions created by organic acid metabolites of LAB [68]. There are also fears that fumonisin binds with starch to form an undetectable complex and besides this, they may react with reducing sugar (D-glucose) to form sugar adducts or are hydrolysed to aminopolyols AP1 and AP2 [68].

The foregoing findings indicate that mycotoxin-reduction in fermented cereal food matrices has not yet been properly elucidated. It is therefore necessary to screen probiotic microbial isolates to find those strains that have a definite potential to degrade aflatoxins during fermentation in food matrices. Such mycotoxin-degrading species need to be fully compatible with the human GIT ecosystem. Some workers recommended the use of probiotic microorganisms with high aflatoxin B1 binding capability in fermented foods [24].

However, binding is not degradation and the binding probiotic cells are consumed along with the food matrix. The fate of bound toxins in fermented food matrices needs to be investigated. Probiotics and/or LAB suitably screened for their biological mycotoxin degradation, among other technological and health benefits could be better applied in human food fermentation, even though, prevention of mycotoxin contamination is the better option. Besides fermentation and contamination-preventive measures, it was noted that processing operations including sorting, winnowing, washing, crushing and dehulling [68] significantly reduced mycotoxin levels in several cereal foods.

3. Cereal-based beverages with a probiotic potential

3.1. Selected non-African cereal foods

Most of the commercial products containing probotics and prebiotics available today are dairy-based [70]. Several workers have, however, endeavoured to develop non-dairy, cereal-based probiotic and/or synbiotic products [4, 57, 70-76]. The following non-African fermented cereal beverages have a probiotic potential or in other words, the potential to be transformed into functional beverages.

3.1.1. Boza

Boza is consumed in countries of the Balkan region including Bulgaria, Romania, Albania and Turkey [4, 77]. Reports indicated that *boza* in Turkey contained 0.03-0.39% (w/v) alcohol but the country's national regulations allow beverages with an alcohol content of not more than 5.0 g/L to be considered non-alcoholic [78].

Boza is a highly viscous traditional fermented product, made from millet, maize, wheat, rye, or rice and other cereals mixed with sugar [79, 78, 80]. In the preparation of *boza*, the milled cereals are mixed in water and then cooked in an open or steam-jacketed boiler. The gruel is cooled and strained to remove the bran and hull. Sugar is added and then fermented at 30 °C for 24 hours by back-slopping or use of sourdough and/or by adding yoghurt starter cultures [78]. Fermented *boza* is then cooled to refrigeration temperatures and distributed into 1L plastic bottles to be consumed within 3-5 days [78]. *Boza* is popularly accepted in the countries referred to above due to its pleasant taste, flavour and nutritional value [4].

Spontaneous fermentation involves LAB and yeasts [80]. Lactic acid bacterial species isolated from *boza* included *Leuconostoc paramesenteroides*, *L. mesenteroides* subsp. *mesenteroides*, *L. mesenteroides* subsp. *dextranicum*, *L. oenus*, *L. raffinolactis* *Lb. coryniformis*, *L. confusus*, *L. sanfrancisco*, *Lb. fermentum* *Lb. plantarum*, *Lb. acidophilus*, *Lb. coprophilus* and *Lb. brevis* [4, 79, 80]. The yeast isolates included *Saccharomyces cerevisiae*, *Candida tropicalis*, *Candida glabrata*, *Geotrichum penicillatum* and *G. candidum* [4, 80]. The microflora in *boza* [4, 80] can vary depending on the region and/or country as well as the combination of cereals used and other factors. Only three species were however recommended for inclusion in a mixed starter culture for *boza* production namely: *S. cerevisiae*, *L. mesenteroides* subsp. *mesenteroides* and *L. confusus* [80].

3.1.2. Kvass

Kvass is a non-alcoholic fermented cereal-based beverage made from rye and barley malt, rye flour, stale rye bread, and sucrose and is most often consumed in Eastern Europe [81]. *Kvass* is manufactured using two techniques. One technique involves the use of stale dough bread in which the sugars for the yeast fermentation are obtained from the bread-making process, while the second technique involves the use of malt enzymes to hydrolyse the gelatinized starch [81]. Before fermentation is initiated by the addition of baker's yeast or back-slopping, sucrose is added to the *kvass* wort [81]. The fermentation process is terminated by cooling the *kvass* to 4 °C and the product contains proteins, amino acids, vitamins and organic acids either from the raw materials or from the activity of the fermenting microorganisms [81].

The *kvass* alcohol content is less than 1% while the carbohydrate components predominantly include maltose, maltotriose, glucose and fructose [81]. Maltose and maltotriose components are categorized as isomalto-oligosaccharides that are not completely broken down by digestive enzymes in the GIT [81]. Isomalto-oligosaccharides can hence serve as bifidogenic (prebiotic) factors for the proliferation of probiotic bifidobacteria in the intestines [81].

The predominant microorganisms in *kvass* fermentation were found to be *Lb. casei*, *L. mesenteroides* and *S. cerevisiae*. *Kvass* is not heat-treated after fermentation and as a result high counts of viable cells can be found in the beverage [81]. The isolation of *Lb. casei* from *kvass* (in which it was highly viable), is indicative of the potential of cereal-based beverages such as this to be used as alternatives to milk products in the delivery of probiotics and other functional ingredients to the consumer in the developing world [81].

3.1.3. Pozol

Pozol is a traditional fermented maize dough consumed in South-eastern Mexico [4]. *Pozol* is made mainly by Indian and Mestizo populations of Mexico [82]. During *pozol* preparation, maize grains are cooked in lime water to obtain nixtamal (nixtamalization is a process in which maize (corn), or other grains are treated by soaking and cooking in limewater). This results, *inter alia*, in the grain being more easily ground and the nutritional value being improved). The nixtamalized product is then cleaned by washing in water to separate the husks. The grains are ground, moulded into balls, then wrapped in banana leaves and spontaneously fermented at room temperature for about 7 days [82]. The pH of *pozol* is usually in the range of 3.7-4.7 after 48 hours of fermentation [82]. *Pozol* balls at different stages of fermentation can be mixed with water to make a gruel of desired viscosity and then consumed as a beverage by adults, children and infants [82]. Although African fermented maize gruels are not nixtamalized, *pozol* is similar to African traditional products such as *mageu/mahewu, ogi, kenkey* and *koko* that will be discussed in the next section of this chapter.

Escherichia coli was isolated from *pozol* after 48 hours of fermentation [82]. This was linked to the high pH in the initial stages of fermentation and the possibility of the presence of high pH-localities in the dough after 48 hours even though the measured pH was 3.4-4.7 [82]. It is also possible that acid fermented doughs can harbor some pathogenic bacterial strains resistant to high acidity and/or strains adapted to low pH [82].

3.2. African traditional fermented foods

In Table 5 a number of African traditional lactic acid-fermented cereal-based foods and beverages and the major lactobacilli involved in fermentation are listed. Cereals including maize, sorghum and millet have been used individually or in combination in the preparation of a variety of fermented beverages in Africa [83].

3.2.1. Ben-saalga

Ben-saalga is a pearl millet (*P. glaucum*)-based fermented beverage mainly consumed in Burkina Faso [41, 43, 84]. It is popularly consumed by the young, elderly, the sick and the general populace [41, 84]. The traditional way of producing *ben saalga* involves washing the pearl millet, soaking, wet-milling, kneading and sieving moistened flour, and fermenting the settled, but diluted slurry prior to cooking. This then becomes the *ben-saalga* beverage [41, 43, 84]. The pH decreases from 6 to to a pH of 3.6 – 4.0 during a 24-hour fermentation period [84, 85]. In terms of the LAB responsible for the fermentation, spontaneously fermented *ben saalga* is dominated by *Lb. fermentum*, *Lb. plantarum* and *Pediococcus pentosaceus* [41]. Ethanol, lactic acid and acetic acid were the main products of fermentation in *ben saalga* [84].

Ben saalga has a solids content of 8-10 g/ 100 mL and like other cereal beverages discussed in this chapter, it has a poor energy density and nutrient content [41]. However, the preparation of *ben-saalga* results in a reduction of millet's antinutritional factors, such as phytic acid, by about 50% [41]. Thirty three of the 99 bacterial isolates from *ben-saalga* showed antimicrobial activity against at least one of the indicator pathogens used in the study [43]. Seven of the isolates, identified as *Lb. plantarum*, were bacteriocinogenic against indicator pathogens which included *Escherichia coli* U-9, *Listeria monocytogenes* CECT 4032, *L. innocua*, *Salmonella typhimurium*, *S. aureus* CECT 192 and *B. cereus* LWL1 [43]. These findings indicate the probiotic and/or the prophylactic and the therapeutic potential of intake of this fermented cereal beverage. These characteristics may even be improved by using selected starter cultures that can benefit the health of the consumer and enhance the preservation and safety of the food.

3.2.2. Dégué

Dégué is a millet-based fermented food consumed in Burkina Faso [86]. Preparation of *dégué* involves dehulling and grinding of the millet grains, modeling into balls with water and steam cooking to produce gelatinized balls. The balls are then stored to allow a further 24-hour spontaneous fermentation [86]. The pH of *dégué* is usually in the range of 4.57-4.72 and the following microorganisms have been found in the product: *Lb. fermentum*, *Lb. brevis*, *Lb. gasseri*, *Lb. casei*, *E. coli* and *Enterococcus* sp. [86].

Fermented food product name	Raw materials	Lactobacilli involved	Nature of use	Country or region	References
Ogi, Ogi-baba	Maize, millet or sorghum	*Lb. plantarum*	Paste as staple, breakfast or weaning food	Nigeria, W. Africa	[11, 26, 99]
Uji	Maize, millet or sorghum	*Lb. plantarum*	Porridge	Uganda, Kenya, Tanzania	[11]
Koko	Maize	*Lb. plantarum, Lb. brevis*		Ghana	[11]
Kenkey	Maize	*Lb. fermentum Lb. reuteri*	Mush steamed, eaten with vegetables	Ghana	[11]
Kwunu-Zaki	Millet, sorghum or maize	LAB*	Paste used as breakfast cereal	Northern Nigeria	[37]
Mahewu	Maize, sorghum, millet	*Lb.delbrueckii, Lb. bulgaricus Strep. lactis*	Gritty gruels, Solid staple	S. Africa	[28, 99]
Mawe	Maize	LAB*	Basis of preparation of many dishes	S. Africa, Togo	[11]
Mangisi	Millet	Unknown	Sweet-sour non-alcoholic drink	Zimbabwe	[11]
Munkoyo	Sorghum, millet or maize plus munkoyo roots	Unknown	Liquid drink	Zambia, Africa	[11]
Mutwiwa	Maize	LAB*	Porridge	Zimbabwe	[11]
Tobwa	Maize	LAB*	Non-alcoholic drink	Zimbabwe	[11]
Togwa	Sorghum, millet, maize		Acid fermented gruel for refreshment and weaning	Tanzania	[34]
Liha	Maize	Unknown	Sweet-sour non-alcoholic drink	Ghana, Togo, Benin, Nigeria	[118]

Table 5. African acid-fermented non-alcoholic cereal-based foods and beverages and the lactic acid bacteria involved in the fermentation (LAB*, lactic acid bacteria)

3.2.3. Kanun-Zaki

Kanun-zaki is a non-alcoholic fermented cereal-based beverage consumed in Northern Nigeria [11, 37]. *Kanun-zaki* can be prepared from pearl millet, sorghum or maize ([37]:49). This product is popularly served as a breakfast dish [25]. In the preparation of *Kanun-zaki*, the kernels are washed and dried in the sun, then coarsely ground in a mortar and pestle. The flour is then is mixed with hot water to form a paste which is spontaneously fermented for 1-3 days resulting in a sour beverage [25]. It was reported that this beverage is nutritionally, medically and economically important in the regions where it is widely consumed [39].

3.2.4. Kenkey

Kenkey is a fermented maize dough product eaten by the people of Ghana, primarily the Gas, Fantis and Ewes [38, 41]. The preparation of the two main types of *kenkey* (Ga-*kenkey* and Fanti-*kenkey*) was described in reference [41].The Fanti people's name for *kenkey* is *dokon* interpreted to mean 'mouth-watering' because of its pleasant odour and flavour [38]. Similar products to *kenkey* made from sour maize dough include *akasa, koko, banku, abele, akple,* and *kpekpe* though these are not as popular as *kenkey* [38]. *Kenkey* fermentation is spontaneous and is dominated by lactic acid bacteria, particularly *Lb. fermentum* and *Lb. reuteri,* and yeasts that include *C. krusei (Issatchenkia orientalis)* as the dominant yeast species, while *S. cerevisiae* also contributes to the flavour [11, 41]. Apart from improvement in the protein content from 1.3 to 3.3 g per 16 g nitrogen in ready-to-eat *kenkey*, the *kenkey* flavour is attributed to the formation of flavour compounds, during fermentation, such as 2,3-butanediol, butanoic acid, lactic acid, 3-methylbutanoic acid, octanoic acid, 2-phenylethanol, and propanoic acid [41].

3.2.5. Koko

Koko is a millet-based spontaneously fermented beverage mainly consumed in Northern Ghana [44]. The predominant microbial species during fermentation are *Lb. fermentum* and *Weissella confusa* [44]. It was reported that isolates from *koko* showed good antimicrobial activity, tolerance to 0.3% oxgall bile and acid resistance at pH 2.5, which are characteristics of good probiotic strains [44].

3.2.6. Mageu (mahewu)

Mageu is a non-alcoholic largely maize-based beverage popular among the indigenous people of Southern Africa, but is also consumed in some Arabian Gulf countries [4, 74, 83]. It is consumed at schools and mines and on farms. It is a refreshing drink and a traditional weaning beverage for infants. *Mageu* is prepared by using 8% to 10% (w/v) maize flour as the major solid substrate in aqueous suspension. Wheat flour or maize bran is added to initiate the lactic acid fermentation [32]. Some ethnic groups also use sorghum and millet flours instead of maize flour and *mageu* is known by different names (Table 6) among the ethnic groups in Southern Africa. Acceptable *mageu* contains 0.4 – 0.5% lactic acid corresponding to an average pH of 3.5 [87, 88, 89].

Several studies have been conducted on *mageu*. One of these included an investigation of the survival of bacterial enteric pathogens in fermented *mageu*, from which it was concluded that fermented *mageu* had bacteriostatic and bactericidal properties [33]. Another study targeted the growth and survival of *Bacillus cereus* in fermented *mageu* in which growth inhibition of the organism was observed [32]. Studies on the development of a starter culture for *mageu* [88, 90, 91] led to the production of mahewu on a commercial scale [92].

Ethnic group	Local name of product	Reference
Zulu	Amahewu	[91]
Swazi	Emahewu	[89]
Xhosa	Emarewu	[91]
Venda	Mabundu	[70]
Pedi	Mapotho	[70]
Sotho	Machleu	[89]

Table 6. Local names for sour maize porridge (*mageu*) in Southern Africa

3.2.7. Mawe

This is fermented maize dough consumed in the form of a variety of dishes in Togo, Benin and Nigeria [68]. Making the *mawe* (maize dough) involves washing, wet extraction of the endosperm and kneading to a dough which is then spontaneously fermented for about 3 days [41]. In Bennin, *mawe* dough is used for the preparation of cooked beverages (*koko*), stiff gels (*akassa, agid and, eko*) and steam cooked bread (*ablo*) [41]. The predominant LAB in the fermented *mawe* dough included *Lb. fermentum, Lb. cellobiosus, Lb. brevis, Lb. curvatus, Lb. buchneri* and *Weissella confusa*. Other microorganisms in the dough included pediococci and yeasts such as *Candida krusei, C. kefyr, C. glabrata* and *Saccharomyces cerevisiae* [41]. It was reported that in a study of *mawe* production using starter cultures, *C. krusei*, stimulated the growth of *Lb. fermentum* and *Lb. brevis* [41]. Fermentation of this product offers a number of benefits that include flavour enhancement, nutrient bioavailability (including that of some proteins, minerals and B vitamins) as well as protection against some pathogens due to reduction of the pH to 3.5-4.0 [41]. Maize products are however, deficient in some amino acids such as lysine, tryptophan and methionine, which are found more abundantly in legumes such as cowpeas and sybeans. Co-fermentation with legumes can therefore be expected to improve the quality of the protein and protein levels significantly.

3.2.8. Munkoyo

Munkoyo is a traditional fermented maize-based beverage popularly consumed in Zambia and the Democratic Republic of Congo's Katanga province in the south [93, 94]. In Zambia, tree species of *Eminia, Vigna* and *Rhynchosa*, generally referred to as *munkoyo*, are extracted and the extract, high in α- and β-amylases, is used for the liquefaction of maize porridge gel

[93, 94]. The thinned porridge is then spontaneously Fermented, mainly by LAB, for 24-48 hours at room temperature. The sweet-sour *Munkoyo* flavoured drink has a mean pH of 3.5 due to organic acids produced during fermentation, but alcohol (14-26 g/kg) is also detectable. The beverage is consumed by people of all ages [93].

Introduction of *Rhynchosia heterophylla* root extract, *Lb. confusus* LZ1 and *Sacchromyces cerevisiae* YZ20 to the fermentation mix, resulted in a *munkoyo* beverage of pH 3.3, 60 mmol/l lactic acid and an ethanol content of 320-410 mmol/l [93]. The workers observed that a ratio of not more than 1:1000 (yeast: LAB starter culture) fermented for not more than 24 hours resulted in an acceptable *munkoyo* beverage [93]. *Munkoyo* was found to have antibacterial activities. Total coliforms in the *munkoyo* mash initially were 10 cfu/mL but were absent when tested after 15 hours of fermentation due to acidification of the product [94]. The microorganisms in *munkoyo* were not recognised probiotics and it was therefore recommended that the incorporation of probiotic starter cultures producing D (+) lactate be investigated to improve the nutritional, sensory and health benefits of *munkoyo* [94].

3.2.9. Obushera (bushera)

Obushera fermented spontaneously from malted sorghum or millet flour is consumed by young people and adults in Western Uganda [95]. *Obushera* is prepared using sorghum or millet flour. The flour is mixed with water and cooked into a thin porridge and then mixed with a portion of previously fermented porridge. The added fermented portion acts as a 'starter culture' for fermentation to commence and the result is the '*obushera*' beverage consumed by people of any age [48]. Obushera, produced on a small commercial scale, can be used as a thirst quencher, social drink, energy drink and weaning food [95]. The household *bushera*, with a pH in the range 3.7-4.5, had LAB counts varying from 7.1 to 9.4 log$_{10}$ cfu/mL and coliform counts that were in the range of <1 to 5.2 log$_{10}$ cfu/mL [96]. The LAB species from household *bushera* included *Lb. plantarum*, *Lb. paracasei* subsp. *paracasei*, *Lb. fermentum*, *Lb. brevis*, *Lb. delbrueckii* subsp. *delbrueckii* and *Streptococcus thermophilus*. The isolates from laboratory fermented *bushera* belonged to the genera *Lactococcus*, *Leuconostoc*, *Lactobacillus*, *Weissella* and *Enterococcus* [96]. This is indicative of the probiotic potential of *obushera*.

3.2.10. Ogi

Ogi is another traditional African acid-fermented cereal gruel prepared from maize, although sorghum and millet flours are also used [11, 25]. During fermentation, *Lb. plantarum* is the predominant microorganism although bacteria such as *Corynebacterium* spp hydrolyse the corn-starch following which yeast genera such as *Saccharomyces* and *Candida* contribute to the flavour [11, 27]. *Ogi* is traditionally produced by washing the grains, steeping for 12 to 72 hours, wet-milling, wet-sieving and sedimenting the filtrate for 1-3 days to obtain sour *ogi* [64, 97]. The pH of *ogi* is 3.0 – 4.0 after fermentation depending on the time of fermentation and the presence of LAB [64, 68]. *Ogi* has a sour flavour and a characteristic aroma [25, 38, 98]. In Nigeria the name of '*ogi*' depends on the locality and the type of cereal. *Ogi* is the generic name in the Western states of Nigeria where it is usually processed from white maize. *Ogi* from sorghum is known as *'ogi*-baba' [99] while 'ogi-gero' is prepared from millet. In Northern Nigeria, *ogi* is known as 'akamu' or 'eko gbona', while in the Republics of Togo, Benin and Ghana, *ogi* from maize is known as *'koko'* [38, 98]. *Ogi* is the major traditional weaning food commonly served to babies in West Africa. It is also eaten as a breakfast meal and it is a food of choice for the sick [25, 31, 64].

It was observed that use of *Lb. brevis* alone to ferment sterile maize slurry for *ogi* production rapidly reduced the pH to 3.0 in 48 hours compared to the sterile slurry fermented by *S. cerevisiae* [64]. In this study, it was illustrated that it is possible to use starter cultures, such as *Lb. brevis*, to produce *ogi* without compromising its acceptability [64]. The use of starter cultures results in rapid drop in the pH of the food matrix [40]. Rapid pH decline may imply significant increase in the *Lactobacillus* population and increased concentration of organic acids can be indicative of the anti-pathogenic and/or prophylactic and therapeutic potential of *ogi* or other fermented cereal beverages.

3.2.11. Poto poto

This is a traditional fermented maize dough used in homes by the people of the Congo for weaning and for other purposes [86, 100]. *Poto poto* is prepared by soaking maize kernels for about 55 hours followed by milling and sedimentation of the paste in water [86]. The paste is fermented for about 11 hours and then cooked to produce maize gruel [86, 100]]. The fermented paste can be made into *poto poto* balls for selling to make *poto poto* gruel through addition of water and sugar [86, 100]. The pH of *poto poto* samples was found to be in the range 3.48-3.66 [86].

When DNA bands from TTGE gels of *poto poto extracts* were sequenced, the following microorganisms were observed to be present in the fermented product namely: *Lb. plantarum* (predominant), *Lb. gasseri, Enterococcus* sp., *E. coli, Lb. acidophilus, Lb. delbrueckii, Lb. reuteri* and *Lb. casei* [86]. It was established that *Lb. plantarum* and *Lb. fermentum* isolated from *poto poto* produced bacteriocins that were variably inhibitive against strains of *E. coli, Salmonella typhi, Enterobacter aerogenes, Bacillus cereus, Staphylococcus aureus, Listeria monocytogenes* and *Enterococcus faecalis* [100]. The *E. coli, B. cereus* and other food pathogens reported to be in *poto poto* can consequently be inactivated by the bacteriocin-producing LAB from the same food source and make it safer for human consumption [86, 100].

3.2.12. Thobwa

This is a non-alcoholic thin porridge drink prepared from sorghum in Malawi and is popularly consumed by people of all demographics in the country. It is important to note however, that there is an alcoholic version of the *thobwa* in Malawi [67]. *Thobwa* may be similar to *togwa* reportedly made from maize or cassava flour and finger millet malt and consumed in Southern Tanzania [4].

3.2.13. Ting

Ting is a fermented traditional sorghum food of Botswana and South Africa [101, 102]. Ting is prepared by combining sorghum flour (40-45%, w/v) with warm water and the slurry formed is kept in a warm place (~30-37 °C) for spontaneous fermentation to take place over a period of 2-3 days [102]. Bogobe and motogo (stiff and soft porridge respectively) are the two types of porridge that can be prepared and/or cooked from ting previously soured to pH 3.5-4.0 mainly by LAB and yeasts [102]. Motogo (soft) is usually consumed for breakfast and administered to weaning infants while bogobe (stiff) is consumed at lunchtime and supper by adults [101, 102]. In recent studies, the dominant microbiota during ting fermentation consisted of Lb. reuteri, Lb. fermentum, Lb. harbinensis, Lb. plantarum, Lb. parabuchneri, Lb. casei and Lb. coryniformis, Lb. rhamnosus, Lb. curvatus and Weissella cibaria [101, 102]. The presence of these microorganisms and the low pH (3.5-4.0) inhibits proliferation of a number of pathogens, in this manner maintaining the safety of the food. Fermentation of sorghum for ting production improves nutrient levels and reduces antinutritional factors thus increasing the bioavailability of macro-and micronutrients as well as enhancing the sensory attributes [101].

3.2.14. Uji

Uji is a non-alcoholic beverage consumed widely in East Africa (Uganda, Kenya and Tanzania). It is usually prepared from maize [41, 103] although sorghum and/or millet could be mixed with the maize flour [35, 41]. There are two types of uji, fermented and unfermented. The unfermented uji is prepared by boiling water and adding the flour while stirring to obtain the desired drinkable viscosity [41]. Fermented Uji can be obtained by fermenting before or after cooking the porridge [38, 41].

Finely ground cereal is slurried with water at a concentration of about 30% w/v. The slurry is spontaneously fermented for two to five days at room temperature (25 °C). During fermentation of uji, Lb. plantarum has been found to be the dominant Lactobacillus species [35] while Lb. fermentum, Lb. cellobiosus and Lb. buchneri, Pediococcus acidilactici and P. pentosaceus are also reported to be part of the fermenting microorganisms in uji [41]. The pH of uji decreases to 3.5 to 4.0 whereas total acidity (as lactic acid) reaches 0.3 to 0.6% in 32 to 40 hours [38]. After fermentation, uji is diluted to about 8 to 10% solids and brought to boil. It is further diluted to 4-5% solids and then sweetened by the addition of 6% sucrose and consumed while still warm [38]. Like other maize beverages, uji is of low energy density and is deficient in essential amino acids. Fortification with legumes can improve the protein quality and content while the involvement of α-amylase-rich malt flour and/or fermenting with starch-hydrolyzing starter cultures can increase the rate of fermentation [41]. Fermented and non-fermented uji is mainly consumed by rural and urban housewives. Non-fermented cooked uji is also consumed in boarding schools, hospitals and hostels. As is the case with mageu in South Africa [89], uji is also known by different names in different localities in Kenya (see Table 7).

Ethnic group	Local name of product
Embu	Ucuru
Kamba	Uccu
Luo	Nyuka
Luhya	Obusera
Swahili	Uji[a]

Source: reference [38], [a] the common name of sour porridge in East Africa

Table 7. Local names for sour porridge in Kenya

4. Microorganisms involved in cereal-based food fermentations

4.1. Lactic acid bacteria (LAB) involved in African food fermentations

Microorganisms of major importance in lactic acid fermentations belong to the genera *Lactobacillus, Lactococcus, Leuconostoc* and *Pediococcus* [30, 31]. Others include *Streptococcus, Aerococcus, Carnobacterium, Enterococcus, Tetragenococcus, Weisella* and *Vagococcus* [42]. These genera are lactic acid bacteria (LAB) that are widely used in the production of fermented food [39, 52]. The LAB are described as Gram positive, catalase-negative non-sporing rods and cocci, which are usually non-motile [31]. The LAB starter cultures are significant in the production of desired preservative organic acids in the food product during food fermentation [52]. Starter cultures are, however, not usually employed in food fermentations in Africa. Table 8 below shows the lactic acid bacterial species that are dominant in the spontaneous fermentations of several African traditional foods.

Product name	Dominant bacteria	Reference
Fufu	*Lb. plantarum*	[26]
Gari	*Lb. plantarum*	[27]
Mageu	*Lactococcus lactis*	[99]
Mawe	*Lb. fermentum, Pediococcus pentosaceus, Lactococcus lactis*	[31]
Ogi	*Lb. plantarum*	[26]
Ogi-baba	*Lb. plantarum, Lactococcus lactis*	[99]
Togwa	*Lb. plantarum*	[34]
Uji	*Lb. plantarum*	[35]

Table 8. Lactic acid bacteria (LAB) dominant in the spontaneous lactic acid fermentation of African traditional foods

Strains of *Lb. plantarum, Lb. fermentum, Lb. brevis, Pediococcus pentosaceus* and *P. acidilactici* are reported to be among the most predominant species in most African cereal-based fermented beverages [23, 39]. The strains of some of these species have several reported probiotic properties and/or characteristics. Species such as *Lb. plantarum* and *Lb. fermentum* are characterized by being less fastidious, relatively acid resistant, bile tolerant and can thrive on the substances provided in the cereal matrices [39]. It was reported that *Lb. plantarum* showed rapid acidification and produced inhibitory compounds that were active against *Penicillium* and *Aspergillus* strains [40].

Although most of the lactobacilli are generally poor starch fermenters [104], *Lb. plantarum* and *Lb. fermentum* are reported to be the most dominant bacterial species in acid-fermented cereal-based foods. This can be attributed to the degree of acid tolerance and superiority of these species in the utilization of starchy substrates [34, 39]. *Lactobacillus plantarum* isolates from starchy foods such as 'togwa' [34], 'ogi' [104] and cassava [34, 104] have been shown to have good starch-fermenting abilities. The fact that several cereal-based beverages are high in starch, has resulted in several α-amylase-containing lactic acid bacteria, termed amylolytic LAB, becoming sought-after in Africa and elsewhere globally. It has been reported that several strains of *Lb. plantarum*, *Lb. fermentum*, and *Lb. manihotivorans* with amylolytic capabilities have been isolated from maize-, cassava-, sorghum- and millet-based fermentations [39, 42]. Such strains can ferment starch from a variety of different sources.

4.2. Other microorganisms and combinations of microbial species involved in cereal based food fermentations

Besides LAB, *Saccharomyces cerevisiae* is notable as a predominant yeast species involved in food fermentation in Africa [45]. However, it is important to note that there are several factors determining the predominant microbial species and these include the type of cereal, the geographical location or region, conditions in the fermentation medium, moisture content and the season of the year. Yeast species isolated from an ogi maize fermention mix included *Geotrichum fermentans*, *G. candidum*, *Rhodotorula graminis*, *Saccharomyces cerevisiae*, *Candida krusei*, and *C. tropicalis* [97]. Further investigations revealed that *Candida krusei* was better than *S. cerevisiae*, but both species improved the growth of *Lb. plantarum* in maize slurry when each of the yeast species were in combination with the lactobacilli [97]. This was attributed to the capability of the two yeast strains to produce amylolytic enzymes which enabled starch breakdown into simpler sugars for the lactobacilli to metabolise into organic acids [97]. For the same reason, during the mixed culture fermentation of *mawe*, *Candida krusei* improved the growth of *Lb. fermentum* and *Lb. brevis* [23, 41]. During yeast and *Lactobacillus* mixed culture fermentation, the yeasts were also able to provide vitamins and other nutrients for the metabolic activities of the lactobacilli [40].

Certain yeasts were important in producing enzymes such as lipase, esterase and phytase [97]. The lipolytic activity resulted in fatty acids which are precursors of flavour while esterase activity determined aroma and flavour. On the other hand, phytase, produced by these organisms, lowers phytic acid which can form complexes with minerals that in turn can negatively affect protein digestibility [97]. A mixture of *Lb. fermentum* and *Saccharomyces cerevisiae* as starters in the fermentation of *kenkey* and *koko* achieved more rapid pH reduction in 24 hours than spontaneously fermented preparations in 48 hours [39].

4.3. Safety concerns around the use of bacterial strains that could be used as probiotics

The cereal fermented foods and the predominant LAB are generally regarded as safe (GRAS, [23]. Some of the LAB in the fermented food beverages are of human origin and have been used for centuries knowingly or unknowingly [30]. The dominant microorganisms involved in the fermentation of cereal-based beverages have no reported health risk to human life [23]. It was however, noted that some strains of *Enterococcus faecium, E. faecalis*, and *Lb. rhamnosus* were in isolated, highly questionable, cases linked to endocarditis [30]. *Escherichia coli Nissle, Saccharomyces boulardii, Streptococcus thermophilus, Enterococcus francium, Propionibacterium, Pediococcus* and *Leuconostoc* have also been categorized as probiotic species or genera [10].

Most of the bacteria used as probiotics, such as *Lactobacillus* and *Bifidobacterium*, are of human or animal origin and are generally recognized as safe [105]. Apart from *Lactobacillus* and *Bifidobacterium*, other genera such as *Enterococcus* have safety concerns as some of the species are pathogenic [10]. It was reported that even though some enterococci are of technological importance in cheese making, some clinical isolates are regarded as opportunistic pathogens [105]. On that basis LAB, but not enterococci, are generally regarded as safe (GRAS, [105] and can be used in the preparation of cereal-based probiotic beverages.

4.4. Concerns relating to the isomeric type of lactic acid produced by lactic acid bacteria

The organic acids contribute to preservation and food safety, however, it is important to note the concerns relating to L (+) and D (-) lactic acid isomers. The LAB predominantly found in spontaneously fermented African cereal beverages produce lactic acid as one of the major organic acids. Lactic acid contributes to preservation, taste and safety of the fermented foods and beverages [46]. However, lactic acid can occur in two isomers namely L (+) and D (-) isomers and it is only the former isomer that can be degraded in the human system due to the presence of L-lactate dehydrogenase in the gastro-intestinal canal [27, 42, 94]. The genera *Streptococcus, Enterococcus, Lactococcus* and *Carnobacterium* mainly produce the L(+) isomer while *Leuconostoc* spp. and all subspecies of *Lb. delbrueckii* produce the D (-) isomer [23]. The *Weissella* species, *Lb. sakei* and heterofermentative lactobacilli produce a racemate (DL) of isomers [23]. Reports indicate that industrial production of mahewu, a fermented maize beverage, using *Lb. delbrueckii*, creates a challenge of D (-) lactate production [94]. The D (-) lactate producing *Lb. delbrueckii* (ID12441) was also the major fermenting organism isolated from *munkoyo* (see section 3.2.8) [94]. This is a concern since the organisms involved in spontaneous fermentation and the major lactic acid isomer produced in cereal beverages for weaning infants and children may not be known. Lactobacilli and pediococci produce lactic acid isomers that are species specific [23, 30]. In beverages used for weaning purposes, it needs to be established whether LAB strains produce the D (-) or the L (+) lactic acid isomer [53]. An acid-base imbalance can be induced in children consuming excessive amounts of beverages containing D (-) lactic acid and therefore L (+) lactic acid is the most recommended isomer for man [94]. It is therefore necessary to screen any probiotic cultures used in foods due to the disadvantages (possible acidosis) of offering children foods containing D (-) lactic acid [53].

5. Probiotic cereal-based beverages

5.1. Introduction

It is estimated that over 60 million people use sorghum and millet as part of their staple food in Africa in the fermented or unfermented form [63]. This is in addition to maize which is a staple cereal for the majority of the people in Africa and elsewhere in the world. This extensive consumption of cereals is partially the basis for the mounting research into the development of non-dairy cereal-based probiotic beverages. Consumers are becoming more aware of the need to eat food for health reasons. This implies that apart from good taste and nutrients provided, food needs to impart additional health benefits to the consumer. Such benefits can be realized by processing the food in such a way that its functionality is improved, for example by incorporating ingredients such as prebiotics and probiotics.

Probiotic bacteria have several reported potential health benefits [70]. Besides probiotics, prebiotic oligosaccharides also impart reported health benefits to the consumer [70]. However, in terms of foods that are used to deliver probiotic bacteria to the consumer, milk and milk products are almost exclusively used for this purpose [4, 10]. Such dairy products however have limitations that include cost (especially in the developing world), allergens, cultural food taboos against milk consumption, requirement of cold-chain facilities, the need to use beverages that form part of the people's daily diets as well as the need to maintain viability of the probiotic bacterial population in excess of the physiologically required therapeutic minimum of 10^6 -10^7 cfu/mL viable cells in the product when consumed [106].

Probiotic microorganisms need to be consumed regularly and adequately (10^6 cfu/mL per serving) to maintain the intestinal population and to ensure that health benefits will be derived by the consumer [105]. The increasing need to eat food for health reasons, the demand for vegetarian probiotic foods, the growing lactose intolerance in the world population, and the arguable concern about the cholesterol content of fermented dairy products, are other factors that increase the need for the development of non-dairy cereal-based foods [4, 10, 105]. The following paragraphs illustrate the investigations that have been directed towards cereal- and/or legume-based probiotic beverage development.

5.2. Oats-based probiotic beverages

5.2.1. Proviva

Proviva is known to be the first commercial oats-based probiotic food beverage [4]. *Proviva* is produced by Skane Dairy and it has been a commercial product in Sweden since 1994. *Proviva* has malted barley added as liquefying agent and the active probiotic component is

Lactobacillus plantarum 299v. The final product which is a mixture of fruit juice and 5% oat meal has a probiotic bacterial population count in the region of 5 x 10^{10} cfu/L [4, 76].

5.2.2. Yosa

Yosa is a probiotic oat snack food marketed in Finland and other Scandinavian countries. *Yosa*, which has a flavour and texture comparable to that of dairy yoghurt, is made by cooking the oat bran pudding in water and fermenting with lactic acid bacteria and bifidobacteria. The probiotic species are reported to be *Lb. acidophilus* LA5 and *Bf. lactis* Bb12 [11, 76]. Apart from probiotic bacteria, *yosa* also contains oat fibre, a source of β-glucan that has the potential to lower blood cholesterol and so reduce the chances of heart disease [11, 49].

5.2.3. Other experimental probiotic oats products

Several workers have endeavoured to develop non-dairy cereal-based probiotic food products. An oats-based synbiotic functional drink made by fermenting an oats substrate with *Lactobacillus plantarum* B28 was developed [4]. At the end of 21 days of refrigerated storage the bacterial cell counts were still at a level of 7.5 x 10^{10} cfu/ml. The drink was referred to as synbiotic due to the presence of β-glucan, a functional component in cereals and usually highest in oats and barley in addition to the probiotic organism [4, 105]. Oats therefore appears to be a suitable substrate for the growth of probiotic bacteria [71].

It is important, however, to take the probiotic species into consideration when developing cereal based probiotic beverages. The probiotic bacterial population levels were studied in an envisaged synbiotic oats beverage consisting of 5% oats, 2% inulin, 0.5% whey protein concentrate and 4% sugar [107]. After a storage period of 10 weeks at 4 °C the population levels for two probiotic species (*Lb. plantarum* B-28 and *Lb. paracasei* ssp. *casei* B-29) were 1.77 x 10^6 – 1.29 x 10^7 cfu/mL and 7.39 x 10^7 – 4.49 x 10^8 cfu/mL respectively. However when *Lb. acidophilus* ATCC 521 was inoculated into the same oats beverage, the initial population level of 6.77 x 10^7 cfu/mL declined to 1.55 x 10^5 cfu/mL by the 4th week of storage at 4 °C. This decline gradually continued during a subsequent storage period [107]. This tendency was confirmed by other workers [71] who also found that, *Lb. acidophilus* showed slower rates of pH reduction and lower viable counts in oats due to its higher requirement for nutrients in comparison with *Lb. plantarum* and *Lb. reuteri*. To be referred to as a probiotic beverage at the time of consumption such beverages should have a population level of at least 10^6 cfu/mL viable cells [107]. These findings illustrated that the survival of probiotics in cereal beverages is species and strain specific and this should be kept in mind in developing such products.

5.3. Probiotic beverages incorporating malted cereals and hidrolysates

The potential of four bifidobacterial species of human origin to ferment a barley malt hidrolysate similar to that obtained in the brewery was investigated [76]. These species included *Bf. adolescentis* NCIMB 702204, *Bf. infantis* NCIMB 702205, *Bf. breve* NCIMB 702257 and *Bf. longum* NCIMB 702259. The workers found that the addition of yeast extract to the malt hidrolysate as a growth promoter was necessary for the population levels to increase by 1.5 - 2.0 log$_{10}$ cycles to 8.73 – 9.00 log$_{10}$ cfu/ml after 24 hours of fermentation at 37 °C. Their work illustrated the potential of using bifidobacteria to develop a probiotic malt-based beverage by way of looking at the population levels attained in the study [76]. The study did not include product characterisation to establish its sensory attributes neither was the acceptance of the product tested among the target consumers. In addition to this, shelf-life studies in terms of viable bacterial cells were not conducted. On the other hand the barley-malt hidrolysate used as the substrate may not be commercially feasible for use in the developing world and if it were, its protein deficiencies would have malnutrition implications for the African consumer [76].

In another study relating to barley malt, the potential of using *Lactobacillus reuteri* (probiotic) and yeast to develop a cereal-based probiotic drink by fermenting a 5% (w/v) malt suspension was investigated [75]. The workers observed that using a mixed culture of *Lb. reuteri* and yeast resulted in a better decrease in pH, increased lactic acid production and increased ethanol production compared to that observed with pure cultures.The protective effect of extracts of malt, barley and wheat on the bile tolerance of *Lactobacillus reuteri*, *Lb. acidophilus* and *Lb. plantarum* has also been investigated [108]. It was illustrated that the cereal extracts, particularly from malt, exerted a protective effect, against bile salts, on the studied lactobacilli. The protection was attributed to the presence, in cereal malt extracts, of non-reducing sucrose and soluble oligosaccharides (non-digestible carbohydrates) that have been reported to improve bile tolerance. The study indicated the potential of malt, barley and wheat extracts to offer protection against bile to the probiotics when ingested together.

The factors that influence the growth of selected potential probiotic lactobacilli (e.g. *Lb. fermentum, Lb. reuteri, Lb. acidophilus* and *Lb. plantarum*) in selected cereal substrates as a way of assessing the potential of producing a probiotic cereal-based beverage was investigated [72]. In their study, a malt medium enabled the tested lactobacilli to attain higher counts (8.10 – 10.11 log$_{10}$ cfu /mL) than in non–malted barley and wheat media (7.20 – 9.43 log10 cfu /mL). The differences in counts were attributed to a higher level of sugars (15 g/L total fermentable sugars) and an increased free amino nitrogen concentration (80 mg/L) in malt medium than in the non-malted barley or wheat media (3 – 4 g/L total fermentable sugars and free amino nitrogen concentration of 15.3 – 26.6 mg/L). The sugars were present in the form of maltose, sucrose and also in the form of their monomeric components (glucose and fructose). Growth limitation was a result of either a low pH or a substrate deficiency. In malt medium, where sugars were abundant, the microbial growth was limited by low pH (3.40 – 3.77) while in barley and wheat media, growth was limited by insufficient fermentable sugars and free amino nitrogen. This was based on the observation that growth was halted at a higher pH (3.73 – 4.88) in barley and wheat media than in malt medium [72]. Barley is not abundant in the developing world and therefore a barley-malt probiotic beverage production would not be feasible [72] in this part the world.

5.4. Maize (corn)-based probiotic beverages

5.4.1. Synbiotic mahewu (mageu)

Mageu is commercially produced in South Africa which provides it with the potential to deliver probiotic bacteria to the consumers for whom it is part of their daily diets. The commercial *mageu* is prepared using *Lactobacillus delbrueckii* and the product is pasteurized after fermentation and it is therefore not a probiotic product. The possible enhancement of the functional quality of *mageu* was investigated [70]. To this end, six pure probiotic *Lactobacillus* starter cultures and prebiotic oligosaccharides in developing six fermented synbiotic maize-based *mageu*-like beverages were tested. The strains included *Lb. casei* BGP93, *Lb. casei* (Shirota strain), *Lb. rhamnosus* LRB, *Lb. paracasei* BGPI, *Lb. plantarum* BG112, *Lb. acidophilus* PRO and *Lb. delbrueckii* subsp. *lactis* C09 (used to prepare the control). The suitable prebiotic ingredient and the factors affecting the growth of these organisms in the maize gruel, as well as the sustained viability of these organisms in the product during extended refrigerated storage were investigated [70].

The viability of the probiotic strains, in terms of population level, in the fermented synbiotic maize-based beverages at the end of a 90-day storage period at 5 °C exceeded 7.5 $\log_{10}$ cfu/mL [70]. This was well above the recommended therapeutic minimum of 6 $\log_{10}$ cfu/mL at the time of consumption [109, 110]. Intake of a portion of 200 – 300 ml of the experimental synbiotic *mageu* products would potentially enable the consumer to derive 7 to 10.5 g d^{-1} of prebiotic Raftiline® GR (inulin) and $2 \times 10^{10} - 3 \times 10^{11}$ viable probiotic bacterial cells d^{-1}. A trained sensory panel found that the synbiotic maize-based beverages fermented by *Lb. acidophilus* PRO and *Lb. rhamnosus* LRB were the most similar to the control (*Lb. delbrueckii*). This was confirmed by a larger consumer acceptance panel [111]. This illustrated that *mageu* can be converted to an acceptable synbiotic beverage and that it was able to sustain a population of viable probiotic cells, exceeding the therapeutic minimum level, during an extended storage period.

5.4.2. Mahewu (mageu) with bifidobacteria

The survival of probiotic *Bifidobacterium lactis* DSM 10140 as harvested and inoculated free cells or as microencapsulated cells in mahewu (*mageu*) was studied [74]. The workers observed that the counts of free cells of *B. lactis* reduced significantly during the 21day storage at 4 °C and 22 °C both in the presence or absence of oxygen. Poor viability of *Bf. lactis* in mahewu was attributed to exposure to the low pH (3.5) of mahewu and the inadequate buffering capacity as a result of a low protein content (5.2 g/L) in a medium containing 78.4 g/L of carbohydrates [74]. The workers then recommended the use of microencapsulation coupled with storage at 4 °C as being optimal for the delivery of *Bf. lactis* to the consumer [74]. However, microencapsulation is not without its technological challenges and added cost. *Bifidobacterium lactis* has also been said to be closely related to *Bf. animalis* which is a probiotic of animal origin [112]. It is therefore important that the potential of using bifidobacteria of human origin as starters in combination with lactobacilli are investigated in providing a probiotic enhanced *mageu* product.

5.4.3. Fermented maize weaning porridge

In a fermented "maize porridge" (18.5% w/w maize meal) mixed with malted barley (1.5% w/w), the growth and metabolism of four strains of probiotic lactobacilli (*Lb. reuteri* SD 2112, *Lb. rhamnosus* GG, *Lb. acidophilus* LA5 and *Lb. acidophilus* 1748) were studied in terms of cell counts, pH and metabolites [73]. Bacterial cell counts attained maximum levels of 7.2-8.2 $\log_{10}$ cfu within 12 hours of fermentation at 37 °C [73]. The lowest pH range attained after 24 hour fermentation period at 37 °C was 3.1-3.7 [73]. The products were of low viscosity that could be attributed to the use of the barley malt expected to be the source of amylase for the enzymatic hydrolysis of maize starch. Whereas the malt may have increased the level of fermentable sugars, it also led to a product of low viscosity (too watery) that may not have consumer appeal in the developing world either as porridge or a beverage. This product was not subjected to sensory evaluation, consumer preference evaluation or shelf-life testing. 'Maize weaning porridge' as it was referred to by the workers would not be nutritionally suitable for this purpose due to the inherent protein deficiency of maize that was the principal ingredient. It should also be noted that barley malt may not be readily available in the developing world.

5.5. Probiotic soy-based probiotic beverages

Soybeans and rice fermentation media are also reported to be suitable substrates for the growth of certain probiotic lactobacilli and bifidobacteria [49]. Soybean usage is however hampered by the presence of raffinose and stachyose, which can cause flatulence [105]. The non-inactivated lipoxygenase enzyme in the soybean is the causative agent of the beany off-flavour (as perceived in Western societies) in soy-containing products [105]. These limiting factors can, however, be significantly reduced by fermenting with technologically suitable LAB. Soy yoghurt and/or "sogurt" developed using soymilk, is characterized by a hard and coarse texture in addition to a beany "off-flavour". Coupled with inadequate acid development, this has resulted in a lower sensory appeal of these products [105]. Reports indicate that inclusion of fructose, calcium, cheese whey proteins, gelatin and lactose as well as probiotic bacteria improved the textural and sensory properties of sogurt [105].

Soymilk is suitable for the growth of lactobacilli and bifidobacteria and a probiotic soymilk and soybean yoghurt with added prebiotic oligofructose and inulin was developed [4]. This was found to be the case with several lactobacilli that included *Lb. casei*, *Lb. fermentum*, *Lb. reuteri*, and *Lb. acidophilus* [49]. Probiotic bacteria were also introduced into a non-fermented vegetarian frozen soy dessert. This product was composed of a soymilk beverage, sugar, oil, stabilizer and salt. The probiotic organisms introduced included *Lactobacillus acidophilus*, *Lb. rhamnosus*, *Lb. paracasei* ssp. *paracasei*, *Saccharomyces boulardi* and *Bifidobacterium lactis*. Bacterial population levels after 6 months' storage exceeded 10^7 cfu/g for all species except for *S. boulardi* [49]. The population level of the yeast species was below the therapeutic minimum of 10^6 cfu/g and this was attributed to the absence of 'cell shielding'.

In summary it can be stated that generally speaking, cereals are good growth-substrates of probiotic bacteria [108]. This is illustrated by the Yosa oats-based product, which to date is the only cereal-based commercial product known to contain both LAB and bifidobacteria. Since cereal-nutrient components vary, growth rates of probiotic organisms may also vary. Further research is therefore imperative to investigate the growth factors that may enhance the growth and survival of lactobacilli and bifidobacteria in cereal-based gruels. The indigestible variable fractions of the cereals can be utilised as prebiotics by probiotics in the GIT of the host upon ingestion of the fermented cereal-based beverage and these should also be defined and tested.

5.6. Therapeutic minimum levels of bacterial species in probiotic beverages

The therapeutic minimum population level for bacterial species in probiotic beverages is recommended to be 10^6 cfu ml^{-1}. This is the lowest probiotic bacterial count in a probiotic product that may adequately impart prophylactic and therapeutic benefits to the host. In order to realize therapeutic effects of probiotic bacteria in a product, the bacterial counts should exceed 10^6 cfu ml^{-1} [113]. Such a dose should be consumed regularly to ensure permanent colonisation in the small intestines. These high bacterial cell counts of probiotic bacteria are proposed to allow for the possible reduction in numbers during passage through the stomach and the intestines [114]. The need to have live probiotic cultures in products claimed to be probiotic has resulted in the formation of regulatory bodies and food legislation in some countries.

The Swiss Food Regulation and the International Standard of FIL/IDF require probiotic products to contain at least 10^6 cfu ml^{-1} [115]. The Fermented Milks and Lactic Acid Bacteria Beverages Association of Japan specifies a minimum of 10^7 cfu ml^{-1} to be present in fresh probiotic dairy products [114, 115]. Japan has the FOSHU (Foods for Specified Health Use) programme for approving functional foods for marketing. A product with a "FOSHU" tag is defined as a food, which is expected to have certain functional benefits and has been licensed to bear a label to that effect [1]. The USA's National Yoghurt Association (NYA) specifies a population level of 10^8 cfu/g of lactic acid bacteria, at the time of manufacture, before placing a "Live and Active Culture" logo on the containers of the product [14]. However, in the USA, no indication is given as to what the viable count should be at the end of shelf-life. In the South African context, the South African Food and Health Draft Regulation (regulation 63) stipulates that selected probiotic microbes must be present at levels of at least 10^6 cfu ml^{-1} of product in order to exert a beneficial effect [110].

6. Conclusions and recommendations

Cereals and fermented cereal beverages can be advocated for use as delivery vehicles of health-benefiting functional ingredients such as probiotics and prebiotics. However, it is important to note some of the challenges associated with cereal grains and how they may be circumvented in improving probiotic cereal food delivery to masses in Africa and the developing world. It was noted that there is no known distribution channel for starter cultures to small scale or household scale processers of cereal-based fermented beverages in Africa and the developing world [30]. The other bottleneck is the fact that probiotic strains that have been technologically used successfully in dairy products may not exhibit similar acceptable growth and viability in cereal beverages. This accentuates the need for doing further screening [105]. The developed plant-cereal-based synbiotic beverages may also not have the necessary acceptable sensory attributes [3, 105, 116]. In a recent study, the use of a strain of *Lb. paracasei* BGP1 in a maize based fermented synbiotic experimental product resulted in off-flavours detected by a trained sensory panel [70, 111].

The use of probiotic strains in a combination of cereals and legumes in fermented products needs to be based on a number of considerations including technological and functional properties; sensory properties, growth rate; capability to deal with antinutritional factors; reduction of toxic substances in cassava; reduction of mycotoxins in cereals; reduction of flatulence causing compounds in legumes; pathogen inhibitory capabilities; co-existence and growth in mixed cultures [30]. These determinations however are hampered by the lack of facilities, expertise and the cost-benefit ratio that, in most cases, is not favourable to small scale and household scale cereal beverage producers in the developing world [30].

Author details

R. Nyanzi and P.J. Jooste*
*Department of Biotechnology and Food Technology,
Tshwane University of Technology, Pretoria, South Africa*

7. References

[1] Berner LA., O'Donnell JA. Functional foods and health claims legislation: application to dairy foods. International Dairy Journal 1998;8, 355-362.

[2] Marchand J., Vandenplas Y. Microorganisms administered in the benefit of the host: myths and facts. European Journal of Gastroenterology and Hepatology 2000;12(10), 1077-1088.

[3] Tuorila H., Cardello AV. Consumer responses to an off-flavour in the presence of specific health claims. Food Quality and Preference 2002;13, 561-569.

[4] Prado FC., Parada JL., Pandey A., Soccol CR. Trends in non-dairy probiotic beverages. Food Research International 2008;41, 111-123.

[5] Siró IN., Kápolna E., Kápolna BT., Lugasi A. Functional food. Product development, marketing and consumer acceptance-A review. Appetite, 2008;51(3), 456-467.

[6] Goldberg, I. Introduction. In: Goldberg, I. (Ed.) Functional Foods. Chapman and Hall; 1994. pXV-XVII, 6-13.

* Corresponding Author

[7] Salminen S., Roberfroid M., Ramos P., Fonden R. 1998. Prebiotic substrates and lactic acid bacteria. In: Salminen, S., van Wright A. (Eds.) Lactic acid bacteria: microbiology and functional aspects. Marcel Dekker; 1998. p343 - 358.

[8] Niness KR. Inulin and Oligofructose: what are they? Journal of Nutrition 1999;129, 1402S-1406S.

[9] Sanz Y. Ecological and functional implications of the acid-adaptation ability of *Bifidobacterium*: away of selecting improved probiotic strains. International Dairy Journal 2007;17, 1284-1289.

[10] Ranadheera RDCS., Baines SK., Adams MC. Importance of food in probiotic efficacy. Food Research International 2010;43(1), 1-7.

[11] Blandino A., Al-Aseeri ME., Pandiella SS., Cantero D., Webb, C. Cereal-based fermented foods and beverages. Food Research International 2003;36(6), 527-543.

[12] Manning TS., Gibson GR. Prebiotics. Best practice and research. Clinical Gastroenterology 2004;18(2), 287–298.

[13] Commane D., Hughes R., Shortt C., Rowland J. The potential mechanisms involved in the anticarcinogenic action of probiotics. Mutation Research 2005;591, 276–289.

[14] Kailasapathy K., Rybka S. *L. acidophillus* and *Bifidobacterium spp.*- their therapeutic potential and survival in yoghurt. The Australian Journal of Dairy Technology 1997;52(April), 28-35.

[15] Zeimer CJ., Gibson GR. An overview of probiotics, prebiotics and synbiotics in functional food concept: perspectives and future strategies. International Dairy Journal 1998;8, 473-479.

[16] Franz CMAP., Stiles ME., Schleifer KH., Holzapfel WH. Enterococci in foods - a conundrum for food safety. International Journal of food Microbiology 2003;88, 105–122.

[17] Collins JK., Thornton G., Sullivan GO. Selection of probiotic strains for human Applications. International Dairy Journal 1998;8, 487-490.

[18] Young J. European Market Development in prebiotic- and probiotic- containing foodstuffs. British Journal of Nutrition 1998;80(Supp 2), S231-233.

[19] Bosscher D., Van Loo J., Franck A. Inulin and oligofructose as functional ingredients to improve bone mineralization. International Dairy Journal 2006;16, 1092–1097.

[20] Modler HW., Mckeller RC., Yaguchi M. Bifidobacteria and bifidogenic factors. Canadian Institute of Food Science and Technology Journal 1990;24(1), 29-41.

[21] Gibson RG., Willis CL., Van Loo J. Non-digestible oligosaccharides and bifidobacteria: implications for health. International Sugar Journal 1994;96(1150), 381-387.

[22] Nout MJR., Rombouts FM. Fermentative preservation of plant foods. Journal of Applied Bacteriology 1992;73, 136-147.

[23] Holzapfel WH. Appropriate starter culture technologies for small-scale fermentation in developing countries. International Journal of Food Microbiology 2002;75, 197-212.

[24] Shetty PH., Jespersen L. *Saccharomyces cerevisiae* and lactic acid bacteria as potential mycotoxin decontaminating agents. Trends in Food Science & Technology 2006;17, 48-55.

[25] Iwuoha CI., Eke OS. Nigerian indigenous fermented foods: their traditional process of operation, inherent problems, improvements and current status. Food Research International 1996;29(5/6), 527-540.

[26] Adegoke GO., Babalola AK. Characterisation of microorganisms of importance in the fermentation of fufu and ogi , two Nigeria foods. Journal of Applied Bacteriology 1988;65, 449-453.

[27] Caplice E., Fitzgerald GF. Food fermentations: role of microorganisms in food production and preservation. International Journal of Food Microbiology 1999;50, 131-149.

[28] Sanni AI. The need for process optimisation of African fermented foods and beverages. International Journal of Food Microbiology 1993;18, 85-95.

[29] Campbell-Platt G. Fermented foods - a world perspective. Food Research International 1994;27, 253-257.

[30] Holzapfel WH. Use of starter cultures in fermentation on a household scale. Food Control 1997;8(5/6), 241-258.

[31] Oyewole OB. Lactic fermented foods in Africa and their benefits, Food Control 1997;8(5/6), 289-297.

[32] Byaruhanga YB., Bester BH., Watson TG. Growth and survival of *Bacillus cereus* in *mageu*, a sour maize beverage. World Journal of Microbiology & Biotechnology 1999;15, 329-333.

[33] Simango C., Rukure G. Survival of bacterial enteric pathogens in traditional fermented food. Journal of Applied Bacteriology 1992;73, 37-40.

[34] Mugula JK., Narvhus JA., Sørhaug T. Use of starter cultures of lactic acid bacteria and yeasts in the preparation of *togwa*, a Tanzanian fermented food. International Journal of Food Microbiology 2003;83(3), 307-318.

[35] Onyango C., Bley T. Raddatz H., Henle T. Flavour compounds in backslop fermented uji (an East African sour porridge). European Food Research & Technology 2004;218, 579-583.

[36] Nout MJR. Ecology of accelerated natural lactic fermentation of sorghum-based infant food formulas. International Journal of Food Microbiology 1991;12, 217-224.

[37] Efiuvwevwere BJ., Akona O. The microbiology of 'Kunun-Zaki', a cereal beverage from Northern Nigeria, during the fermentation (production) process. World Journal of Microbiology & Biotechnology 1995;11, 491-493.

[38] Steinkraus KH. Handbook of Indigenous Fermented Foods. Marcel Dekker; 1983. p1-667.

[39] Ezeogu LI. Research in ethnic West African fermented cereal-based foods. In: Taylor JRN., Cracknell RL. (Eds.) The ICC book of ethnic cereal-based foods and beverages across the continents. The University of Pretoria, Pretoria, South Africa; 2009. p 63-92.

[40] Edema MO., Sanni AI. Functional properties of selected starter cultures for sour maize bread. Food Microbiology 2008;25(4), 616-625.

[41] Nout MJR. Rich Nutrition from the poorest - Cereal fermentations in Africa and Asia. Food Microbiology 2009;26, 685-692.

[42] Reddy G., Altaf M., Naveena BJ., Venkateshwar M., Kumar E.V. Amylolytic bacterial acetic acid fermentation - A review. Biotechnology Advances 2008;26(1), 22-34.

[43] Omar NB., Abriouel H., Lucas R., Martinez-Cañamero, M., Guyot, J., Gálvez A. Isolation of bacteriocinogenic *Lactobacillus plantarum* strains from ben saalga, a traditional fermented gruel from Burkina Faso. International Journal of Food Microbiology 2006;112, 44-50.

[44] Lei V., Friis H., Michaelsen KF. Spontaneously fermented millet product as a probiotic treatment for diarrhea in young children: An intervention study in Northern Ghana. International Journal of Food Microbiology 2006;110, 246-253.

[45] Shetty PH., Hald B., Jespersen L. Surface binding of aflatoxin B1 by *Saccharomyces cerevisiae* strains with potential decontaminating abilities in indigenous fermented foods. International Journal of Food Microbiology 2007;113, 14-46.

[46] Chelule PK., Mbongwa HP., Carries S., Gqaleni N. Lactic acid fermentation improves the quality of amahewu, a traditional South African maize-based porridge. Food Chemistry 2010;122(3), 656-661.

[47] Towo E., Matuschek E., Svanberg U. Fermentation and enzyme treatment of tannin sorghum gruels: effects on phenolic compounds, phytate and in vitro accessible iron. Food Chemistry 2006;94(3), 369-376.

[48] Mensah P. Fermentation-the key to food safety assurance in Africa? Food Control 1997;8(5/6), 271-278.

[49] Rivera-Espinoza, Y., Gallardo-Navarro Y. Non-dairy probiotic products. Food Microbiology 2010;27(1), 1-11.

[50] Cook PE. Fermented foods as biotechnological resources. Food Research International 1994;27, 309-316.

[51] Olasupo NA., Olukoya, DK., Odunfa SA. Studies on bacteriocinogenic *Lactobacillus* isolates from selected Nigerian fermented foods. Journal of Basic Microbiology 1995;35(5), 319-324.

[52] Hansen EB. Commercial bacterial starter cultures for fermented foods of the future. International Journal of Food Microbiology 2002;78, 119-131.

[53] Leroy FDR., De Vuyst L. Lactic acid bacteria as functional starter cultures for the food fermentation industry. Trends in Food Science & Technology 2004;15(2), 67-78.

[54] Westby A., Reilly A., Bainbridge Z. Review of the effect of fermentation on naturally occurring toxins. Food Control 1997;8(5/6), 329-339.

[55] Onyekwere OO., Akinrele IA., Koleoso OA., Heys G. Industrialisation of gari fermentation. In: Steinkraus K.H. (Ed.). Industrialisation of Indigenous Fermented Foods. Marcel Dekker; 1989. p363-389.

[56] Claver IP., Zhou H.-M., Zhang H.-H., Zhu K.-X., Li Q., Murekatete N. The Effect of Soaking with Wooden Ash and Malting upon Some Nutritional Properties of Sorghum Flour Used for Impeke, a Traditional Burundian Malt-Based Sorghum Beverage. Agricultural Sciences in China 2011;10(11), 1801-1811.

[57] Reddy NR., Pierson MD. Reduction of antinutritional and toxic components in plant foods by fermentation. Food Research International 1994;27, 284-290.

[58] Ologhobo AD., Fetuga BL. Investigations on the trypsin inhibitor, hemagglutinin, phytic and tannic acid contents of cowpea *Vigna unguiculata*. Food Chemistry 1983;12, 249-254.

[59] Frontela C., García-Alonso FJ., Ros G., Martínez C. Phytic acid and inositol phosphates in raw flours and infant cereals: The effect of processing. Journal of Food Composition and Analysis 2008;21, 343-350.

[60] Dykes L., Rooney LW. Sorghum and millet phenols and antioxidants. Journal of Cereal Science 2006;44, 236 – 251.

[61] Dlamini NR., Taylor JRN., Rooney, LW. The effect of sorghum type and processing on the antioxidant properties of African sorghum-based foods. Food Chemistry 2007;105(4), 1412-1419.

[62] Chethan S., Sreerama YN., Malleshi N.G. Mode of inhibition of finger millet malt amylase by the millet phenolics. Food Chemistry 2008;111, 187-191.

[63] Correia MITD., Liboredo JC., Consoli MLD. The role of probiotics in gastrointestinal surgery. Nutrition 2010; 28(3), 230-234.

[64] Teniola OD., Odunfa SA. The effects of processing methods on the levels of lysine, methionine and the general acceptability of *ogi* processed using starter cultures. International Journal of Food Microbiology 2001;63, 1-9.

[65] Bvochora JM., Zvauya R. Biochemical changes occurring during the application of high gravity fermentation technology to the brewing of Zimbabwean traditional opaque beer. Process Biochemistry 2001;37(4), 365-370.

[66] Wagacha JM., Muthomi JW. Mycotoxin problem in Africa: Current status, implications to food safety and health and possible management strategies. International Journal of Food Microbiology, 2008;124(1), 1-12.

[67] Matumba L., Monjerezi M., Khonga EB., Lakudzala DD. Aflatoxins in sorghum, sorghum malt and traditional opaque beer in southern Malawi. Food Control 2011;22(2), 266-268.

[68] Fandohan P., Zoumenou D., Hounhouigan DJ., Marasas WFO., Wingfield MJ., Hell K. Fate of aflatoxins and fumonisins during the processing of maize into food products in Benin. International Journal of Food Microbiology 2005;98(3), 249-259.

[69] Alberts JF., Engelbrecht Y., Steyn PS., Holzapfel WH., Van Zyl WH. Biological degradation of aflatoxin B1 by *Rhodococcus erythropolis* cultures. International Journal of Food Microbiology 2006;109, 121-126.

[70] Nyanzi R. Enhancing the functional quality of mageu. MTech *dissertation*. Tshwane University of Technology. Pretoria; 2007.

[71] Charalampopoulos D., Wang R., Pandiella SS., Webb C. Application of cereal components in functional foods: a review. International Journal of Food Microbiology 2002;79, 131-141.

[72] Charalampopoulos D., Pandiella SS., Webb C. Growth studies of potentially probiotic lactic acid bacteria in cereal-based substrates. Journal of Applied Microbiology 2002;92, 851-859.

[73] Helland MH., Wicklund T., Narvhus J. Growth and metabolism of selected strains of probiotic bacteria, in maize porridge with added malted barley. International Journal of Food Microbiology 2004;91, 305-313.

[74] Mcmaster LD., Kokott SA., Reid SJ., Abratt VR. Use of traditional African fermented beverages as delivery vehicles for *Bifidobacterium lactis* DSM 10140. International Journal of Food Microbiology 2005;102(2), 231-237.

[75] Kedia G., Wang R., Patel H., Pandiella SS. Use of mixed cultures for the fermentation of cereal-based substrates with potential probiotic properties. Process Biochemistry 2007;42, 65-70.

[76] Rozada-Sánchez R., Sattur AP., Thomas K., Pandiella SS. Evaluation of *Bifidobacterium* spp. For the production of a potentially probiotic malt-based beverage. Process Biochemistry 2008;43, 848-854.

[77] Todorov SD., Dicks LMT. Screening for bacteriocin-producing lactic acid bacteria from boza, a traditional cereal beverage from Bulgaria: Comparison of the bacteriocins. Process Biochemistry 2006;41(1), 11-19.

[78] Yeğin SR., Üren A. Biogenic amine content of boza: A traditional cereal-based, fermented Turkish beverage. Food Chemistry 2008;111(4), 983-987.

[79] Hancioğlu Ö., Karapinar M. 1997. Microflora of Boza, a traditional fermented Turkish beverage. International Journal of Food Microbiology 1997;35, 271-274.

[80] Zorba M., Hancioglu O., Genc M., Karapinar M., Ova G. The use of starter cultures in the fermentation of boza, a traditional Turkish beverage. Process Biochemistry 2003;38(10), 1405-1411.

[81] Dlusskaya E., Jänsch A., Schwab C., Gänzle MG. 2008. Microbial and chemical analysis of kvass fermentation. European Food Research & Technology 2008;227, 261-266.

[82] Sainz T., Wacher C., Espinoza J., Centurión D., Navarro A., Molina, J., Inzunza A., Cravioto A., Eslava C. Survival and characterization of Escherichia coli strains in a typical Mexican acid-fermented food. International Journal of Food Microbiology 2001;71, 169-176.

[83] Bvochora JM., Reed JD., Read JS. & Zvauya R. Effect of fermentation processes on proanthocyanidins in sorghum during preparation of mahewu, a non-alcoholic beverage. Process Biochemistry 1999;35, 21-25.

[84] Tou EH., Mouquet-Rivier C., Rochette I., Traoré AS., Tréche S., Guyot JP. Effect of different process combinations on the fermentation kinetics, microflora and energy density of ben-saalga, a fermented gruel from Burkina Faso. Food Chemistry 2007;100(3), 935-943.

[85] Tou EH., Guyot JP., Mouquet-Rivier C., Rochette I., Counil E., Traoré, AS., Tréche S. Study through surveys and fermentation kinetics of the traditional processing of pearl millet (*Pennisetum glaucum*) into ben-saalga, a fermented gruel from Burkina Faso. International Journal of Food Microbiology 2006;106(1), 52-60.

[86] Abriouel H., Omar NB., López, RL., Martinez-Cañamero M., Keleke S., Gálvez A. Culture-independent analysis of the microbial composition of the African traditional fermented foods *poto poto* and *dégué*. International Journal of Food Microbiology 2006;111, 228-233.

[87] Schweigart F., De Wit JP. 1960. Favourite beverages of the Bantu: preparing and drying of mahewu and its nutritional value. National Nutritional Research Institute, CSIR. Pretoria (May 1960).

[88] Schweigart F. The drying of lactic acid bacteria cultures for mahewu production. Lebensm.Wiss.u. Technology 1971;4(1):20-23.

[89] Holzapfel WH. Industrialization of mageu fermentation in South Africa. In: Steinkraus KH. (Ed.). Industrialization of Indigenous Fermented Foods. Marcel Dekker; 1989. p285-328.

[90] Schweigart F., Fellingham SA. A study of fermentation in the production of mahewu, an indigenous sour maize beverage of Southern Africa. Milchwissenschaft 1963;18, 241-246.

[91] Van Noort G., Spence C. The mahewu industry. South African Food Review 1976;October, 129-133.

[92] Edwards C. Mageu – where to for Africa's energy drink? South African Food Review 2003;30 (3), 25-27.

[93] Zulu RM., Dillon VM., Owens JD. 1997. Munkoyo beverage, a traditional Zambian fermented maize gruel using *Rhynchosia* root as amylase source. International Journal of Food Microbiology 1997;34(3), 249-258.

[94] Foma RK., Destain J., Mobinzo PK., Kayisu K., Thonart P. Study of physicochemical parameters and spontaneous fermentation during traditional production of *munkoyo*, an indigenous beverage produced in democratic Republic of Congo. Food Control 2012;25, 334-341.

[95] Mukisa IM., Nsiimire DG., Byaruhanga YB., Muyanja CMBK., Langsrud T., Narvhus JA. Obushera: Descriptive sensory profiling and consumer acceptance. Journal of Sensory Studies 2010;25, 190-214.

[96] Muyanja CMBK., Narvhus JA., Treimo J., Langsrud T. Isolation, characaterisation and identification of lactic acid bacteria from *bushera*: a Ugandan traditional fermented beverage. International Journal of Food Microbiology 2003;80, 201-210.

[97] Omemu AM., Oyewole OB., Bankole MO. Significance of yeasts in the fermentation of maize for ogi production. Food Microbiology 2007;24(6), 571-576.

[98] Onyekwere OO., Akinrele IA., Koleoso OA. Industrialisation of ogi fermentation. In: Steinkraus KH. (Ed.) Industrialisation of Indigenous Fermented Foods. Marcel Dekker; 1989. p329-362.

[99] Odunfa SA., Adeyele S. Microbiological changes during the traditional production of ogi-baba, a West African fermented sorghum gruel. Journal of Cereal Science 1985;3, 173-180.

[100] Omar NB., Abriouel H., Keleke S., Venuezela AS., Martinez-Cañamero M., López RL., Ortega E., Gálvez A. Bacteriocin-producing *Lactobacillus* strains isolated from *poto poto*, a Congolese fermented maize product, and genetic fingerprinting of their plantaricin operons. International Journal of Food Microbiology 2008;127, 18-25.

[101] Madoroba E., Steenkamp ET., Theron J., Scheirlinck I., Cloete TE., Huys G. Diversity and dynamics of bacterial populations during spontaneous sorghum fermentations

used to produce ting, a South African food. Systematic and Applied Microbiology, 2011;34(3), 227-234.

[102] Sekwati-Monang B., Gänzle MG. Microbiological and chemical characterisation of ting, a sorghum-based sourdough product from Botswana. International Journal of Food Microbiology 2011;150, 115-121.

[103] Mbugua SK. Microbial growth during spontaneous Uji fermentation and its influence on the end product. East African Agriculture and Forestry Journal 1985;50(4), 101-110.

[104] Johansson M-L., Sanni A., Lonner C., Molin G. 1995. Phenotypically based taxonomy using API 50 CH of Lactobacilli from Nigerian ogi and the occurrence of starch fermenting strains. International Journal of Food microbiology 1995;25, 159-168.

[105] Peres CTM., Peres CL., Hernández-Mendoza AN., Malcata FX. Review on fermented plant materials as carriers and sources of potentially probiotic lactic acidbacteria – With an emphasis on table olives. Trends in Food Science & Technology 2012; in press.

[106] Lavermicocca P. Highlights on new food research. Digestive and Liver Disease 2006;38(Suppl. 2), S295-S299.

[107] Gokavi S., Zhang L., Zhang L., Huang M.-K, Zhao X., Guo M. Oat-based synbiotic beverage fermented by Lactobacillus plantarum, Lactobacillus paracasei ssp. casei, and Lactobacillus acidophilus. Journal of Food Science 2005;70(4), 216-223.

[108] Patel HM., Pandiella SS., Wang RH., Webb C. Influence of malt, wheat and barley extracts on the bile tolerance of selected strains of lactobacilli. Food Microbiology 2004;21, 83-89.

[109] Shah NP., Lankaputhra WEV. Improving viability of Lactobacillus acidophilus and Bifidobacterium spp. in yoghurt. International Dairy Journal 1997;7, 349-356.

[110] Theunissen J., Witthuhn C. Probiotic content: truth or fiction? South African Food Review 2004;31 (5):15-17.

[111] Nyanzi R., Jooste PJ., Abu JO., Beukes EM. Consumer acceptability of a synbiotic version of the maize beverage mageu. Development Southern Africa 2010;27 (3), 447-463.

[112] Gomes AMP., Malcata FX 1999. Bifidobacterium spp. And Lactobacillus acidophilus: biological, biochemical, technological and therapeutical properties relevant for use as probiotics. Trends in Food Science & Technology, 1999;10, 139-157.

[113] Kailasapathy K., Supriadi D. Effect of whey protein concentrate on the survival of Lactobacillus acidophilus in lactose hydrolysed yoghurt during refrigerated storage. Milchwissenschaft 1996;51(10), 565-568.

[114] Shah NP. Probiotic bacteria: selective enumeration and survival in dairy foods. Journal of Dairy Science 2000;83, 894-907.

[115] Shin HS., Lee JH., Pestka JJ., Ustunol, Z. Viability of Bifidobacteria in commercial dairy products during refrigerated storage. Journal of Food Protection 2000;63(3), 327-331.

[116] Luckow T., Delahunty C. Consumer acceptance of orange juice containing functional ingredients. Food Research International 2004;37, 805-814.

[117] Taylor JRN., Schober TJ., Bean SR. Novel food and non-food uses for sorghum and millets. Journal of Cereal Science 2006;44, 252-271.

[118] Tagbor AAK. Shelf-life extension and fortification of *Liha,* a fermented Ghanaian maize malt beverage. MTech *dissertation*, Technikon Pretoria; 2001.

[119] Chaitow L., Trenev N. Probiotics: the revolutionary 'friendly bacteria' way to vital health and well-being. Thorsons Publishers Ltd., England; 1990.

Chapter 11

Probiotics and Lactose Intolerance

Roel J. Vonk, Gerlof A.R. Reckman,
Hermie J.M. Harmsen and Marion G. Priebe

Additional information is available at the end of the chapter

1. Introduction

Lactose is the main sugar in milk and therefore the main energy source for the newborn. Milk contains 4,8% lactose [1]. Lactose is a disaccharide consisting out of glucose and galactose.

In normal physiological conditions lactose is hydrolyzed by lactase also known as lactase-phlorizin hydrolase and under its systemic name lactose- galactosehydrolase (EC 3.2.1.108), which is a brush-border membrane bound enzyme. Glucose and galactose are taken up by the intestinal cells and transported into the bloodstream (Fig. 1). A considerable part of glucose and most galactose is cleared by the liver after the first pass. Lactose which is not hydrolyzed in the small intestine is passing into the colon where it is fermented. Lactose itself and its metabolites are osmotic active products causing an osmotic pressure; excessive amounts present in the colon are related to the development of clinical symptoms as diarrhea.

The apparent lactase enzyme activity is affected by various factors like a. age, b. genetic background, c. integrity of the small intestinal membrane and d. the small-intestinal transit time

a. The activity of the enzyme lactase is age dependent. The activity is high in the first year of age and declines until adulthood is reached. It is not clear what the physiological advantage is of the age dependency of the lactase activity in relation to the disaccharide glucose-galactose.

Several remarkable aspects can be brought up in this respect:

-   Galactose has a higher hepatic clearance than glucose, which prevents a significant postprandial increase in blood glucose in the systemic circulation.
-   Galactose does not lead to an induction of the pancreatic insulin response.

- Lactase might have a variable and limited capacity which leads to a regulated spill over of lactose into the colon. There lactose might act as a primer (prebiotic) for the colonic microbiota in the first period of life (See also the subchapter of colonic fermentation of lactose).

b. The role of the genetic background of the lactase activity has been described in detail elsewhere [2].

c. The lactase activity is strongly affected by the integrity of the small intestinal membrane. This is the reason why in patients with celiac disease, which have not been treated optimally, symptoms of lactose intolerance may appear [3].

d. Finally, the turnover of lactose by the enzyme is dependent on the small intestinal transit time (apparent enzyme activity).

Fermented milk products can alleviate symptoms by delaying gastric emptying, orocecal transit time, or both. Delay of gastric emptying is due to the higher viscosity of the fermented milk product as compared to milk. Decrease of orocecal transit time is due to the metabolic products of probiotics or a lower osmotic force due to improved lactose digestion. A longer passage time in lactose maldigesters aids in hydrolyzing as much lactose as possible before spill over into the colon occurs. These findings support that pasteurized yogurt already provides alleviation of symptoms and that yogurt containing living probiotics improves this alleviation [4]. The effect of sugars, including lactose, on the small intestinal transit time is not well documented [5]. Changes in intestinal transit time due to the sugar molecules might especially play a role in other pathological conditions like irritable bowel disease.

Lactose intolerance is the pathophysiological situation in which the small intestinal digestion and / or colonic fermentation is altered which leads to clinical symptoms.

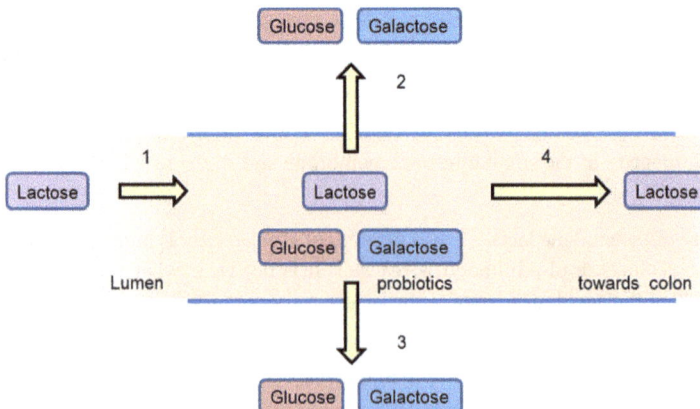

Figure 1. Small intestinal metabolism of lactose. Lactose enters the small intestine (1), lactose is then coverted by lactase from the host (2) or by probiotics (3). Excess amounts of lactose spill over into the colon (4).

2. Colonic fermentation of lactose

Lactose which is spilled over into the colon can be hydrolyzed by the colonic bacterial enzyme β-galactosidase resulting in the formation of glucose and galactose. Glucose and galactose are subsequently converted into lactate as well as into the short chain fatty acids (SCFA) acetate, propionate and butyrate (see Fig. 2). Additionally, microbial biomass will be formed. The original substrate lactose, the intermediate products glucose and galactose and the final products can all contribute to the osmotic load in the colon. This might lead to increased colonic transit time, altered fermentation profiles and ultimately to diarrhea.

The central question is which molecule contributes most to the pathological symptoms, like diarrhea: the original substrate lactose and / or one of the metabolites.

As indicated in Fig. 2 the number of molecules is doubled after the first conversion by β-galactosidase and tripled after the second conversion. A rapid conversion to the final metabolites enhances the osmotic force considerable.

We first analyzed the role of lactose itself assuming that β-galactosidase is the rate limiting step. In a recent paper of us [6], we describe that inducing the colonic β-galactosidase by administration of yogurt and additional probiotics alleviates the clinical symptoms of lactose intolerance in an adult Chinese population. This suggests a specific role of lactose itself in the development of clinical symptoms. Our observation was confirmed by [7], who observed in post-weaning Balb/c mice that symptoms of diarrhea were reduced by inducing the β-galactosidase activity by administration of a recombinant *Lactococcus lactis* MG1363/FGZW strain expressing β-galactosidase.

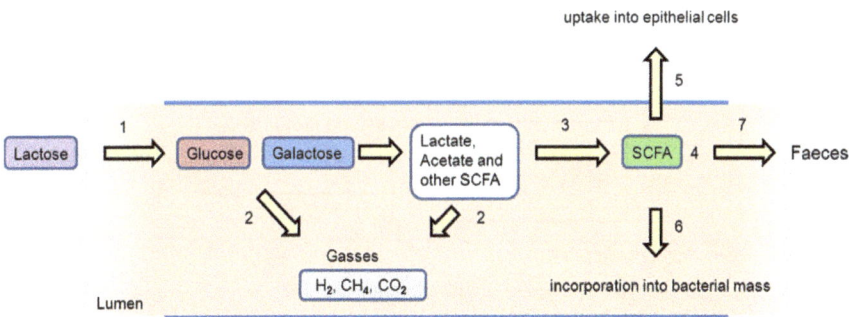

Figure 2. Colonic metabolism of lactose. Lactose enters the colon (1) and is fermented by the microbiota into glucose and galactose. Gasses such as hydrogen, methane and carbondioxide are formed (2). Lactate is also formed and converted into short chain fatty acids (SCFA)(3,4), also in this stage gasses are formed (2). These SCFAs can be taken up by epithelial cells (5) or can be used by the microbiota (6) or excreted in the faeces (7).

In contrast with these observations is the fact that β-galactosidase is an abundant enzyme in the colonic microbiota. It is present in many phylogroups of bacteria which in total might contribute to more than 40% of the total population of the colonic microbiome (Table 1). However, relative abundance and composition of bacteria with β-galactosidase in the distal colon do not seem to be related to lactose intolerance [8]. Another argument to consider is that the conversion of lactose into glucose, galactose and subsequently SCFA / lactate doubles and triples respectively the osmotic pressure. This aspect will be discussed in more detail under the chapter administration of pre- and probiotics.

Domain	Phylum	Order	Family
Bacteria (1718)			
	CFB group bacteria (1006)		
		Bacteroidales (994)	
			Bacteroidaceae (830)
			Porphyromonadaceae (102)
			more… (62)
		Flavobacteriales (12)	
	Firmicutes (394)		
		Clostridiales (327)	
			Lachnospiraceae (146)
			Clostridiaceae (86)
			more… (95)
		Erysipelotrichales (36)	
		Lactobacillales (29)	
		Selenomonadales (2)	
	Proteobacteria (190)		
		g-proteobacteria (182)	
			Enterobacteria (176)
			more… (6)
		more… (8)	
	Actinobacteria (95)		
		Bifidobacteriales (74)	
		Coriobacteriales (15)	
		Actinomycetales (6)	
	Spirochetes (32)		
	more… (1)		
unclassified (4)			

Table 1. Overview of all bacteria known to produce β-galactosidase.

Considering the physiological aspects of lactose digestion and fermentation it is clear that sufficient small intestinal hydrolysis of lactose related to the dose consumed will prevent symptoms of lactose intolerance. In case of relative insufficient lactase activity in the small intestine, spillover into the colon will occur. Adequate removal of osmotic active molecules, however, can prevent development of clinical symptoms of diarrhea.

3. Clinical symptoms of lactose intolerance

Symptoms of intestinal discomfort, abdominal pain and / or diarrhea can occur in case of lactose intolerance. These complaints are, however, not specific and can also be noticed in several other clinical conditions (for example irritable bowel syndrome, coeliac disease, Crohn's disease). For proper treatment and correct interpretation of interventions accurate diagnosis of the underlying pathophysiology is therefore very important.

4. Diagnostics of lactose intolerance

The most direct diagnosis is the analysis of lactase activity. However, the enzyme activity derived from a small intestinal biopsy does not reflect the overall lactase activity in the small intestine because of the patchy character of the distribution of this enzyme. This can lead to false positive and negative estimation of the overall physiological capacity to hydrolyze lactose.

Screening the genotype of people with lactose intolerant-like symptoms can aid in the correct diagnosis of lactose intolerance. The lactase gene can contain single-nucleotide polymorphisms (SNP) in the promotor region which leads to a high capacity to digest lactose. The most common SNP C/T-13910 is found in many Northwest European people. Several methods have been developed to detect this most common SNP. Järvelä et al. [2] sum up in their review the different methods for detection: minisequencing, enzyme digest, polymerase chain reaction-restriction fragment length polymorphism and pyrosequencing. For detection of all known SNPs, sequencing is the most reliable technique. Because there is a poor correlation between abdominal symptoms and lactase activity, genetics alone is not sufficient for a correct clinical diagnosis of adult lactose intolerance.

For congenital lactase deficiency genetic screening is effective, mutations occur in the lactase gene itself and symptoms start shortly after birth [2]. The prevalence of this syndrome however, is very low.

The analysis of the capacity to digest lactose in vivo by using two stable isotopes might be theoretically the best diagnostical method [9]. This test consists of the administration of ^{13}C-lactose and ^{2}H-glucose and calculation of the ratio of the ^{13}C-glucose/^{2}H-glucose concentrations measured in plasma. This test can be used to analyze the effect of interventions and to demonstrate changes in the capacity to digest lactose. However, as a routinely used diagnostic tool this test is not applicable because of its complex character.

The most commonly used diagnostic method for lactose intolerance is the hydrogen breath test. This test is easy to apply in clinical practice, but as discussed in detail by us [12] others [11] this test leads to false positive and false negative results.

A way to improve the precision of the breath test is to use ^{13}C-lactose as a substrate and measure both H_2 and $^{13}CO_2$ in breath as first described by Hiele et al. [12]. This might be the best applicable test in daily practice.

5. Application of pre- and probiotics to improve the clinical symptoms of lactose intolerance

An effect of an intervention with probiotics can be expected at two levels:

a. hydrolysis of lactose in the milk product and in the small intestine
b. at the level of colonic fermentation

a. The hydrolytic capacity of probiotic strains can be used to reduce the actual amount of lactose in the product, as occurs in yogurt. It can also be used to increase the overall hydrolytic capacity in the small intestine. The probiotic strain can be alive or can be lysed in the intestinal tract for its effect. *Lactobacillus acidophilus* is a bile-salt tolerant bacterium which hardly increases lactose digestion. However, sonication of *Lactobacillus Acidophilus* milk weakens their membranes and improves lactose-intolerance symptoms [4]. *Lactobacillus delbrüeckii* in a milk product can deliver β-galactosidase activity. These microorganisms do not have to be alive as long as their membranes are intact which helps to protect β-galactosidase during gastric passage [4]. Yogurt improves the lactose intolerance due to the presence of a group of lactobacillus bacteria it contains, i.e., *Lactobacillus acidophilus* [13]. Kinova et al. [14] described the beneficial effects of *Lactobacillus* present in fermented milk products. In [15] is described that consumption of yogurt containing *Lactobacillus bulgaricus* and *Streptococcus thermophiles* alleviate the lactose intolerance through their enzyme lactase when the product reaches the intestinal tract. Also Masood et al. [16] describe the beneficial effects of lactic acid bacteria in their review. From these findings it is inferred that lactose intolerance can be reduced by regularly consuming the fermented dairy products due to the production of β-galactosidase enzyme by lactic acid bacteria present in them.

In general, it can be stated that in yogurt several probiotic strains are present which results in a better tolerance of lactose in lactose intolerant persons.

b. Application of probiotics to manipulate the colonic fermentation.

As suggested before [17], one of the problems in studies concerning this topic is that it is difficult to prove that the intervention only has an effect at the level of the colon and not at the level of the small intestine.

As discussed before it is not clear which compound, lactose or one of its fermentation metabolites contributes most to the development of symptoms of lactose intolerance. The hypothesis is that removal of these product(s) can reduce the clinical symptoms.

1. Removal of lactose

Lactose is hydrolyzed by β-galactosidase. We recently published [6] that a mix of probiotics in yogurt together with *Bifidobacterium longum* capsules could increase the β-galactosidase activity in faeces and alleviate the complaints of lactose intolerance.

Together with the observation that the capacity to digest lactose, which was measured by the 13C-lactose/2H-glucose test, was not changed, it could be concluded that this intervention has an effect on colonic metabolism, possibly by enhancing the β-galactosidase activity. A study with mice [7] suggested the same mechanism. However, after analyzing the presence of β-galactosidase in the common bacterial strains in humans it can be concluded that β-galactosidase is abundantly present and it seems that administration of exogenous β-galactosidase from probiotics is not important. Alleviation of complaints and enhanced β-galactosidase concentration in stool therefore might have been a coincidence in our study.

2. Removal of glucose and galactose

Glucose is a preferred substrate for many bacterial strains and it is not likely that enhanced glucose removal by probiotic administration might play a role in alleviation of symptoms. Also galactose is easily consumed by most bacteria. Our in vitro studies [18] also indicated that accumulation of glucose and galactose does not occur during the breakdown of lactose, which confirms that these molecules once formed are subsequently metabolized very fast.

3. Removal of acetate, propionate, butyrate and lactate

As illustrated in Fig. 2 removal of SCFA takes place at the epithelium by uptake in the colonocytes and through the uptake and metabolism by various bacteria ("bacterial mass").

Uptake of SCFA into the epithelial cells is very effective because of co-transport of fluid which reduces the osmotic force [19]. The maximal epithelial uptake rate is not known and it is not known if this varies in persons with hypolactasia with and without symptoms after lactose consumption.

Another major way by which SCFA are removed is via the uptake and metabolism by bacteria. SCFA serve as a carbon and energy source for the anaerobic bacteria and this may increase the "bacterial mass". In the presence of sulphate, lactate may be metabolized by sulphate-reducing bacteria, producing toxic sulphide as byproduct [20]. On the other hand lactate together with acetate can be converted by different groups of bacteria into butyrate; for instance by bacteria such as *Eubacterium hallii* and *Anaerostipes cacca* [21]. Butyrate is thought to be beneficial for colonic health. Also *Bacteroides* several subspecies are capable of metabolizing lactate, but produce propionate. The metabolism of intermediates like lactate and acetate are an important step in the breakdown of sugars by gut bacteria [22]. For gut health it is important that from lactate a balanced mixture of SCFA are formed and for this correct conditions should be present. The hypothesis that for the prevention of diabetes type 1 butyrate production is preferred over propionate production is stated by [23]. They stated this because butyrate production enforces the barrier function of the gut. Therefore, conditions that stimulates these metabolic associations should be enforced. This implies that a mixture of pro- and prebiotics as occurs in yogurt might be an efficient approach, since it favors acetate and lactate formation, and in this way stimulate butyrate formation. If lactate removal via for instance butyrate production, does not occur this may impact functioning of the epithelium. It then can be speculated that an impaired epithelial function will hamper the uptake of lactate, and causes an increased osmotic pressure in the gut.

Several other studies have reported the beneficial effect of a probiotic intervention on symptoms of lactose intolerance but without describing a precise mechanism. In some of these studies the observation that the specific strains under study survive the small intestinal passage is used as an argument that the effect occurs at the colonic level.

The combination of *Lactobacillus casei* Shirota and *Bifidobacterium breve* Yakult has been shown to survive gastrointestinal transit and to improve symptoms of lactose intolerance. This effect persists after the intervention is ceased [24]. Other probiotic strains have shown beneficial effects on lactose digestion and symptoms in lactase deficient persons [12,25,26]. Further investigation with different strains of *bifidobacteria* or *lactobacilli* on symptoms of lactose intolerance showed contradictory results. [27] observed that 7 day supplementation with *Lactobacillus acidophilus* did not change hydrogen production or symptoms. [28] however found a decrease in hydrogen production after 7 days of milk intake supplemented with *Lactobacillus acidophilus*, but not all individuals had relief of their symptoms. *Bifidobacterium breve* for 5 days did not improve lactose intolerance symptoms, but reduction in breath hydrogen was measured [29]. Overall these contradictions have not led to a general acceptance of probiotics as a efficient treatment for lactose intolerance [30-32].

The observation of adaptation seen in lactose intolerant persons consuming regularly small amounts of dairy products might be in accordance with the concept of adaptation of the colonic metabolism by increased lactate metabolizing populations in the gut. This allows efficient metabolism of increased amounts of lactose [33]. The observation that lactulose fermentation is impaired during ingestion of ampicillin (2g / day) gives rise to the idea that antibiotics can disrupt the microbiota in the colon. There is no evidence in the literature that antibiotics have a negative effect on the fermentation of lactose, however it would not be surprising if such a phenomenon was found [34].

6. Conclusion

There is evidence that probiotics can alleviate symptoms of lactose intolerance. This can occur by increased hydrolysis of lactose in the dairy product and in the small intestine. It can also be achieved by manipulation of the colonic metabolism. However, the precise mechanism how colonic metabolism influences lactose intolerance symptoms is not yet known. The reported studies are not consistent in their experimental set-up, results and conclusions.

The diagnosis of lactose maldigestion and the relation to complaints is highly complex. For an effective treatment of lactose intolerance and a correct interpretation of the effects of an intervention, knowledge of the underlying mechanisms of lactose intolerance is essential. Development of new strategies concerning the treatment with probiotics should therefore include an analysis of the relevant intermediate endpoints. In this way applications of probiotics for treatment of lactose intolerance could lead to a promising strategy.

Author details

Roel J. Vonk [*], Gerlof A.R. Reckman, Hermie J.M. Harmsen and Marion G. Priebe
Dept. of Cell Biology, Centre for Medical Biomics and Dept. of Medical Microbiology, UMCG, Groningen, The Netherlands

7. References

[1] Chandan R. Dairy-based ingredients. Eagan Press, St. Paul, MN; 1997.
[2] Järvelä I, Torniainen S, Kolho K. Molecular Genetics of Human Lactase Deficiencies. Annals of Medicine 2009;41 568-575.
[3] Koetse HA, Vonk RJ, Gonera-De Jong GBC, Priebe MG, Antoine JM, Stellaard F, Sauer PJJ. Low Lactase Activity in a Small-Bowel Biopsy Specimen: Should Dietary Lactose Intake Be Restricted in Children with Small Intestinal Mucosal Damage? Scandinavian Journal of Gastroenterology 2006;41(1) 37-41.
[4] de Vrese M, Stegelmann A, Richter B, Fenselau S, Laue C, Schrezenmeir J. Probiotics-Compensation for Lactase Insufficiency. The American Journal of Clinical Nutrition 2001;73(suppl) 421S-429S.
[5] He T, Priebe MG, Welling GW, Vonk RJ. Effect of Lactose on Oro-Cecal Transit in Lactose Digesters and Maldigesters. European Journal of Clinical Investigation 2006;36(10) 737-742.
[6] He T, Priebe MG, Zhong Y, Huang C, Harmsen HJM, Raangs GC, Antoine JM, Welling GW, Vonk RJ. Effects of Yogurt and Bifidobacteria Supplementation on the Colonic Microbiota in Lactose-Intolerant Subjects. Journal of Applied Microbiology 2008;104 595-604.

---

[*] Corresponding Author

[7] Li J, Zhang W, Wang C, Yu Q, Dai R, Pei X. Lactococcus Lactis Expressing Food-grade β-galatosidase Alleviates Lactose Intolerance Symptoms in Post-weaning Balb/c Mice. Applied Microbiology and Biotechnology 2012;DOI 10.1007/s00253-012-3977-4.

[8] He T, Priebe MG, Vonk RJ, Welling GW. Identification of Bacteria with β-galactosidase Activity in Faeces from Lactas Non-Persistent Subjects. FEMS Microbiology Ecology 2005;54(3) 463-469.

[9] Vonk RJ, Stellaard F, Priebe MG, Koetse HA, Hagedoorn RE, De Bruijn S, Elzinga H, Lenoir-Wijnkoop I, Antoine J-M. The 13C/2H-glucose Test for Determination of Small Intestinal Lactase Activity. European Journal of Clinical Investigation 2001;31(3) 226-233.

[10] He T, Venema K, Priebe MG, Welling GW, Brummer R-JM, Vonk RJ. The Role of Colonic Metabolism in Lactose Intolerance. European Journal of Clinical Investigation 2008;38(8) 541-547.

[11] Ojetti V, LaMura R, Zocco MA, Cesaro P, De Masi E, La Mazza A, Cammarota G, Gasbarrini G, Gasbarrini A. Quick Test: New Test for the Diagnosis of Duodenal Hypolactasia. Digestive Diseases and Sciences. 2008;53(6) 1589-1592.

[12] Hiele M, Ghoos Y, Rutgeerts P, Vantrappen G, Carchon H, Eggermont E. 13CO2 Breath Test Using Naturally 13C-Enriched Lactose for Detection of Lactase Deficiency in Patients with Gastrointestinal Symptoms. Journal of Laboratory and Clinical Medicine 1988;122(2) 193-200.

[13] Fuller R. Probiotics in Human Medicine. Gut 1991;32 439-442.

[14] Kinová Sepová H, Bilková A, Bukovský M. Lactobacilli and their Probiotic Properties. Ceska Slov Farm. 2008;57(2) 95-98.

[15] Schaafsma G. Lactose Intolerance and Consumption of Cultured Dairy Products — a Review. International Dairy Federation Newsletter 1993;2 15–16.

[16] Masood MI, Qadir MI, Shirazi JH, Khan IU. Beneficical Effects on Lactic Acid Bacteria on Human Beings. Critical Reviews in Microbiology 2011;37(1) 91-98.

[17] Priebe MG, Vonk RJ, Sun X, He T, Harmsen HJM, Welling GW. The Physiology of Colonic Metabolism. Possibilities for Interventions with Pre- and Probiotics. European Journal of Nutrition 2002;41(s1) 2-10.

[18] He T, Priebe MG, Harmsen HJM, Stellaard F, Sun X, Welling GW, Vonk RJ. Colonic Fermentation May Play a Role in Lactose Intolerance in Humans. The Journal of Nutrition 2006;136(1) 58-63.

[19] Binder HJ. Role of Colonic Short-Chain Fatty Acid Transport in Diarrhea. Annual Review of Physiology 2010;72 297-313.

[20] Marquet P, Duncan SH, Chassard C, Bernalier-Donadille A, Flint HJ. Lactate Has the Potential to Promote Hydrogen Sulphide Formation in the Human Colon. FEMS Microbiology Letters 2009;299(2) 128-134.

[21] Muñoz-Tamayo R, Laroche B, Walter E, Doré J, Duncan SH, Flint HJ, Leclerc M. Kinetic Modelling of Lactate Utilization and Butyrate Production by Key Human Colonic Bacterial Species. FEMS Mircobiology Ecology 2011;76(3) 615-624.

[22] Flint HJ, Bayer EA, Rincon MT, Lamed R, White BA. Polysaccharide Utilization by Gut Bacteria: Potential for New Insights from Genomic Analysis. Nature Reviews Microbiology. 2008;6(2) 121-31.

[23] Brown CT, Davis-Richardson AG, Giongo A, Gano KA, Crabb DB, Mukherjee N, Casella G, Drew JC, Ilonen J, Knip M, Hyöty H, Veijola R, Simell T, Simell O, Neu J, Wasserfall CH, Schatz D, Atkinson MA, Triplett EW. Gut Microbiome Metagenomics Analysis Suggests a Functional Model for the Development of Autoimmunity for Type 1 Diabetes. PLoS ONE. 2011;6(10) e25792.

[24] Almeida CC, Lorena SLS, Pavan CR, Akasaka HMI, Mesquita MA. Beneficial Effects on Long-Term Consumption of a Probiotic Combination of *Lactobacillus casei* Shirota and *Bifidobacterium breve* Yakult May Persist After Suspension of Therapy in Lactose-Intolerant Patients. Nutrition in Clinical Practice 2012;27(2) 247-251.

[25] Lin M-Y, Dipalma JA, Martini MC, Gross CJ, Harlander SK, Savaiano DA. Comparative Effects of Exogenous Lactase (β-galactosidase) Preparations on in Vivo Lactose Digestion. Digestive Diseases and Sciences 1993;38(11) 2022-2027.

[26] Rabot S, Rafter J, Rijkers GT, Watzl B, Antoine J-M. Guidance for Substantiating the Evidence for Beneficial Effects of Probiotics: Impact of Probiotics on Digestive System Metabolism. Journal of Nutrition 2010;140(3) 677S-689S.

[27] Saltzman JR, Russell RM, Golner B, Barakat S, Dallal GE, Goldin BR. A Randomized Trial of *Lactobacillus acidophilus* BG2FO4 to Treat Lactose Intolerance. The American Journal of Clinical Nutrition. 1999;69(1) 140-146.

[28] Kim HS, Gilliland SE. *Lactobacillus acidophilus* as a Dietary Adjunct for Milk to Aid Lactose Digestion in Humans. Journal of Dairy Science 1983;66 959-966.

[29] Park MJ, Lee JH, Kim KA, Kim JS, Jung HC, Song IS, Kim CY. The Changes in the Breath Hydrogen Concentration After the Ingestion of *Bifidobacterium breve* KY-16 in the Lactose Malabsorbers. The Korean Journal of Gastroenterology. 1999;34(6) 741-748.

[30] Levri KM, Ketvertis K, Deramo M, Merenstein JH, D'amico F. Do Probiotics Reduce Adult Lactose Intolerance? The Journal of Family Practice. 2005;54 613-620.

[31] Shaukat A, Levitt MD, Taylor BC, MacDonald R, Shamliyan TA, Kane RL, Wilt TJ. Systematic Review: Effective Management Strategies for Lactose Intolerance. Annals of Internal Medicine. 2010;152(12) 797-803.

[32] Wilt TJ, Shaukat A, Shamliyan T, Taylor BC, MacDonald R, Tacklind J, Rutks I, Schwarzenberg SJ, Kane RL, Levitt M. Lactose Intolerance and Health. Evidence Report – Technology Assesment 2010;192 1-410.

[33] Rong Q, Cheng Yu H, HuiZhang D, Guo Z, Ling LI, Sheng YE. Milk Consumption and Lactose Intolerance in Adults. Biomedical and Environmental Sciences 2011;24(5) 512-517.

[34] Rao SS, Edwards CA, Austen CJ, Bruce C, Read NW. Impaired Colonic Fermentation of Carbohydrate After Ampicillin. Gastroenterology 1988;94(4) 928-932.

Permissions

The contributors of this book come from diverse backgrounds, making this book a truly international effort. This book will bring forth new frontiers with its revolutionizing research information and detailed analysis of the nascent developments around the world.

We would like to thank Prof. Dr. Everlon Cid Rigobelo, for lending his expertise to make the book truly unique. He has played a crucial role in the development of this book. Without his invaluable contribution this book wouldn't have been possible. He has made vital efforts to compile up to date information on the varied aspects of this subject to make this book a valuable addition to the collection of many professionals and students.

This book was conceptualized with the vision of imparting up-to-date information and advanced data in this field. To ensure the same, a matchless editorial board was set up. Every individual on the board went through rigorous rounds of assessment to prove their worth. After which they invested a large part of their time researching and compiling the most relevant data for our readers. Conferences and sessions were held from time to time between the editorial board and the contributing authors to present the data in the most comprehensible form. The editorial team has worked tirelessly to provide valuable and valid information to help people across the globe.

Every chapter published in this book has been scrutinized by our experts. Their significance has been extensively debated. The topics covered herein carry significant findings which will fuel the growth of the discipline. They may even be implemented as practical applications or may be referred to as a beginning point for another development. Chapters in this book were first published by InTech; hereby published with permission under the Creative Commons Attribution License or equivalent.

The editorial board has been involved in producing this book since its inception. They have spent rigorous hours researching and exploring the diverse topics which have resulted in the successful publishing of this book. They have passed on their knowledge of decades through this book. To expedite this challenging task, the publisher supported the team at every step. A small team of assistant editors was also appointed to further simplify the editing procedure and attain best results for the readers.

Our editorial team has been hand-picked from every corner of the world. Their multi-ethnicity adds dynamic inputs to the discussions which result in innovative outcomes. These outcomes are then further discussed with the researchers and contributors who give their valuable feedback and opinion regarding the same. The feedback is then collaborated with the researches and they are edited in a comprehensive manner to aid the understanding of the subject.

Apart from the editorial board, the designing team has also invested a significant amount of their time in understanding the subject and creating the most relevant covers. They scrutinized every image to scout for the most suitable representation of the subject and create an appropriate cover for the book.

The publishing team has been involved in this book since its early stages. They were actively engaged in every process, be it collecting the data, connecting with the contributors or procuring relevant information. The team has been an ardent support to the editorial, designing and production team. Their endless efforts to recruit the best for this project, has resulted in the accomplishment of this book. They are a veteran in the field of academics and their pool of knowledge is as vast as their experience in printing. Their expertise and guidance has proved useful at every step. Their uncompromising quality standards have made this book an exceptional effort. Their encouragement from time to time has been an inspiration for everyone.

The publisher and the editorial board hope that this book will prove to be a valuable piece of knowledge for researchers, students, practitioners and scholars across the globe.

List of Contributors

Danfeng Song, Salam Ibrahim and Saeed Hayek
Department of Family and Consumer Science, North Carolina Agricultural and Technical State University, Greensboro, NC, USA

A. Krastanov
University of Food Technologies, Department "Biotechnology", Plovdiv, Bulgaria

Z. Denkova
University of Food Technologies, Department "Organic Chemistry and Microbiology", Plovdiv, Bulgaria

Alice Maayan Elad and Uri Lesmes
Department of Biotechnology and Food Engineering, Technion, Israel Institute of Technology, Haifa, Israel

Carina Paola Van Nieuwenhove
CERELA-CONICET, S. M. de Tucumán, Argentina
Facultad de Ciencias Naturales e IML- Universidad Nacional de Tucumán, S. M. de Tucumán, Argentina

Victoria Terán
CERELA-CONICET, S. M. de Tucumán, Argentina

Silvia Nelina González
CERELA-CONICET, S. M. de Tucumán, Argentina
Facultad de Bioquímica, Química y Farmacia- Universidad Nacional de Tucumán, S. M. de Tucumán, Argentina

Emiliane Andrade Araújo
Universidade Federal de Viçosa, Campus Rio Paranaíba, Rio Paranaíba, MG, Brazil

Ana Clarissa dos Santos Pires and Antônio Fernandes de Carvalho
Departamento de Tecnologia de Alimentos, Universidade Federal de Viçosa, Viçosa, MG, Brazil

Maximiliano Soares Pinto
Instituto de Ciências Agrárias, Universidade Federal de Minas Gerais, Montes Claros, MG, Brazil

Gwénaël Jan
INRA, UMR1253 Science et Technologie du Lait et de l'OEuf, Rennes, France

Fariborz Akbarzadeh
Faculty of Medicine, Tabriz University of Medical Sciences, Tabriz, I.R. Iran
Cardiovascular Research Center, Tabriz University of Medical Sciences, Tabriz, Iran

Aziz Homayouni
Department of Food Science and Technology, Faculty of Health and Nutrition, Tabriz
University of Medical Sciences, Tabriz, I.R. Iran

Gabriel-Danut Mocanu and Elisabeta Botez
Department of Food Science, Food Engineering and Applied Biotechnology, Faculty of
Food Science and Engineering, "Dunarea de Jos" University of Galati, Romania

Aziz Homayouni
Department of Food Science and Technology, Faculty of Health and Nutrition, Tabriz
University of Medical Sciences, Tabriz, I.R. Iran

Maedeh Alizadeh
Pediatric Nursing, Faculty of Nursing and Midwifery of Maragheh, Tabriz University of
Medical Sciences, Tabriz, I.R. Iran

Hossein Alikhah
Faculty of Medicine, Tabriz University of Medical Sciences, Tabriz, I.R. Iran

Vahid Zijah
Department of Dentistry, Behbood Hospital, Tabriz University of Medical Sciences, Tabriz,
I.R. Iran

Esteban Boza-Méndez, Rebeca López-Calvo and Marianela Cortés-Muñoz
National Research Center of Food Science and Technology (CITA), University of Costa
Rica, San José, Costa Rica

R. Nyanzi and P.J. Jooste
Department of Biotechnology and Food Technology, Tshwane University of Technology,
Pretoria, South Africa

Roel J. Vonk, Gerlof A.R. Reckman, Hermie J.M. Harmsen and Marion G. Priebe
Dept. of Cell Biology, Centre for Medical Biomics and Dept. of Medical Microbiology,
UMCG, Groningen, The Netherlands